Cardiac MR Imaging

Editors

CLERIO F. AZEVEDO
ROBERTO C. CURY

MAGNETIC RESONANCE IMAGING CLINICS OF NORTH AMERICA

www.mri.theclinics.com

Consulting Editors
SURESH K. MUKHERJI
LYNNE S. STEINBACH

August 2019 • Volume 27 • Number 3

ELSEVIER

1600 John F. Kennedy Boulevard • Suite 1800 • Philadelphia, Pennsylvania, 19103-2899

http://www.mri.theclinics.com

MRI CLINICS OF NORTH AMERICA Volume 27, Number 3
August 2019 ISSN 1064-9689, ISBN 13: 978-0-323-68245-9

Editor: John Vassallo (j.vassallo@elsevier.com)
Developmental Editor: Meredith Madeira

Magnetic Resonance Imaging Clinics of North America (ISSN 1064-9689) is published quarterly by Elsevier Inc., 360 Park Avenue South, New York, NY 10010-1710. Months of issue are February, May, August, and November. Business and Editorial Offices: 1600 John F. Kennedy Blvd., Ste. 1800, Philadelphia, PA 19103-2899. Customer Service Office: 3251 Riverport Lane, Maryland Heights, MO 63043. Periodicals postage paid at New York, NY and additional mailing offices. Subscription prices are $404.00 per year (domestic individuals), $736.00 per year (domestic institutions), $100.00 per year (domestic students/residents), $437.00 per year (Canadian individuals), $959.00 per year (Canadian institutions), $545.00 per year (international individuals), $959.00 per year (international institutions), and $275.00 per year (international and Canadian students/residents). International air speed delivery is included in all *Clinics* subscription prices. All prices are subject to change without notice. **POSTMASTER:** Send address changes to *Magnetic Resonance Imaging Clinics*, Elsevier Health Sciences Division, Subscription Customer Service, 3251 Riverport Lane, Maryland Heights, MO 63043. Customer Service (orders, claims, online, change of address): Elsevier Health Sciences Division, Subscription **Customer Service, 3251 Riverport Lane, Maryland Heights, MO 63043. Tel:**1-800-654-2452 **(U.S. and Canada); 314-447-8871 (outside U.S. and Canada). Fax: 314-447-8029. E-mail: journalcustomer service-usa@elsevier.com (for print support); journalsonlinesupport-usa@elsevier.com (for online support).**

Reprints. For copies of 100 or more of articles in this publication, please contact the Commercial Reprints Department, Elsevier Inc., 360 Park Avenue South, New York, NY 10010-1710. Tel.: 212-633-3874; Fax: 212-633-3820; E-mail: reprints@elsevier.com.

Magnetic Resonance Imaging Clinics of North America is covered in the *RSNA Index of Imaging Literature, MEDLINE/PubMed (Index Medicus),* and *EMBASE/Excerpta Medica.*

Contributors

CONSULTING EDITORS

SURESH K. MUKHERJI, MD, MBA, FACR
Professor, Department of Radiology,
Michigan State University, East Lansing,
Michigan, USA

LYNNE S. STEINBACH, MD, FACR
Professor of Radiology and Orthopaedic
Surgery, Department of Radiology and
Biomedical Imaging, University of California,
San Francisco, San Francisco, California, USA

EDITORS

CLERIO F. AZEVEDO, MD, PhD
Diagnósticos da America (DASA), São Paulo,
São Paulo, Brazil; Division of Cardiology, Duke
Cardiovascular Magnetic Resonance Center,
Duke University Medical Center, Duke
Medicine Pavilion, Durham, North Carolina,
USA

ROBERTO C. CURY, MD, PhD
Diagnósticos da America (DASA), São Paulo,
São Paulo, Brazil

AUTHORS

AMNA ABDEL-GADIR, MBBS, MRCP
Institute of Cardiovascular Science, University
College London, Barts Heart Centre, St
Bartholomew's Hospital, London, United
Kingdom

HÉLDER JORGE ANDRADE GOMES, MD
Cardiologist and Cardiac Imaging,
Hospital Samaritano de São Paulo,
São Paulo, Brazil

CLERIO F. AZEVEDO, MD, PhD
Diagnósticos da America (DASA),
São Paulo, São Paulo, Brazil; Division
of Cardiology, Duke Cardiovascular
Magnetic Resonance Center, Duke
University Medical Center, Duke Medicine
Pavilion, Durham, North Carolina, USA

DAHLIA BANERJI, MD
Cardiac MR PET CT Program, Department of
Radiology (Cardiovascular Imaging), Division of
Cardiology, Massachusetts General Hospital,
Harvard Medical School, Boston,
Massachusetts, USA

RONG BING, MBBS
British Heart Foundation Centre for
Cardiovascular Science, University of
Edinburgh, Edinburgh, United Kingdom

**MARCIO SOMMER BITTENCOURT, MD,
MPH, PhD**
Delboni - DASA, Hospital Israelita Albert
Einstein and School of Medicine, Faculdade
Israelita de Ciência da Saúde Albert Einstein,
Center for Clinical and Epidemiological
Research, University Hospital and São Paulo
State Cancer Institute, University of São Paulo,
São Paulo, Brazil

FILIPE PENNA DE CARVALHO, MD
Diagnósticos da America (DASA), Rio de
Janeiro, Brazil

JOÃO L. CAVALCANTE, MD, FACC, FSCMR
Valve Science Center, Minneapolis Heart
Institute Foundation, Associate Cardiologist,
Director, Cardiac MRI and Structural CT and
Cardiovascular Imaging Core Lab, Minneapolis
Heart Institute, Abbott Northwestern Hospital,
Minneapolis, Minnesota, USA

OTÁVIO R. COELHO-FILHO, MD, PhD, MPH
Faculdade de Ciências Médicas - Universidade
Estadual de Campinas, Assistant Professor of
Medicine, Division of Cardiology, Department
of Medicine, Hospital das Clínicas, State
University of Campinas (UNICAMP), São
Paulo, Brazil

VINÍCIUS DE PADUA VIEIRA ALVES, MD
Radiology Department, Universidade Federal
Fluminense, Niterói, Rio de Janeiro, Brazil

MARC DWECK, MD, PhD
British Heart Foundation Centre for
Cardiovascular Science, University of
Edinburgh, Edinburgh, United Kingdom

FERNANDA ERTHAL, MD
Diagnósticos da America (DASA), Rio de
Janeiro, Brazil

**JULIANO LARA FERNANDES, MD, PhD,
MBA**
Jose Michel Kalaf Research Institute,
Radiologia Clinica de Campinas, Campinas,
São Paulo, Brazil

THIAGO FERREIRA DE SOUZA, MD, MSc
Faculdade de Ciências Médicas - Universidade
Estadual de Campinas, São Paulo, Brazil

MIHO FUKUI, MD, PhD
Valve Science Center, Minneapolis Heart
Institute Foundation, Minneapolis, Minnesota,
USA

BRIAN B. GHOSHHAJRA, MD, MBA
Cardiac MR PET CT Program, Department of
Radiology (Cardiovascular Imaging), Division of
Cardiology, Massachusetts General Hospital,
Harvard Medical School, Boston,
Massachusetts, USA

SANDEEP S. HEDGIRE, MD
Cardiac MR PET CT Program, Department of
Radiology (Cardiovascular Imaging), Division of
Cardiology, Massachusetts General Hospital,
Harvard Medical School, Boston,
Massachusetts, USA

EDWARD HULTEN, MD, MPH
Cardiopulmonary Clinic Chief,
Cardiopulmonary Clinic, Department of
Medicine, Evans Army Community Hospital,
Fort Carson, Colorado, USA; Uniformed

Services University School of Health Sciences,
Bethesda, Maryland, USA

MICHAEL JEROSCH-HEROLD, PhD
Noninvasive Cardiovascular Imaging Program,
Department of Radiology, Brigham and
Women's Hospital, Boston, Massachusetts,
USA

KRISTOPHER D. KNOTT, MA, MBBS, MRCP
Barts Heart Centre, The Cardiovascular
Magnetic Resonance Imaging Unit and The
Inherited Cardiovascular Diseases Unit,
St Bartholomew's Hospital, London, United
Kingdom

GABRIELA LIBERATO, MD
Heart Institute (InCor), Clinical Hospital
HCFMUSP, University of São Paulo Medical
School, Brazil, São Paulo, São Paulo,
Brazil

KATIA MENACHO, MD
Institute of Cardiovascular Science, University
College London, Barts Heart Centre, St
Bartholomew's Hospital, London, United
Kingdom

DEXTER MENDOZA, MD
Thoracic Imaging and Intervention,
Department of Radiology, Massachusetts
General Hospital, Harvard Medical
School, Boston, Massachusetts, USA

JAMES C. MOON, MB, BCh, MRCP, MD
Barts Heart Centre, The Cardiovascular
Magnetic Resonance Imaging Unit
and The Inherited Cardiovascular
Diseases Unit, Institute of Cardiovascular
Science, University College London,
St Bartholomew's Hospital, London, United
Kingdom

NEGAREH MOUSAVI, MD
Assistant Professor of Medicine,
McGill University Health Centre, Royal
Victoria Hospital, Montreal, Quebec,
Canada

ZORANA MRSIC, MD
Instructor of Medicine, Department of
Cardiology, Walter Reed National Military
Medical Center, Bethesda, Maryland,
USA

MARCELO SOUTO NACIF, MD, PhD
Programa de Pós-Graduação em Ciências Cardiovasculares, Hospital Universitário Antônio Pedro, Universidade Federal Fluminense, Niterói, Rio de Janeiro, Brazil; Unidade de Radiologia Clínica, Hospital viValle (Rede D'or-São Luiz), São José dos Campos, São Paulo, Brazil

TOMAS G. NEILAN, MD, MPH
Cardio-oncology Program and Cardiac MR PET CT Program, Massachusetts General Hospital, Harvard Medical School, Boston, Massachusetts, USA

DAVID R. OKADA, MD
Postdoctoral Fellow, Division of Cardiology, Department of Medicine, Johns Hopkins Hospital, Johns Hopkins Medicine, Baltimore, Maryland, USA

THIAGO QUINAGLIA, MD, PhD
Faculdade de Ciências Médicas, Universidade Estadual de Campinas, São Paulo, Brazil

CARLOS EDUARDO ROCHITTE, MD, PhD
Associate Professor of Cardiology, Academic Coordinator of Cardiovascular Magnetic Resonance and Computed Tomography Sector, Heart Institute (InCor), University of São Paulo Medical School, Brazil, Director of Cardiovascular Magnetic Resonance and Computed Tomography Sector, Heart Hospital (HCOR), Hospital do Coracão, São Paulo, São Paulo, Brazil

MARLY CONCEIÇÃO SILVA, MD, PhD
Axial Diagnostic Center, Belo Horizonte, Minas Gerais, Brazil

KATHERINE C. WU, MD
Associate Professor, Department of Medicine, Division of Cardiology, Johns Hopkins Hospital, Johns Hopkins Medicine, Baltimore, Maryland, USA

Contents

Cardiac MR (CMR) imaging contributes uniquely to the comprehensive assessment and management of aortic stenosis (AS), beyond the information provided by transthoracic echocardiography. The severity of AS and subsequent ventricular remodeling response can be assessed using cine images and phase-contrast mapping. CMR imaging also identifies myocardial tissue characteristics, which are valuable markers of left ventricular decompensation and adverse outcomes in AS. CMR imaging may be used as an alternative modality for transcatheter aortic valve replacement (TAVR) planning and post-TAVR management. This article explores the clinical utility of CMR imaging evaluation.

T2* mapping techniques has evolved significantly since their introduction in the early 2000s and a significant amount of evidence has been gathered to support their clinical routine use for iron overload assessment. This article focuses on the most important aspects of how to perform T2* imaging, from acquisition, to postprocessing, to analyzing the data with clinical concentration. Newer techniques have made T2* mapping more robust and accurate, allowing a broader use of this technique for noncontrast ischemia imaging based on blood oxygen levels, in addition to evaluation of intramyocardial hemorrhage and microvascular obstruction.

Despite recent advancements in newer biomarkers development and improved imaging techniques, the diagnosis of cardiac amyloidosis (CA) remains a frequent clinical challenge. In this setting, cardiac MR (CMR) imaging has emerged as a powerful tool to assess heart morphology and function, with the unique advantage of noninvasive tissue characterization. This article summarizes the CMR imaging common findings in CA and the latest research in this field, including delayed enhancement, native T1 mapping, and extracellular volume quantification.

Muscular dystrophy is a group of genetically inherited diseases with irreversible and progressive muscle loss and is associated with cardiac involvement. Particularly in Duchenne and Becker dystrophies, cardiac disorders are the leading causes of mortality. Cardiovascular magnetic resonance imaging (CMR) can detect even incipient myocardial fibrosis (late gadolinium enhancement), which has prognostic significance in patients with preserved left ventricular function by echocardiogram and before the onset of symptoms. Early detection of cardiac abnormalities by CMR enables early cardioprotective treatment, leading to a better prognosis.

Chemotherapy is associated with cardiovascular injury, including the development of a cardiomyopathy and vascular remodeling. Cardiac magnetic resonance (CMR) is sensitive to detect not only established morphologic and functional abnormalities but also early, potentially reversible, signs of myocardial injury. It robustly detects and quantifies myocardial edema, inflammation, and focal fibrosis, as well as interstitial fibrosis and vascular remodeling. These capabilities support the role of CMR as an excellent tool for evaluating cardiotoxicity. Novel CMR markers may even enhance patient management by facilitating the early detection of reversible myocardial tissue remodeling before classic morphologic and functional changes appear.

Late gadolinium enhancement (LGE) has become a standard clinical tool to evaluate myocardial fibrosis to define myocardial viability in the context of ischemic myocardial disease. More recently, LGE has also been used to characterize the presence and pattern of fibrosis in nonischemic cardiomyopathies. It yields unique and valuable diagnostic and prognostic insights for myriad nonischemic clinical indications and has become a key part of routine cardiac MR imaging, and a tool to guide treatment. This article reviews the technical aspects of LGE performance and its diagnostic and prognostic implications in nonischemic cardiomyopathy.

Cardiac fibrosis, characterized by net accumulation of extracellular matrix in the myocardium, is a common final pathway of heart failure. This myocardial fibrosis (MF) is not necessarily the primary cause of dysfunction; it often results from a reparative process activated in response to cardiomyocyte injury. In light of currently available treatments, late-identified MF could be definitive or irreversible, associated with worsening ventricular systolic function, abnormal cardiac remodeling, and increased ventricular stiffness and arrhythmia. T1 mapping should be used to detect incipient changes leading to myocardial damage in several clinical conditions and also in subclinical disease. This article reviews available techniques for MF detection, focusing on noninvasive quantification of diffuse fibrosis and clinical applications.

MAGNETIC RESONANCE IMAGING CLINICS OF NORTH AMERICA

SERIES OF RELATED INTEREST

Neuroimaging Clinics of North America
Available at: www.Neuroimaging.theclinics.com
PET Clinics
Available at: www.pet.theclinics.com
Radiologic Clinics of North America
Available at: www.Radiologic.theclinics.com

VISIT THE CLINICS ONLINE!
Access your subscription at:
www.theclinics.com

PROGRAM OBJECTIVE

The goal of *Magnetic Resonance Imaging Clinics of North America* is to keep practicing physicians up to date with current clinical practice by providing timely articles reviewing the state of the art in patient care.

TARGET AUDIENCE

All practicing physicians and healthcare professionals who provide patient care utilizing findings from Magnetic Resonance Imaging.

LEARNING OBJECTIVES

Upon completion of this activity, participants will be able to:

1. Review the current role of CMR in the assessment of patients with aortic stenosis.
2. Discuss clinical applications of CMR and its role in the assessment of patients with cardiac amyloidosis, as well as patients with malignant ventricular arrhythmias.
3. Recognize the value of CMR techniques for evaluating cardiotoxicity.

ACCREDITATION

The Elsevier Office of Continuing Medical Education (EOCME) is accredited by the Accreditation Council for Continuing Medical Education (ACCME) to provide continuing medical education for physicians.

The EOCME designates this enduring material for a maximum of 11 *AMA PRA Category 1 Credit*(s)™. Physicians should claim only the credit commensurate with the extent of their participation in the activity.

All other healthcare professionals requesting continuing education credit for this enduring material will be issued a certificate of participation.

DISCLOSURE OF CONFLICTS OF INTEREST

The EOCME assesses conflict of interest with its instructors, faculty, planners, and other individuals who are in a position to control the content of CME activities. All relevant conflicts of interest that are identified are thoroughly vetted by EOCME for fair balance, scientific objectivity, and patient care recommendations. EOCME is committed to providing its learners with CME activities that promote improvements or quality in healthcare and not a specific proprietary business or a commercial interest.

The planning committee, staff, authors and editors listed below have identified no financial relationships or relationships to products or devices they or their spouse/life partner have with commercial interest related to the content of this CME activity:

Amna Abdel-Gadir, MBSS, MRCP; Hélder Jorge Andrade Gomes, MD; Clerio F. Azevedo, MD, PhD; Dahlia Banerji, MD; Rong Bing, MBBS; Marcio Sommer Bittencourt, MD, MPH, PhD; Filipe Penna de Carvalho, MD; João L. Cavalcante, MD, FACC, FSCMR; Otávio R. Coelho-Filho, MD, PhD, MPH; Roberto C. Cury, MD, PhD; Vinícius de Padua Vieira Alves, MD; Marc Dweck, MD, PhD; Fernanda Erthal, MD; Juliano Lara Fernandes, MD, PhD, MBA; Thiago Ferreira de Souza, MD, MSc; Miho Fukui, MD, PhD; Brian B. Ghoshhajra, MD, MBA; Sandeep S. Hedgire, MD; Edward Hulten, MD, MPH; Michael Jerosch-Herold, PhD; Alison Kemp; Kristopher D. Knott, MA, MBBS, MRCP; Pradeep Kuttysankaran; Gabriela Liberato, MD; Katia Menacho, MD; Dexter Mendoza, MD; James C. Moon, MB, BCh, MRCP, MD; Negareh Mousavi, MD; Zorana Mrsic, MD; Suresh K. Mukherji, MD, MBA, FACR; Marcelo Souto Nacif, MD, PhD; Tomas G. Neilan, MD, MPH; David R. Okada, MD; Thiago Quinaglia, MD, PhD; Carlos Eduardo Rochitte, MD, PhD; Marly Conceição Silva, MD, PhD; Lynne S. Steinbach, MD, FACR; John Vassallo; Katherine C. Wu, MD.

UNAPPROVED/OFF-LABEL USE DISCLOSURE

The EOCME requires CME faculty to disclose to the participants:

1. When products or procedures being discussed are off-label, unlabelled, experimental, and/or investigational (not US Food and Drug Administration [FDA] approved); and
2. Any limitations on the information presented, such as data that are preliminary or that represent ongoing research, interim analyses, and/or unsupported opinions. Faculty may discuss information about pharmaceutical agents that is outside of FDA-approved labelling. This information is intended solely for CME and is not intended to promote off-label use of these medications. If you have any questions, contact the medical affairs department of the manufacturer for the most recent prescribing information.

TO ENROLL

To enroll in the *Magnetic Resonance Imaging Clinics of North America* Continuing Medical Education program, call customer service at 1-800-654-2452 or sign up online at http://www.theclinics.com/home/cme. The CME program is available to subscribers for an additional annual fee of USD 260.

METHOD OF PARTICIPATION

In order to claim credit, participants must complete the following:
1. Complete enrolment as indicated above.

2. Read the activity.
3. Complete the CME Test and Evaluation. Participants must achieve a score of 70% on the test. All CME Tests and Evaluations must be completed online.

CME INQUIRIES/SPECIAL NEEDS

For all CME inquiries or special needs, please contact elsevierCME@elsevier.com.

Foreword

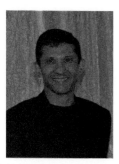

Suresh K. Mukherji, MD, MBA, FACR
Consulting Editor

Cardiac magnetic resonance (MR) has been a challenging topic for many years. The technology has been available since I was a resident...in the last century! The growth potential is obvious, and numerous vendors focused on developing new MR techniques that would help facilitate greater utilization. Unfortunately, the promise of widespread acceptance of cardiac MR never fully materialized for a variety of reasons. However, there are some specific clinical applications for cardiac MR, and these important topics are the foundation for this issue of *Magnetic Resonance Imaging Clinics of North America*.

Drs Azevedo and Cury have done a remarkable job in creating an issue that provides state-of-the art updates on accepted clinical applications of cardiac MR and also summarizes some rapidly evolving techniques that may soon be used clinically. I wish to personally thank them for their efforts in creating such an innovative issue. I also want to thank the authors for creating their wonderful articles that are beautifully illustrated.

I have no doubt that Drs Azevedo and Cury have succeeded in their mission to create an issue that is clinically oriented and practical. This important contribution will benefit all physicians who use cardiac imaging to help improve the lives of their patients afflicted with these complex cardiac disorders.

Suresh K. Mukherji, MD, MBA, FACR
Department of Radiology
Michigan State University
846 Service Road
East Lansing, MI 48824, USA

E-mail address:
sureshkm@msu.edu

Magn Reson Imaging Clin N Am 27 (2019) xv
https://doi.org/10.1016/j.mric.2019.05.002
1064-9689/19/© 2019 Published by Elsevier Inc.

Preface

Cardiovascular MR Imaging: Current Status and Future Directions

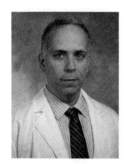 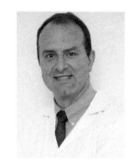

Clerio F. Azevedo, MD, PhD   Roberto C. Cury, MD, PhD

Editors

It has been an honor and a pleasure to serve as Guest Editors for this issue of *Magnetic Resonance Imaging Clinics of North America* with a focus on Cardiovascular Magnetic Resonance (CMR). We would like to thank the authors, all of whom are international experts with vast expertise in clinical CMR, for their outstanding contributions to this issue by providing a succinct yet thorough review of the topics.

The heart is a complex and challenging organ to image. It is constantly moving, not only from cardiac contraction/relaxation cycles but also as a result of respiratory motion. Notwithstanding, technological advancements over the past 20 years have allowed CMR to become the most versatile imaging modality in cardiology today.

Indeed, the time for CMR has come! Once viewed primarily as a research tool with very limited clinical utility, CMR has now become an essential tool in the workup of numerous cardiovascular diseases. In this issue, several of these clinical conditions in which CMR plays a pivotal role are reviewed. Moreover, emerging themes, such as quantification of myocardial perfusion, clinical applications of T1 and T2 mapping, transcatheter aortic valve replacement (TAVR) planning, and CMR applications in electrophysiology, are also visited.

Drs Fukui, Bing, Dweck, and Cavalcante begin by beautifully reviewing the technical aspects and the current role of CMR in the assessment of patients with aortic stenosis, including quantification of flows and myocardial fibrosis, as well as TAVR planning. This is followed by Drs Menacho, Abdel-Gadir, Moon, and Fernandes' comprehensive review of T2* mapping techniques and the assessment of myocardial iron overload by CMR. Drs Carvalho, Erthal, and Azevedo further explore state-of-the-art clinical applications of CMR and discuss its role in the assessment of patients with cardiac amyloidosis. Drs Okada and Wu describe the current state-of-the-art and discuss the future directions of CMR applications in electrophysiology, a growing field in cardiology today. This is brilliantly followed by Drs Banerji, Mendoza, Hedgire, and Ghoshhajra's perspective on the role of CMR in the evaluation of patients with malignant ventricular arrhythmias.

The assessment of myocardial ischemia by stress perfusion CMR, which represents one of the most important clinical applications of CMR in routine practice, is thoroughly reviewed by Drs Silva, Jerosch-Herold, and Coelho-Filho. This is elegantly complemented by Drs Knott, Fernandes, and Moon's description of a novel automated quantitative stress

Magn Reson Imaging Clin N Am 27 (2019) xvii–xviii
https://doi.org/10.1016/j.mric.2019.05.001

mri.theclinics.com

perfusion method that could help introduce quantitative stress CMR into clinical practice. Cardiac involvement represents a major cause of morbidity and mortality in patients with muscular dystrophies. Drs Rochitte, Liberato, and Silva superbly review the role of CMR in the comprehensive assessment of these challenging patients. Cardiotoxicity of cancer chemotherapy represents a major emerging theme in cardiology today. Drs Souza, Silva, Neilan, and Coelho-Filho discuss the value of state-of-the-art CMR techniques for evaluating cardiotoxicity and highlight the potential of CMR to improve patient management by facilitating the early detection of reversible myocardial injury. This is followed by Drs Bittencourt and Hulten's excellent review of the prognostic value of the delayed-enhancement technique in patients with nonischemic heart disease. Last, Drs Gomes, Alves, and Nacif provide a fresh look and reexamine the value of T1 mapping techniques in the assessment of interstitial myocardial fibrosis.

We hope that this issue can be of practical value by serving as a quick reference guide to help answer many routine cardiovascular imaging dilemmas and also stimulate further debate and research into areas where controversy still exists. Enjoy your reading!

Clerio F. Azevedo, MD, PhD
Diagnósticos da America (DASA)
Rua Gilberto Sabino
215 – Pinheiros
São Paulo, SP 05425-020, Brazil

Division of Cardiology
Duke Cardiovascular Magnetic Resonance Center
Duke University Medical Center
Duke Medicine Pavilion
10 Medicine Circle
Room 1E63, DUMC 3934
Durham, NC 27710, USA

Roberto C. Cury, MD, PhD
Diagnósticos da America (DASA)
Rua Gilberto Sabino
215 – Pinheiros
São Paulo, SP 05425-020, Brazil

E-mail addresses:
clerio.azevedo@gmail.com (C.F. Azevedo)
rccury@me.com (R.C. Cury)

Assessment of Aortic Stenosis by Cardiac Magnetic Resonance Imaging
Quantification of Flow, Characterization of Myocardial Injury, Transcatheter Aortic Valve Replacement Planning, and More

Miho Fukui, MD, PhD[a], Rong Bing, MBBS[b],
Marc Dweck, MD, PhD[b], João L. Cavalcante, MD, FSCMR[a,c],*

KEYWORDS

- Aortic stenosis (AS) • Extracellular volume (ECV) • Global longitudinal strain (GLS)
- Late gadolinium enhancement (LGE) • Phase-contrast mapping
- Transcatheter aortic valve replacement (TAVR) • T1 mapping

KEY POINTS

- The severity of aortic stenosis (AS) and subsequent ventricular remodeling can be assessed using cardiac MR (CMR) cine images and phase-contrast mapping.
- CMR can identify myocardial deformation and fibrosis, cornerstones of left ventricular decompensation in AS, using global longitudinal strain analysis, late gadolinium enhancement, and T1 mapping.
- CMR imaging can be a valuable alternative modality in the comprehensive assessment of transcatheter aortic valve replacement (TAVR) planning and post-TAVR management of paravalvular leak.

INTRODUCTION

With an aging population, acquired valvular disease, aortic stenosis (AS) in particular, has become among the most common clinical entities seen in daily practice.[1] Noninvasive cardiac imaging is essential to evaluate the severity of AS and to determine the optimal timing of intervention. Although transthoracic echocardiography (TTE) is the most commonly used and studied imaging modality in this field, advances in cardiovascular magnetic resonance (CMR) imaging provide important contributions to the comprehensive assessment and management of these patients. Currently, CMR imaging techniques are considered the reference standard for left ventricular (LV) anatomic and functional assessment.

Disclosures: The authors have nothing to disclose.
[a] Valve Science Center, Minneapolis Heart Institute Foundation, 920 East 28th Street, Suite 620, Minneapolis, MN 55407, USA; [b] British Heart Foundation Centre for Cardiovascular Science, University of Edinburgh, 47 Little France Drive, Edinburgh, EH16 4TJ, UK; [c] Cardiac MRI and Structural CT and Cardiovascular Imaging Core Lab, Minneapolis Heart Institute, Abbott Northwestern Hospital, 800 East 28th Street, Suite 300, Minneapolis, MN 55407, USA
* Corresponding author. Cardiac MRI and Structural CT and Cardiovascular Imaging Core Lab, Minneapolis Heart Institute, Abbott Northwestern Hospital, 800 East 28th Street, Suite 300, Minneapolis, MN 55407.
E-mail address: Joao.Cavalcante@allina.com

Magn Reson Imaging Clin N Am 27 (2019) 427–437
https://doi.org/10.1016/j.mric.2019.04.004

Importantly, CMR imaging can detect and quantify myocardial deformation, as well as myocardial fibrosis,[2] which is a cornerstone of LV decompensation in AS.

Thus, interest has grown in using CMR imaging in patients with AS, which is recognized as a disease of both the valve and the myocardium. This article summarizes the current CMR imaging techniques used for the comprehensive assessment of patients with AS and describes the clinical utility of CMR imaging in such patients.

AORTIC STENOSIS SEVERITY: CINE IMAGES AND PHASE-CONTRAST MAPPING

The standard measures of aortic valve (AV) severity include AV peak velocity, peak and mean gradients, and anatomic or physiologic AV area (AVA). Although TTE remains the primary imaging technique used to assess these parameters, CMR imaging can also provide the measurements of AS severity, in addition to more accurate quantification of LV volumes, myocardial mass, and function.

Cine imaging allows measurement of the anatomic valve area, using the scout line method to determine the exact leaflet position using orthogonal views (ie, 3-chamber and/or coronal LV outflow tract) (**Fig. 1**). The average of 3 anatomic AVA planimetry measurements at the peak systolic phase (largest orifice area) should be used owing to potential limitations in spatial and temporal resolution. This technique has demonstrated good correlation with echocardiography (TTE or transesophageal echocardiography) as the reference standard.[3,4] Direct planimetry measured by CMR imaging and/or transesophageal echocardiogram measures the anatomic stenosis (anatomic orifice area), whereas TTE and cardiac catheterization measure the physiologic functional stenosis at the vena contracta (effective orifice area), which tends to be slightly smaller.

Measurement of peak AV velocity and mean AV gradient with CMR imaging is possible using phase-contrast velocity mapping techniques, which are reproducible and do not require intravenous gadolinium contrast. To obtain the most accurate phase-contrast velocity, the angle of intercept should be oriented as perpendicular as possible to the orientation of the aortic jet flow through the stenotic AV. Additionally, the encoding velocity should be adjusted carefully to avoid aliasing. The phase-contrast imaging techniques, however, tends to underestimate the peak AV velocity and gradient compared with TTE. This can be explained by several factors: local signal loss (from flow turbulence), background correction, partial volume effects (large intravoxel size), phase

shift errors due to fast acceleration, intravoxel dephasing (particularly with velocities >3.5–4 m/s), and relatively low temporal resolution (20–25 ms) that may not be able to capture high jet velocities of short duration.[5]

MYOCARDIAL TISSUE CHARACTERIZATION

Severe AS causes pressure overload of the LV, resulting in progressive maladaptive ventricular remodeling[6] as a means to counterbalance the increased wall-stress (Laplace's law). This may lead to increased myocyte volume (LV hypertrophy), as well as expansion of the extracellular matrix and development of myocardial fibrosis.[7] Histopathology in patients with severe AS demonstrate both diffuse reactive fibrosis and focal replacement fibrosis.[8–10] Crucially, CMR imaging is currently the only imaging modality able to accurately assess and quantify myocardial fibrosis. Diffuse interstitial fibrosis consists of increased deposition of collagen in interstitial spaces, which can be assessed by T1 mapping techniques.[11,12] Focal replacement fibrosis consists of replacement of myocytes by fibrotic tissue, which can be detected by late gadolinium enhancement (LGE) imaging.[7]

Late Gadolinium Enhancement

LGE imaging is the gold-standard method for noninvasive detection of focal myocardial fibrosis in a broad range of cardiovascular conditions, such as ischemic cardiomyopathy,[13] nonischemic dilated cardiomyopathy,[14] cardiac amyloidosis,[15] hypertrophic cardiomyopathy,[16] and AS.[12,17] Focal myocardial fibrosis detected by LGE has proven to be a powerful independent predictor of mortality and adverse cardiovascular events in many conditions.

In patients with severe AS, nonischemic patterns of LGE are twice as common as ischemic patterns,[18] including punctate or focal, subendocardial (resembling myocardial infarction), midwall, and extensive diffuse fibrosis (**Fig. 2**). A single-center prospective study, including 143 consecutive patients with moderate or severe AS, has shown that focal midwall fibrosis pattern can be observed in the myocardium of up to 38% of patients and is associated with a more advanced hypertrophic response and worse prognosis even after surgical AV replacement (AVR).[17] Barone Rochette and colleagues[19] also showed that the extent of myocardial fibrosis detected by LGE imaging before AVR predicted increased perioperative risk and worse all-cause and cardiovascular-related mortality in 154 patients with severe AS but without prior myocardial infarction.

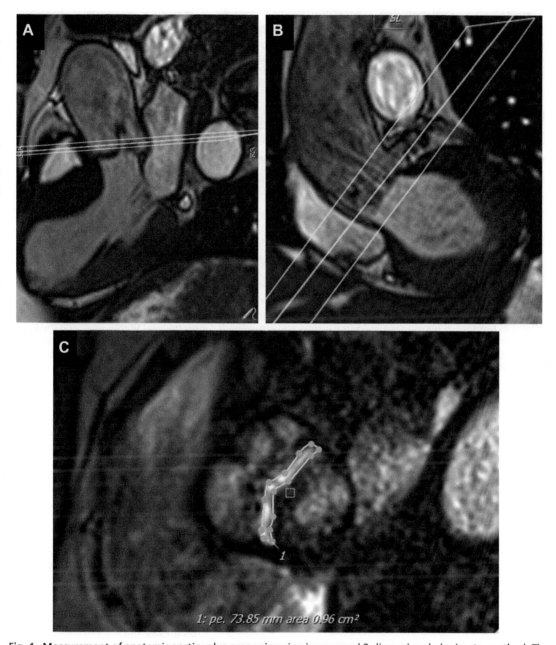

Fig. 1. Measurement of anatomic aortic valve area using cine images and 2-dimensional planimetry method. The scout lines set (*green lines*) at the AV leaflet tips on 2 orthogonal cine views at midsystolic frame measure the anatomic AVA (*yellow dots*) by 2-dimensional planimetry method: (*A*) 3-chamber view and (*B*) coronal view. (*C*) The AVA measurement is 0.96 cm².

Additionally, the poor prognosis associated with nonischemic LGE persists long after AVR. The largest multicenter study of CMR imaging in AS to date included 674 subjects with severe AS and demonstrated that LGE on CMR imaging was observed in 51% of these subjects. Importantly, its presence doubled all-cause mortality and tripled cardiovascular mortality despite

AVR.[18] Furthermore, quantification of LGE demonstrated a strong dose-response association with outcomes. Whether AV intervention should take place before its development deserves further prospective evaluation, which is ongoing.

These adverse associations with the both the presence and amount of LGE are critical because replacement fibrosis in AS progresses quickly and

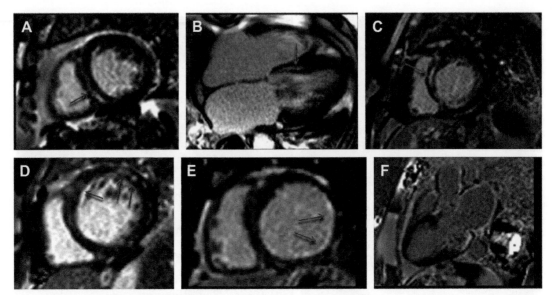

Fig. 2. Focal myocardial fibrosis detected by LGE imaging in AS. Postcontrast LGE imaging performed at 10 to 15 minutes after bolus gadolinium contrast using phase-sensitive inversion recovery sequence. Note the different patterns of myocardial fibrosis seen in AS (*red arrows* and *arrowhead*). Linear midwall fibrosis involving the interventricular septum (*A–C*), patchy midwall fibrosis (*D*), and infarct LGE with a subendocardial pattern (*E, F*). (*From* Cavalcante JL, Lalude OO, Schoenhagen P, Lerakis S. Cardiovascular Magnetic Resonance Imaging for Structural and Valvular Heart Disease Interventions. JACC Cardiovasc Interv 2016;9:399-425, with permission.)

does not regress following AV intervention.[20,21] Interestingly, even in asymptomatic subjects with moderately severe AS, the presence of LGE was associated with LV decompensation.[22] Taken together, these results suggest that early AVR could potentially halt further myocardial fibrosis progression in AS patients presenting with LGE, thereby improving patient outcomes (**Fig. 3**).

T1 Mapping

LGE is the most validated CMR imaging marker of replacement myocardial fibrosis in patients with AS. However, progressive pressure overload and compensatory LV hypertrophy also produce myocyte hypertrophy and interstitial expansion. Focal and diffuse myocardial fibrosis often coexist in

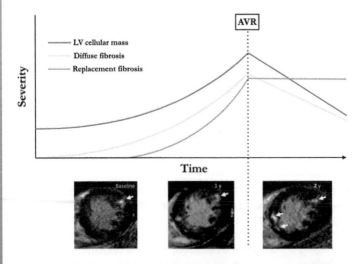

Fig. 3. Myocardial fibrosis progression in AS and response to AVR. With the progression of AS, LV cellular mass gradually increases, followed the development of diffuse fibrosis. Replacement fibrosis occurs later but progresses quickly once established. Although both LV cellular mass and diffuse fibrosis regress following release of pressure-loading conditions after AVR, the burden of replacement fibrosis persists. The insets show LGE imaging in a patient with AS. At baseline, there is focal replacement fibrosis identified by LGE (*white arrows*). At 1 year, there is interval progression of replacement fibrosis (*red arrows*). One year after AVR, despite regression of LV mass, there is no regression of replacement fibrosis (*white arrows*). (*From* Bing R, Cavalcante J, Everett R et al. Imaging and impact of myocardial fibrosis in aortic stenosis. JACC Cardiovasc Imaging 2019;12:283-296, with permission.)

patients with AS. Therefore, although LGE excels at identifying focal fibrosis, it is unable to accurately identify or quantify diffuse interstitial fibrosis, for which the gold standard assessment remains histologic collagen volume fraction.[23] To address this, T1 mapping has emerged as a novel noninvasive imaging modality to detect diffuse fibrosis (Fig. 4). The 3 main parameters are native T1, extracellular volume (ECV) fraction (ECV%), and indexed ECV (iECV). All 3 have been shown to correlate with collagen volume fraction on histology.[12,24–29] Importantly, ECV reflects fibrosis and potential interstitial water limited to the extracellular matrix, whereas native T1 also includes the cardiomyocyte compartment.

Native T1

As fibrosis increases, native T1 values typically increase in patients with AS. Native T1 can detect focal and diffuse fibrosis without the use of contrast agent. Lee and colleagues[30] recently demonstrated that, in a cohort of 127 subjects with moderate or severe AS and 33 healthy volunteers, native T1 was significantly higher in subjects with AS compared with healthy volunteers. Furthermore, native T1 was independently associated with all-cause mortality and heart failure hospitalization, albeit with low numbers of events.

Extracellular volume fraction

ECV can be obtained using postcontrast myocardial T1 mapping values for blood pool, precontrast native T1 and hematocrit: $ECV\% = (\Delta[1/T1_{myo}]/\Delta[1/T1_{blood}]) \times (1 - hematocrit)$, where $\Delta(1/T1)$ is the difference in myocardial or blood pool T1 precontrast and postcontrast.[2] Chin and colleagues[27] showed that ECV% is higher in subjects with AS than in healthy controls. However, there are limited on data assessing the prognostic value of ECV% in subjects with AS.

Indexed extracellular volume

iECV quantifies the total LV ECV (indexed to body surface area): $iECV = ECV\% \times indexed\ LV$ myocardial volume. Chin and colleagues[12] demonstrated that iECV is increased in subjects with AS compared with healthy volunteers and higher iECV identifies subjects with early evidence

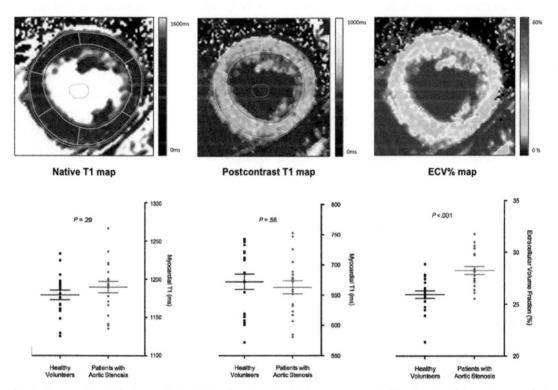

Fig. 4. T1 mapping techniques. Native T1 and postcontrast T1 maps generated by the signal intensity encoded within each voxel, depending on the T1 relaxation time; color coding according to T1 times is applied for visual reference. ECV% maps are generated using the formula $ECV\% = (\Delta[1/T1_{myo}]/\Delta[1/T1_{blood}]) \times (1 - hematocrit)$, where $\Delta(1/T1)$ is the difference in myocardial or blood T1 precontrast and postcontrast. Note that there is significant overlap between health and disease with native and postcontrast T1, in contrast to ECV%. ECV%, extracellular volume fraction; iECV, indexed extracellular volume. (*From* Bing R, Cavalcante J, Everett R et al. Imaging and impact of myocardial fibrosis in aortic stenosis. JACC Cardiovasc Imaging 2019;12:283-296, with permission.)

of LV decompensation and adverse long-term outcome.

iECV and ECV% can be used together to assess the composition of the intracellular and extracellular compartments before and after relief of LV loading conditions, such as in AS patients before and after AVR. As a result of chronic progressive valve obstruction in AS, iECV and LV mass seem to increase relatively proportionally, such that ECV% remains unchanged. After AVR, LV mass (comprising cellular and extracellular mass) and iECV (representing total ECV or mass) decrease, in keeping with the potential for reversal of diffuse fibrosis. However, there is a corresponding increase in ECV% due to a more rapid regression in cellular mass compared with extracellular mass.[20,21]

Importantly, it seems that gender differences exist not only for LV remodeling patterns but also for the magnitude of myocardial fibrosis with men having higher iECV and cell (1-iECV) volumes but the same ECV% as women.[31]

Although the values of T1 mapping are relatively reproducible when using the same sequence and scanner on the same patient, they are influenced by some factors such as age and gender, acquisition sequence, scanner field strength, and postprocessing. Accurate quality control and standardized approaches for T1 mapping are in development, and groups such as the International T1

Multicenter Consortium have now demonstrated reproducible multicenter, multivendor sequences in other conditions. Use of T1 mapping specifically in AS is highly promising and offers the only method of quantifying diffuse fibrosis but does require further research to allow broader clinical application.

Feature-Tracking Global Longitudinal Strain

CMR feature-tracking (FT) allows assessment of global longitudinal strain (GLS) from routine cine images in the clinical setting, thus avoiding the need for dedicated pulse sequences and complex postprocessing analysis (**Fig. 5**). Although CMR-FT–derived GLS has been shown to be a reproducible and independent predictor for mortality in patients with DCM[32] and myocardial infarction over and above LV ejection fraction (LVEF),[33] little has been reported on the prognostic value of CMR-FT–derived GLS in patients with AS. In a small cohort of 63 subjects with severe AS and normal LVEF, baseline CMR-FT–derived GLS was associated with LV mass index regression after AVR.[34] However, the study did not evaluate the association of CMR-FT–derived GLS and hard outcomes such as death and/or hospitalization in AS subjects. Further studies are required to confirm the clinical utility and prognostic value of CMR-FT–derived GLS for subjects with AS.

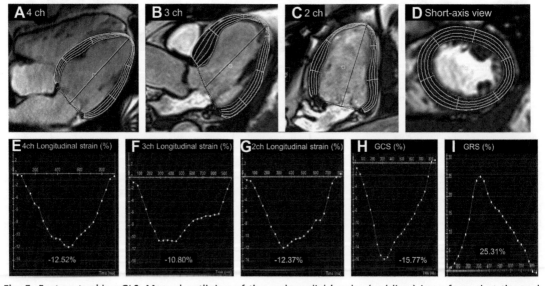

Fig. 5. Feature-tracking GLS. Manual outlining of the endocardial border (*red lines*) is performed at the end-diastolic phase in both long-axis (*A–C*) and short-axis (*D*) cine images. This is followed by automated FT propagation and processing of strain analysis throughout the cardiac cycle. GLS (−11.51%) was calculated from the horizontal long axis (*A, E,* 4-chamber; *B, F,* 3-chamber; and *C, G,* 2-chamber) integrating the average of 18 segments (6 per view). Global circumferential strain (GCS) (*H*) and global radial strain (*I*) were calculated from a single short-axis plane at the level of papillary muscles in the midventricle (*D*). Green lines: epicardial border; blue lines: myocardial tracking; yellow lines: strain curve.

TRANSCATHETER AORTIC VALVE REPLACEMENT PLANNING

Transcatheter AVR (TAVR) has been a breakthrough therapeutic advance in the treatment of patients with severe AS. TAVR teams have embraced multimodality imaging to plan procedures, guide implantation, and evaluate postprocedural outcomes. Although this is typically performed by cardiac computed tomography angiography (CTA), some patients may be unsuitable for the administration of iodinated contrast, such as those with advanced chronic kidney disease. Although 3-dimensional echocardiography may be used,[35] axial imaging is preferable; noncontrast CMR imaging can therefore offer a valuable alternative modality for TAVR planning.

Accurate evaluation of the aortic annulus is essential for appropriate prosthesis sizing to minimize paravalvular leak (PVL) while avoiding potential complications such as coronary artery obstruction or annular rupture. This can be performed by CMR imaging using standard breath-hold cine imaging with the intersection of 2 orthogonal views (3-chamber and coronal). Multiple 6 mm parallel slices, without gaps, are obtained. Verification of the aortic annulus plane is performed using a reference line superimposed over the 2 other views. In the same manner as CTA, aortic annulus area, perimeter, and minimal and maximal annulus diameters are then obtained (**Fig. 6**). Direct comparison of CMR imaging and CTA measurements of the aortic annulus, root, and ascending aorta have shown close agreement and similar ability to predict PVL.[36] CMR imaging may also be used in patients with prosthetic AVs who are being considered for valve-in-valve TAVR, although artifacts can prevent accurate imaging of the aortic root if the original prosthesis has metal struts.[37]

Another alternative for aortic annulus measurement by CMR imaging is to perform an

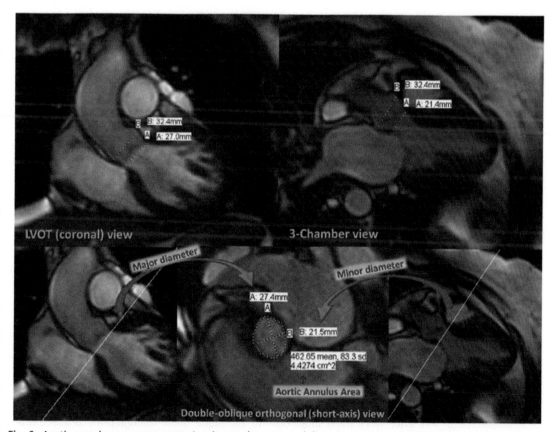

Fig. 6. Aortic annulus measurements. Aortic annulus area and diameter measured using gated breath-hold cines of 2 orthogonal views (3-chamber and coronal views). In the double-oblique orthogonal short-axis view (*bottom center*), A refers to the major annular diameter, 27.4 mm, and B refers to the minor annular diameter, 21.5 mm. LVOT, LV outflow tract. (*From* Cavalcante JL, Lalude OO, Schoenhagen P, Lerakis S. Cardiovascular Magnetic Resonance Imaging for Structural and Valvular Heart Disease Interventions. JACC Cardiovasc Interv 2016;9:399-425, with permission.)

electrocardiogram-gated, free-breathing, 3-dimensional whole-heart navigator non-CMR angiography, which is commonly used for patients with aortopathy. Once the dataset is obtained, double-oblique multiplanar reformats are performed similar to CTA for the evaluation of the aortic annulus. This method has been shown to correlate well against CTA.[38] Importantly, measurement differences in the aortic annulus occur throughout the cardiac cycle with recommendations supporting the use of the best systolic phase in which motion is at a minimum.

Finally, among the recognized limitations of CMR imaging is the difficulty to characterize calcification. Coregistration of a noncontrast-gated CTA dataset allows for detailed visualization of areas where calcification could be problematic (eg, LV outflow tract calcification) while avoiding the need for iodinated contrast administration.

POST–TRANSCATHETER AORTIC VALVE REPLACEMENT ASSESSMENT OF PARAVALVULAR LEAK

PVL remains among the most common complication post-TAVR. Although its prevalence and severity have significantly decreased over the last 5 years, the presence of greater than or equal to moderate PVL has been associated with poor outcomes.[39] Although postprocedure aortography and TTE are the most common methods used for PVL assessment following TAVR, quantification remains challenging[40,41] owing to a variety of reasons: poor acoustic windows, eccentricity of PVL jets, artifact from implanted prosthesis, irregular orifices, and subjectivity and inconsistency with regard to the imaging method and grading.[42,43] In contrast, CMR 2-dimensional phase-contrast imaging potentially offers superior accuracy and reproducibility for quantification of regurgitant volume and regurgitant fraction, which are

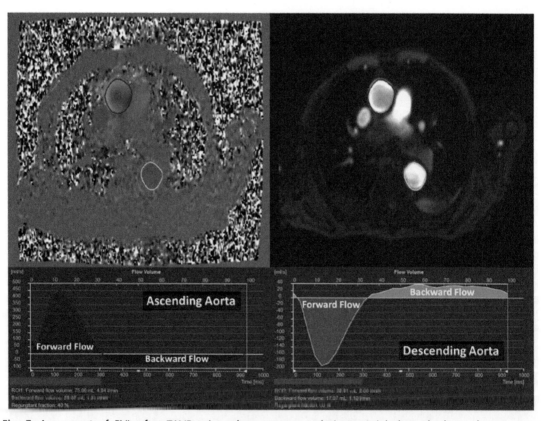

Fig. 7. Assessment of PVL after TAVR using phase-contrast technique. Axial through-plane phase-contrast sequence at the level of the main pulmonary artery used for quantification of forward and backward flow into the ascending (*red circle*) and descending aorta (*green circle*). Automated postprocessing software analysis evaluates holodiastolic flow and reversal in the descending thoracic aorta so that exact calculation of the aortic regurgitant volume and regurgitant fraction is obtained. (*From* Cavalcante JL, Lalude OO, Schoenhagen P, Lerakis S. Cardiovascular Magnetic Resonance Imaging for Structural and Valvular Heart Disease Interventions. JACC Cardiovasc Interv 2016;9:399-425, with permission.)

determined based on the forward flow and reversal of flow, regardless of whether a regurgitant jet has been visually identified (**Fig. 7**).

Previous studies have shown that TTE might underestimate or overestimate the severity of PVL compared with CMR imaging,[40] and a lack of agreement in aortic regurgitation (AR) severity between the 2 techniques has been observed in about 50% of TAVR patients.[44,45] In a recent multicenter study that included 135 subjects treated with TAVR,[46] regurgitant fraction of AR on CMR imaging greater than or equal to 30% performed 40 days after TAVR was associated with higher all-cause mortality, whereas AR grade assessed by TTE at 4 to 5 days after TAVR had no significant capability to discriminate risk. This study suggests that CMR phase-contrast imaging might offer more accurate quantification of PVL, particularly in the presence of difficult imaging and/or ambiguous Doppler evaluation. The ongoing, prospective, multicenter CLASS-CMR (CoreValve Paravalvular Leak Assessment Using Cardiac MRI) study (ClinicalTrials.gov: NCT03195114) will be (1) evaluating the correlation of PVL severity assessed by both cardiac MRI and TTE after TAVR with self-expanding valves, (2) assessing the interobserver and intraobserver variability of both imaging methods, and (3) correlating the severity of PVL with post-TAVR changes in LV remodeling, myocardial fibrosis, and clinical outcomes.

SUMMARY

CMR imaging offers a noninvasive, accurate, and reproducible assessment of cardiac morphology, function, and myocardial tissue characterization. An understanding of these parameters and their interplay in the complex pathophysiology of AS is required to continue improving patient outcomes. Further research and randomized trials will be key to further defining and refining the current applications of this robust imaging technique into the management of patients with valvular heart disease.

REFERENCES

1. Nkomo VT, Gardin JM, Skelton TN, et al. Burden of valvular heart diseases: a population-based study. Lancet 2006;368:1005–11.
2. Messroghli DR, Moon JC, Ferreira VM, et al. Clinical recommendations for cardiovascular magnetic resonance mapping of T1, T2, T2* and extracellular volume: a consensus statement by the Society for Cardiovascular Magnetic Resonance (SCMR) endorsed by the European Association for Cardiovascular Imaging (EACVI). J Cardiovasc Magn Reson 2017;19:75.
3. Cawley PJ, Maki JH, Otto CM. Cardiovascular magnetic resonance imaging for valvular heart disease: technique and validation. Circulation 2009;119: 468–78.
4. Caruthers SD, Lin SJ, Brown P, et al. Practical value of cardiac magnetic resonance imaging for clinical quantification of aortic valve stenosis: comparison with echocardiography. Circulation 2003;108:2236–43.
5. Lotz J, Meier C, Leppert A, et al. Cardiovascular flow measurement with phase-contrast MR imaging: basic facts and implementation. Radiographics 2002;22:651–71.
6. Cavalcante JL. Watchful waiting in aortic stenosis: are we ready for individualizing the risk assessment? Eur Heart J 2016;37:724–6.
7. Mewton N, Liu CY, Croisille P, et al. Assessment of myocardial fibrosis with cardiovascular magnetic resonance. J Am Coll Cardiol 2011;57:891–903.
8. Hein S, Arnon E, Kostin S, et al. Progression from compensated hypertrophy to failure in the pressure-overloaded human heart: structural deterioration and compensatory mechanisms. Circulation 2003;107:984–91.
9. Heymans S, Schroen B, Vermeersch P, et al. Increased cardiac expression of tissue inhibitor of metalloproteinase-1 and tissue inhibitor of metalloproteinase-2 is related to cardiac fibrosis and dysfunction in the chronic pressure-overloaded human heart. Circulation 2005;112:1136–44.
10. Nigri M, Azevedo CF, Rochitte CE, et al. Contrast-enhanced magnetic resonance imaging identifies focal regions of intramyocardial fibrosis in patients with severe aortic valve disease: Correlation with quantitative histopathology. Am Heart J 2009;157:361–8.
11. Treibel TA, Lopez B, Gonzalez A, et al. Reappraising myocardial fibrosis in severe aortic stenosis: an invasive and non-invasive study in 133 patients. Eur Heart J 2018;39:699–709.
12. Chin CWL, Everett RJ, Kwiecinski J, et al. Myocardial fibrosis and cardiac decompensation in aortic stenosis. JACC Cardiovasc Imaging 2017;10:1320–33.
13. Kwong RY, Chan AK, Brown KA, et al. Impact of unrecognized myocardial scar detected by cardiac magnetic resonance imaging on event-free survival in patients presenting with signs or symptoms of coronary artery disease. Circulation 2006;113:2733–43.
14. Becker MAJ, Cornel JH, van de Ven PM, et al. The prognostic value of late gadolinium-enhanced cardiac magnetic resonance imaging in nonischemic dilated cardiomyopathy: a review and meta-analysis. JACC Cardiovasc Imaging 2018;11:1274–84.
15. Raina S, Lensing SY, Nairooz RS, et al. Prognostic value of late gadolinium enhancement CMR in systemic amyloidosis. JACC Cardiovasc Imaging 2016;9:1267–77.

16. Weng Z, Yao J, Chan RH, et al. Prognostic value of LGE-CMR in HCM: a meta-analysis. JACC Cardiovasc Imaging 2016;9:1392–402.

17. Dweck MR, Joshi S, Murigu T, et al. Midwall fibrosis is an independent predictor of mortality in patients with aortic stenosis. J Am Coll Cardiol 2011;58:1271–9.

18. Musa TA, Treibel TA, Vassiliou VS, et al. Myocardial scar and mortality in severe aortic stenosis. Circulation 2018;138:1935–47.

19. Barone-Rochette G, Pierard S, De Meester de Ravenstein C, et al. Prognostic significance of LGE by CMR in aortic stenosis patients undergoing valve replacement. J Am Coll Cardiol 2014;64:144–54.

20. Everett RJ, Tastet L, Clavel MA, et al. Progression of hypertrophy and myocardial fibrosis in aortic stenosis: a multicenter cardiac magnetic resonance study. Circ Cardiovasc Imaging 2018;11:e007451.

21. Treibel TA, Kozor R, Schofield R, et al. Reverse myocardial remodeling following valve replacement in patients with aortic stenosis. J Am Coll Cardiol 2018;71:860–71.

22. Chin CW, Messika-Zeitoun D, Shah AS, et al. A clinical risk score of myocardial fibrosis predicts adverse outcomes in aortic stenosis. Eur Heart J 2016;37:713–23.

23. Schelbert EB, Moon JC. Exploiting differences in myocardial compartments with native T1 and extracellular volume fraction for the diagnosis of hypertrophic cardiomyopathy. Circ Cardiovasc Imaging 2015;8 [pii:e004232].

24. Bull S, White SK, Piechnik SK, et al. Human noncontrast T1 values and correlation with histology in diffuse fibrosis. Heart 2013;99:932–7.

25. Kockova R, Kacer P, Pirk J, et al. Native T1 relaxation time and extracellular volume fraction as accurate markers of diffuse myocardial fibrosis in heart valve disease- comparison with targeted left ventricular myocardial biopsy. Circ J 2016;80:1202–9.

26. Lee SP, Lee W, Lee JM, et al. Assessment of diffuse myocardial fibrosis by using MR imaging in asymptomatic patients with aortic stenosis. Radiology 2015;274:359–69.

27. Chin CW, Semple S, Malley T, et al. Optimization and comparison of myocardial T1 techniques at 3T in patients with aortic stenosis. Eur Heart J Cardiovasc Imaging 2014;15:556–65.

28. White SK, Sado DM, Fontana M, et al. T1 mapping for myocardial extracellular volume measurement by CMR: bolus only versus primed infusion technique. JACC Cardiovasc Imaging 2013;6:955–62.

29. de Meester de Ravenstein C, Bouzin C, Lazam S, et al. Histological Validation of measurement of diffuse interstitial myocardial fibrosis by myocardial extravascular volume fraction from Modified Look-Locker imaging (MOLLI) T1 mapping at 3 T. J Cardiovasc Magn Reson 2015;17:48.

30. Lee H, Park JB, Yoon YE, et al. Noncontrast myocardial T1 mapping by cardiac magnetic resonance predicts outcome in patients with aortic stenosis. JACC Cardiovasc Imaging 2018;11:974–83.

31. Treibel TA, Kozor R, Fontana M, et al. Sex dimorphism in the myocardial response to aortic stenosis. JACC Cardiovasc Imaging 2018;11:962–73.

32. Romano S, Judd RM, Kim RJ, et al. Feature-tracking global longitudinal strain predicts death in a multicenter population of patients with ischemic and nonischemic dilated cardiomyopathy incremental to ejection fraction and late gadolinium enhancement. JACC Cardiovasc Imaging 2018;11:1419–29.

33. Eitel I, Stiermaier T, Lange T, et al. Cardiac magnetic resonance myocardial feature tracking for optimized prediction of cardiovascular events following myocardial infarction. JACC Cardiovasc Imaging 2018;11:1433–44.

34. Hwang JW, Kim SM, Park SJ, et al. Assessment of reverse remodeling predicted by myocardial deformation on tissue tracking in patients with severe aortic stenosis: a cardiovascular magnetic resonance imaging study. J Cardiovasc Magn Reson 2017;19:80.

35. Achenbach S, Delgado V, Hausleiter J, et al. SCCT expert consensus document on computed tomography imaging before transcatheter aortic valve implantation (TAVI)/transcatheter aortic valve replacement (TAVR). J Cardiovasc Comput Tomogr 2012;6:366–80.

36. Jabbour A, Ismail TF, Moat N, et al. Multimodality imaging in transcatheter aortic valve implantation and post-procedural aortic regurgitation: comparison among cardiovascular magnetic resonance, cardiac computed tomography, and echocardiography. J Am Coll Cardiol 2011;58:2165–73.

37. Quail MA, Nordmeyer J, Schievano S, et al. Use of cardiovascular magnetic resonance imaging for TAVR assessment in patients with bioprosthetic aortic valves: comparison with computed tomography. Eur J Radiol 2012;81:3912–7.

38. Ruile P, Blanke P, Krauss T, et al. Pre-procedural assessment of aortic annulus dimensions for transcatheter aortic valve replacement: comparison of a non-contrast 3D MRA protocol with contrast-enhanced cardiac dual-source CT angiography. Eur Heart J Cardiovasc Imaging 2016;17:458–66.

39. Kodali S, Pibarot P, Douglas PS, et al. Paravalvular regurgitation after transcatheter aortic valve replacement with the Edwards sapien valve in the PARTNER trial. characterizing patients and impact on outcomes. Eur Heart J 2015;36:449–56.

40. Ribeiro HB, Le Ven F, Larose E, et al. Cardiac magnetic resonance versus transthoracic echocardiography for the assessment and quantification of aortic regurgitation in patients undergoing

transcatheter aortic valve implantation. Heart 2014; 100:1924–32.

41. Orwat S, Diller G-P, Kaleschke G, et al. Aortic regurgitation severity after transcatheter aortic valve implantation is underestimated by echocardiography compared with MRI. Heart 2014;100: 1933–8.

42. Pibarot P, Hahn RT, Weissman NJ, et al. Assessment of paravalvular regurgitation following TAVR: a proposal of unifying grading scheme. JACC Cardiovasc Imaging 2015;8:340–60.

43. Lerakis S, Hayek SS, Douglas PS. Paravalvular aortic leak after transcatheter aortic valve replacement: current knowledge. Circulation 2013;127: 397–407.

44. Altiok E, Frick M, Meyer CG, et al. Comparison of two- and three-dimensional transthoracic echocardiography to cardiac magnetic resonance imaging for assessment of paravalvular regurgitation after transcatheter aortic valve implantation. Am J Cardiol 2014;113:1859–66.

45. Hartlage GR, Babaliaros VC, Thourani VH, et al. The role of cardiovascular magnetic resonance in stratifying paravalvular leak severity after transcatheter aortic valve replacement: an observational outcome study. J Cardiovasc Magn Reson 2014;16:93.

46. Ribeiro HB, Orwat S, Hayek SS, et al. Cardiovascular magnetic resonance to evaluate aortic regurgitation after transcatheter aortic valve replacement. J Am Coll Cardiol 2016;68:577–85.

T2* Mapping Techniques
Iron Overload Assessment and Other Potential Clinical Applications

Katia Menacho, MD[a], Amna Abdel-Gadir, MBBS, MRCP[b,c],
James C. Moon, MB, BCh, MRCP, MD[d],
Juliano Lara Fernandes, MD, PhD, MBA[e,*]

KEYWORDS

- Parametric mapping • T2* • Iron overload • Blood oxygen level dependent (BOLD) • Hemorrhage

KEY POINTS

- T2* mapping sequences are widely accessible in most commercial scanners and multiple tools to quantify it are available.
- New technical developments have made possible automated and free-breathing acquisition of T2* maps with no major limitations on age.
- Routine T2* assessment of iron overload is recommended in patients with chronic transfusions and has significantly changed prognosis and treatment strategies.
- T1 and T2 maps can be used for iron overload assessment and evidence is rapidly increasing for these alternative methods in this scenario.
- Intramyocardial hemorrhage, microvascular obstruction, and blood oxygen level ischemia assessment are important variables in acute and chronic coronary artery disease that can be evaluated with T2* maps.

Multiparametric mapping of the myocardium has become an area of great interest in the recent year with multiple review articles and recommendation statements.[1] Despite most of the focus initially on T1 mapping and then on T2/edema imaging, T2* mapping was the first clinically useful parametric mapping technique for the heart.[2] Before the introduction of T2* as a diagnostic tool, iron-induced cardiomyopathy was the most common cause of death in transfusion-dependent thalassemic patients. It has been now more than 18 years since the initial applications of T2* images in iron overload assessment began to be performed and the accumulated knowledge gained from that has led to important practical changes in the diagnosis and treatment with chelation. T2* is the current method of choice for the assessment of cardiac iron deposition, with proven evidence in reduction of overall mortality (improvement on life expectancy and fewer cardiovascular complications in transfusion-dependent patients). Moreover, faster protocols

Disclosure: Dr K. Menacho is supported by the Peruvian Scientific, Technological Development and Technological Innovation (FONDECYT) from CONCYTEC, Peru. Dr J.C. Moon is supported by The University College London Hospitals and NIHR Barts Biomedical Research Centre. The remaining authors have nothing to disclose.
[a] Barts Heart Centre, The Cardiovascular Magnetic Resonance Imaging Unit, Institute of Cardiovascular Science, University College London, St Bartholomew's Hospital, 2nd Floor, King George V Block, West Smithfiled, London EC1A 7BE, UK; [b] Institute of Cardiovascular Science, University College London, Gower Street, London WC1E6BT, UK; [c] Barts Heart Centre, St Bartholomew's Hospital, 2nd Floor, King George V Block, London EC1A 7BE, UK; [d] The Cardiovascular Magnetic Resonance Imaging Unit, The Inherited Cardiovascular Diseases Unit, Barts Heart Centre, St Bartholomew's Hospital, 2nd Floor, King George V Block, West Smithfield, London EC1A 7BE, UK; [e] Jose Michel Kalaf Research Institute, Radiologia Clinica de Campinas, Av Jose de Souza Campos 840, Campinas, São Paulo 13092-100, Brazil
* Corresponding author.
E-mail address: jlaraf@terra.com.br

Magn Reson Imaging Clin N Am 27 (2019) 439–451
https://doi.org/10.1016/j.mric.2019.04.008
1064-9689/19/© 2019 Elsevier Inc. All rights reserved.

can make this technology available in developing countries. This article summarizes the most important aspects of T2* mapping when applied in clinical practice, with an additional look into other applications in which T2* maps might also provide unique important data beyond traditional clinical and imaging markers.

T2* TECHNIQUES: FROM ACQUISITION TO POSTPROCESSING
Physical Parameter: T2* Imaging

T2* represents the decay of transverse magnetization caused by a loss of coherence between spins and magnetic field inhomogeneity.[3] This relaxation

is measured using gradient-echo (GRE) imaging. This transverse relaxation is eliminated when a 180° pulse is applied using a spin echo sequence (true T2 relaxation), which removes the magnetic field inhomogeneity,[4] as illustrated in **Fig. 1**. The principle of T2* relaxation is involved in numerous magnetic resonance (MR) applications with GRE sequences, such as perfusion techniques and functional imaging sequences.

T2* Imaging to Assess Iron Loading

A fundamental principle to generate images for iron quantification is to apply a strong magnetic field and radiofrequency signals through GRE

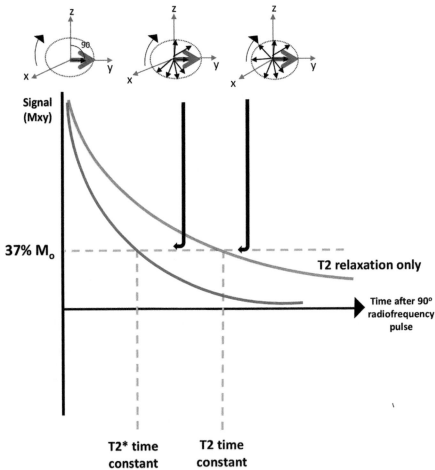

Fig. 1. T2* and T2 decay. Transverse relaxation after an initial 90° radiofrequency pulse. A transverse magnetization (*small red arrow*) has a maximum amplitude as the population of proton magnetic moments (spins) rotate in phase. The amplitude of the net magnetization decays as the proton magnetic moments move out of phase with one another (*small black arrows*). The overall term for the observed loss of phase coherence (dephasing) is T2* relaxation (the combination of T2 relaxation and local variations inhomogeneities in the applied magnetic field). T2 relaxation is the result of spin-spin interactions and this process in irreversible. T2* decay occurs when refocusing pulses are not used and its signal occurs faster (*blue curve*). Both T2 and T2* are exponential processes with time constants T2 and T2* respectively. This constant is the time at which the magnetization has decayed to 37% of its initial value after 90° radiofrequency pulse. (*Adapted from* of John P Ridgway. Cardiovascular magnetic resonance physics for clinicians: part I. J Cardiovasc Magn Reson 2010;12:71; with permission.)

sequences, with time of decay controlled by the MR imaging scanner. The longer the echo time (TE), the darker the resultant image; iron-mediated darkening can be characterized by a half-time constant and is nonlinearly proportional to the level of iron concentrations. Often, this darkening is described as a rate principle (R2*) rather than a time constant. The relaxation rate is just the reciprocal of the time constant, R2* = 1000/T2*. The factor of 1000 is included because T2* is expressed in milliseconds and relation rates in expressed in Hertz (sec^{-1}).[5,6] To calculate T2*, an application of multiple radiofrequency pulses leads to the generation of a series of images with different TEs.[7]

Traditional Sequences to Measure Cardiac Iron Overload

The most updated international expert consensus suggests that, for T2* cardiac iron loading assessment, a multiecho GRE, with 8 equally echo times, ranging from 2 to 18 milliseconds, may be used on a 1.5 T imaging scanner.[1] Fat saturation is needed for the liver but is not essential for heart images. Good shimming of the heart is a requirement for accurate measurements and manual volume shimming may be required in order to reduce potential artifacts. Once adjusting these factors, both bright-blood and dark-blood techniques are validated and widely used clinically.[8,9]

- Bright-blood technique:[8] images are acquired immediately after the R wave to reduce artifacts caused by blood flow and myocardial wall motion.[4]
- Dark-blood technique: a double inversion recovery pulse is used to null the signal from blood; multiecho T2* acquisition is extended to late diastole with minimal cardiac motions technique.[10]

Compared with bright-blood technique, dark blood has been shown to have superior reproducibility, less artifact susceptibility and it is the preferred method to use clinically (**Fig. 2**).[9,10]

Postprocessing and Myocardial T2* Calculation

The measurement of myocardium iron is typically performed in a midventricular short-axis image.[4,10] The septal iron concentration largely reflects the global iron content as shown in biopsy studies,[1,11] so analysis can be restricted to this segment to avoid artifacts caused by susceptibility effects (**Fig. 3**).

One of the most important limitations for postprocessing is the signal plateau, which complicates the

approach to the curve fitting method for evaluation of the T2*.[12] Different approaches have been designed to tackle this. The truncation model discards the late plateau points and then the remaining signal is fitted with a monoexponential equation.[13] The other common method is the offset model, in which an exponential equation plus a constant offset is used to tackle this problem.[7] As a general perspective, the use of offset models may produce underestimation of T2* values on bright-blood data, making it less reproducible compared with the truncation method (**Fig. 4**).[12]

Several approaches have been used to try to improve truncation model accuracy, especially in severe iron stages, in which artifact produces major limitations. Nonlocal means (NLM) providing more accurate pixel-by-pixel MR imaging relaxometry may improve tissue characterization.[14] Moreover, a noise-corrected model has been created, limiting analysis to the region of interest (ROI; base curve fitting) and consistently producing accurate and precise R2* values by correctly assessing the noncentral chi noise.[15] Most clinical vendors and dedicated cardiovascular software have validated methods of interpreting T2* data with both US Food and Drug Administration and Conformité Européene approval.[16–19] Open-source software is also available and validated against commercial tools,[20–23] resulting in a large number of options for sites to choose from in order to quantify T2* with high accuracy.

Breath-hold Versus Free-breathing Techniques

The pixel-wise mapping technique involves curve fitting on individual pixels; it offers a more spatial context than ROI-based methods for the delineation of adjacent tissues with different tissue values[24] and therefore provides a surrogate measure of the iron distribution.[7,11,25,26] This technique covers the entire field of view and provides important information to identify artifacts that may be less apparent. Moreover, pixel-wise mapping is automatic, reduces time of analysis,[27] and the median values calculated from the partial interventricular septum region provide lower intraobserver and interobserver variabilities compared with conventional techniques.[28] However, the main limitation with breath-held mapping is noise and the possibility of artifacts caused by the long breath-hold times. As an alternative, a free-breathing T2* mapping method was developed with full automation, truncation of long TE, and low signal/noise ratio (SNR) images after motion correction with highly accelerated multi-GRE acquisition and multiple averages to improve SNR. This method resulted in consistently good-quality maps, especially when

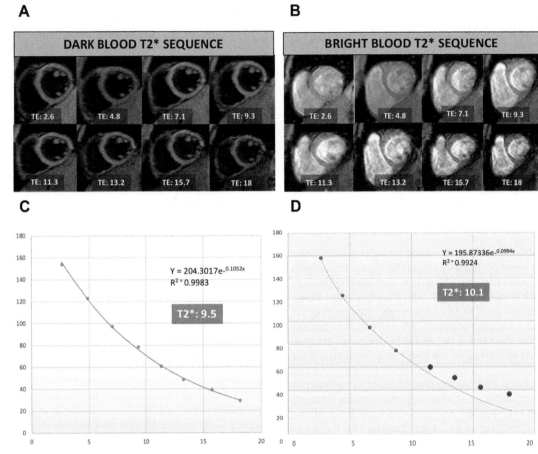

Fig. 2. (*A, B*) Midventricular short-axis image at different TE between 2 and 18 milliseconds in a patient with β-thalassemia. Image quality of black-blood sequence is superior (less artifact susceptibility) compared with bright-blood image. (*C*) Dark-blood image analysis. Background noise is reduced and curve shows a good fit for the 8 GRE time without the use of truncation ($R^2 = 0.9983$, $T2* = 9.5$ milliseconds). This technique reduces the risk of errors during analysis. (*D*) Bright-blood image analysis. The last 4 points (*red circle*) are below the background noise and are removed to improve the curve fit using the truncation method ($R^2 = 0.9924$, $T2* = 10.1$ milliseconds).

respiratory motion and arrhythmias are present and with the same time of acquisition as breath-hold techniques.[27] Other free-breathing methods also showed accurate results in the heart, with improved temporal resolution using single-shot GRE echo-planar imaging (EPI) enabling accurate myocardial measurement and being insensitive to respiratory motion.[29] **Fig. 5** shows examples of different imaging techniques, including breath-hold and free-breathing approaches.

Clinical Application of Iron Overload Assessment with T2*

Since its introduction in early 2001, the use of T2* imaging to guide therapy in patients with iron overload, coupled with improvement in chelator options and advances in other coadjuvant management strategies, resulted in significant

reduction in cardiovascular death and disability in patients with thalassemia major.[30,31] T2* Cardiac Magnetic Resonance (CMR) is a recommended examination in practically all clinical guidelines relating to iron overload treatment[32–34] and its use has been summarized in specific recommendation statements as well.[35]

From a practical standpoint, transfusion-dependent patients should start monitoring myocardial T2* at the age of 10 years if they are routinely followed and have a history of being well chelated.[36] However, patients in whom the treatment follow-up is unclear, or who have irregular chelation or very high liver iron concentrations (LICs), may perform their first MR imaging scan at ages as early as 7 years because significant myocardial iron concentrations (MICs) have been described at this early age.[37] Although initial T2* techniques performed poorly

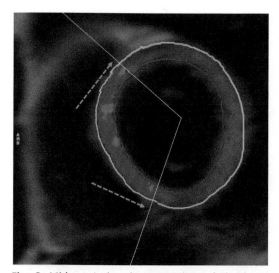

Fig. 3. Midventricular short-axis slice of the heart showing the correct assessment of iron quantification with T2* method. Full-thickness region of interest is defined by limiting the epicardial and endocardial border (gradient infiltration starting at epicardium). Analysis is restricted to the septum (*yellow lines*), in order to avoid artifacts from anterior and posterior cardiac veins (*orange arrows*) and the lung.

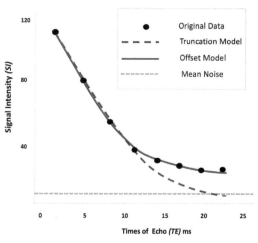

Fig. 4. Patient data fitted using both the offset and truncation models. The offset model fits all the data points well (R2 = 0.996, T2* = 4.4 milliseconds, *red line*), whereas the truncation model fitted the first 4 points only (R2 = 0.999, T2* = 6.9 milliseconds, *blue dotted line*). The mean noise as measured from a background region (*green dotted line*). (*From* He T, Gatehouse PD, Smith GC, et al. Myocardial T2* measurements in iron-overloaded thalassemia: An in vivo study to investigate optimal methods of quantification. Magn Reson Med 2008;60(5):1082–9; with permission.)

in very young children because of lack of breath holding or movement, the newer free-breathing technique copes with these difficulties fairly easily and provides good-quality images, making age restrictions no longer a limitation to when to begin scanning patients, as shown in **Fig. 6.**

Once started, routine follow-up of MICs should be performed yearly in most patients, with this interval varying from 6 months to 2 years depending on specific clinical conditions and service availability.[38] Note that removal of cardiac iron in the heart is a slow process and, especially in acute settings (ie, acute heart failure), the clinical condition sometimes improves significantly, whereas T2* changes will not be proportional.[39] The main reason for this disparity is that T2* measures mostly chronically stored iron in lysosomes, whereas the iron being mobilized by intensive chelation is in labile form, with limited T2* effects.[35] Nevertheless, monitoring the effects of iron chelation or accumulation is a primary target of routine MR imaging scans in these patients and any changes greater than the coefficient of variation of 4% for black-blood images and 8% for bright-blood images should be considered significant changes.[40]

Another important clinical aspect of using T2* for iron overload assessment involves the correlation of T2* values and MIC. Although, T2* values and

LIC correlations were established for the liver at a very early stage in the development of the technique, , T2* was the main variable used for the heart for quantification until Carpenter and colleagues[11] performed the comparison of this MR imaging value with MIC-measured biopsied hearts. Because T2* and MIC are not linearly related, this must be taken into account when assessing longitudinal changes in T2* values because significant changes in MIC occur when small variations are seen at low T2* values. The correlation of T2* and MIC can be seen in **Fig. 7** using the equation MIC = 45 × T2*$^{-1.21}$, as published by Carpenter and colleagues.[11]

When reporting the iron concentrations obtained with various T2* techniques, the value of 20 milliseconds has been traditionally associated with the normal cutoff for non–iron-overloaded myocardial tissue based on the initial Anderson and colleagues[2] data, which showed that almost all patients with T2* greater than these levels did not develop reductions in left ventricular ejection fraction. However, despite the popularity of this number, other investigators have shown that iron deposition is frequently found in patients with septal T2* greater than these levels.[41] Therefore, it would be more appropriate to consider the normal myocardial T2* levels according to measurements performed in normal volunteers,

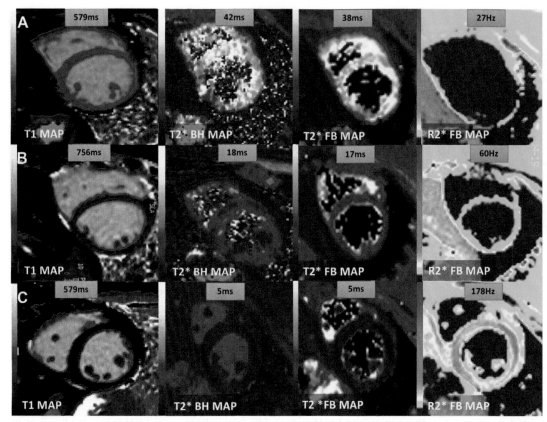

Fig. 5. Mappings techniques for T1 and T2* in (*A*) a normal patient, (*B*) a patient with mild myocardial iron overload, and (*C*) a patient with severe liver iron overload. Note that in patients in (*B*) and (*C*), there is transmural gradient of iron distribution. BH, breath hold; FB, free breathing.

in whom normality was established at 36.1 ± 4.5 milliseconds.[42] Nevertheless, traditional reporting tables for iron overload using T2* have used cutoffs based on clinical management strategies and prognostic data. **Table 1** lists the values of myocardial T2*, MIC, and the reporting levels for iron overload in the heart. Note that although T2* levels less than 10 milliseconds are considered severe, risk increases dramatically as T2* decreases further from 10 to 8 to 6 and even 4 milliseconds.[43] As for normal values, correlations with T1 suggest that 26 milliseconds would be a more appropriate cut point for T2*, and several centers worldwide report potential early iron in the range of 20 to 26 milliseconds.[44] Although not the focus of this article, the authors have also included the corresponding liver reference values because usually both measurements are performed in the same patient with the corresponding calibration curves.[45] A more thorough review of liver iron concentration measurements can be found elsewhere.[38] Despite the main recommendations being for iron overload assessment to be performed at 1.5 T, many studies have now also

performed correlations of iron overload at 3 T, and these values are reported in **Table 1** as well using one of the reference studies with this field strength.[46]

ALTERNATIVE METHODS AND COMPARISONS (T1 AND T2 MAPPING)

As shown in the previous paragraphs, the CMR T2* parameter has transformed the management of patients with iron loading conditions, allowing robust, noninvasive quantification of myocardial iron.[2] It provides tailored and personalized approaches to chelator dosing, which has been linked to improved survival.[30] To further improve diagnostic accuracy there has been an increasing interest in alternative MR imaging methods in the way of native (noncontrast) T1 and T2 mapping to aid the diagnosis of myocardial iron in patients with equivocal disease. Ferritin and hemosiderin alter the behavior and properties of hydrogen nuclei in water within tissue, shortening both T1 and T2 times, similar to T2*. The adoption of CMR parametric mapping techniques in the

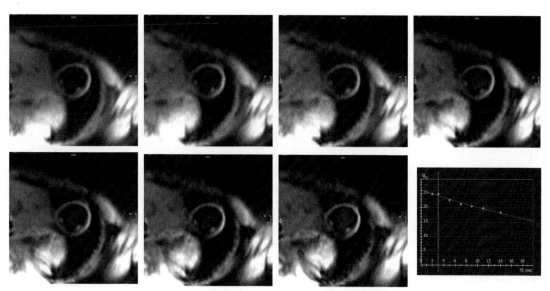

Fig. 6. A T2* series of 7 images acquired in a 4-year-old boy using a free-breathing GRE-EPI sequence with TE varying from 1.97 milliseconds to 14.0 milliseconds. The corresponding decay curve is shown as well and the calculated T2* was normal at 36.5 milliseconds. This series has motion correction already applied and generates clear images of the septum using the black-blood technique allowing accurate placement of a region of interest and T2* calculation.

diagnosis of myocardial diseases, including cardiac amyloidosis and Fabry disease, has been supported by the Society for Cardiovascular Magnetic Resonance Consensus Statement[1] and reflected in the development of commercially available mapping sequences by all major CMR scanner manufacturers. Mapping sequences allow the measurement and display of relaxation times in color on a pixel-by-pixel basis without the need for complex postprocessing.[47–50] For the measurement of myocardial iron using T1 and T2 mapping, as with T2*, an ROI is recommended in the interventricular septum using a short-axis slice.[1] By removing complex analysis, abbreviated mapping

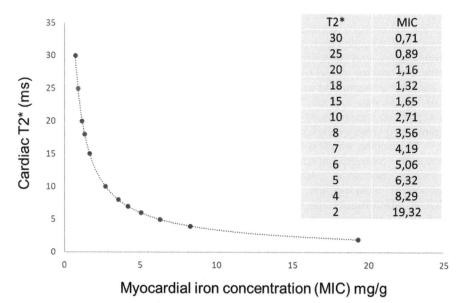

T2*	MIC
30	0,71
25	0,89
20	1,16
18	1,32
15	1,65
10	2,71
8	3,56
7	4,19
6	5,06
5	6,32
4	8,29
2	19,32

Fig. 7. Correlation of myocardial T2* and MIC with the corresponding curve and some calculated examples. From this graph, it is important to appreciate that changes in T2* greater than 30 milliseconds do not significantly change the final MIC values, whereas small changes in T2* (ie, <10 milliseconds) significantly increase MIC.

Table 1
Reference values for liver and myocardial iron concentrations for MR imaging

T2* (ms) 1.5 T	R2* (Hz) 1.5 T	T2* (ms) 3.0 T	R2* (Hz) 3.0 T	MIC/LIC (mg/g dw)	Classification
Myocardium					
≥20	≤50	≥12.6	≤79	≤1.16	Normal
10–20	51–100	5.8–12.6	80–172	>1.16–2.71	Mild to moderate
<10	>100	<5.8	>172	>2.71	Severe
Liver					
≥15.4	≤65	≥8.4	≤119	≤2.0	Normal
4.5–15.4	66–224	2.3–8.4	120–435	>2.0–7.0	Mild
2.1–4.5	225–475	1.05–2.3	436–952	>7.0–15	Moderate
<2.1	>475	<1.05	>952	>15	Severe

T2* and R2* values at 3 T are included but the authors advise caution and recommend normality is defined locally if 3 T has to be used.
Abbreviation: dw, dry weight.
Data from Refs.[11,45,46]

protocols can be performed, as shown by Abdel-Gadir and colleagues,[51] who performed noncontrast CMR for iron overload in Bangkok in 8 minutes per examination, 50 patients per day on 1 magnet, reducing costs 4-fold and showing the clinical and economic advantages.

T1 Mapping for Iron

T1 is an intrinsic magnetic property that represents longitudinal recovery time after excitation of hydrogen atoms. At selected magnetic field strengths, each tissue has its own characteristic range of values, and deviation from these values implies disease. T1 values are increased with the expansion of the extracellular compartment by fibrosis, edema, and amyloid, and reduced in iron, lipid accumulation, and hemorrhage.[52] T2* is more specific and only influenced by the presence of iron, although unrecognized use of gadolinium contrast agents may reduce T2*. In the liver, 1 case report has shown cobalt-chromium from a degenerating metal-on-metal hip as reducing T2*.[53] T1 mapping was first introduced using the inversion recovery–based modified look-locker imaging sequence (MOLLI), with further developments including the shortened MOLLI (ShMOLLI), which requires an acquisition time greater than 9 heartbeats.[48,49] Newer sequences, including saturation recovery single-shot acquisition and saturation pulse prepared heart-rate independent inversion recovery, yield higher accuracy, lower precision, and similar reproducibility compared with MOLLI and ShMOLLI.[50,54] However, means that different sequences have differing normal ranges. This difference is less important than it sounds because

tissue iron, if present, dominates measured T1; deceases in T1 of up to 20 standard deviations have been reported with severe myocardial iron.

The role of T1 mapping in the detection of iron has been promising to date at both 1.5 T and 3 T, and has been shown to correlate with cardiac iron in vitro.[55] Early data by Sado and colleagues[56] were the first to show that myocardial T1 mapping has excellent reproducibility and correlates well with T2* in a group of 88 patients with suspected iron overload. Using the ShMOLLI sequence, T2* was lower in patients than in healthy volunteers (836 ± 138 milliseconds vs 968 ± 32 milliseconds, P<.0001), and no patient with a low T2* value had normal T1 values. This study also showed superior interstudy reproducibility of T1, particularly when low levels of iron are present, and reclassified a significant proportion of patients as having mild cardiac siderosis, doubling the number of patients identified with iron, although almost all of this is mild. These findings were further explored in larger international studies using different T1 mapping sequences.[44,57] A key unknown question is whether using T1 mapping would detect changes in iron loading better than T2* for individual patients (smallest detectable difference) or in studies (increased power). An example and comparison of myocardial T1 images with T2* is shown in **Fig. 5.**

The increase in clinical use of 3 T scanners for noncardiac conditions may provide diagnostic challenges for patients requiring iron quantification because T2* mapping is not routinely recommended at 3 T. The second mapping consensus statement specifically recommends that T2* mapping for iron overload currently should be performed at 1.5 T only.[1] T1 mapping may be used as a method to quantify iron at 3 T where T2* measurements are not possible.[58] Alam and colleagues[58] showed the feasibility of T1 at both 1.5 T and 3 T, and its superiority to T2* when assessing reproducibility.

The administration of contrast and acquisition of a postcontrast T1 map allows the generation of an extracellular volume (ECV) map wherein pixel values represent the interstitial volume. In a small single-center study, ECV was increased in patients with thalassemia major with prior myocardial iron overload, whereas patients without historical iron loading had no evidence of increased ECV. The association between iron and ECV remained significant after controlling for patient age, gender, and cardiovascular risk factors.[59]

Despite the advantages of T1 mapping as a complementary diagnostic tool, there are challenges facing its clinical use. There is a known variation of absolute T1 values between sequences and scanners, and it is susceptible to alteration in a large number of diseases of the heart muscle.[60] Nevertheless, T1 seems to be a more precise measurement of myocardial iron.[44,56,57]

T2 Mapping for Iron

T2 relaxation time reflects the time for the MR signal to decay in the transverse plane and is commonly used to assess myocardial inflammation and edema.[1] As with T1 and T2*, iron deposition in the myocardium causes shortened T2 values. Very little work is available in the literature on the use of T2 for the diagnosis of myocardial iron loading. In a study of 200 patients with thalassemia in Thailand, at 1.5 T, T2 mapping correlated strongly with T2* in patients with myocardial iron loading (r = 0.951, $P<.001$) and with T1 (r = 0.973, $P<.001$).[61] Feasibility at 3 T has also been shown, because myocardial T2 values correlated with T2* in a small 8-patient study ($P = .93$, $P<.0001$).[62]

OTHER POTENTIAL CLINICAL USES FOR T2* MAPPING

Despite the large literature and references to T2* mapping and iron overload assessment, there has been increased interest in applying this technique to other cardiovascular disorders, especially now, given the newer methods with automated maps and free-breathing acquisitions.

The first particular area of interest is the ability of T2* to identify changes in myocardial oxygenation and perfusion under stress, a concept first shown in humans as early as 1996 through blood oxygen level–dependent (BOLD) imaging using T2*.[63,64]

As vasodilation takes place, the consumption of oxygen is lower because of lower oxygen extraction rates, resulting in a decrease in the concentration of paramagnetic deoxyhemoglobin and increase in diamagnetic oxyhemoglobin. Therefore, an increase in T2* values is seen under stress, with magnitudes of 10% to 17%.[65,66] The ability to detect significant changes in myocardial oxygenation led to the possibility of detection of areas of the myocardium with altered blood oxygen/supply balance in coronary artery disease, and adenosine T2* imaging showed a high sensitivity but low specificity in the correlation with angiographically determined stenosis.[67] At 3 T, the BOLD effects with T2* are more pronounced given the faster decay ratios, which affect the signal intensity, and using this field strength other investigators have shown more pronounced changes in ΔT2* in patients with normal coronary arteries compared with nonstenotic lesions and severely obstructive disease.[68] The same principle at 3 T was also applied, showing an increase in T2* in areas of the myocardium perfused by normal coronaries versus no changes in stenotic lesions.[69] The main problems with these studies have been the large number of segments not analyzed because of artifacts, resulting in approximately 25% loss of data. Given the technical developments in T2* mapping sequences, these limitations might be overcome and application of this technique in clinical routine can be applied. **Fig. 8** shows an example of the T2* maps in a patient with normal coronaries undergoing pharmacologic stress test and identifying the vasodilatory effects precontrast, with comparative myocardial blood flow images and splenic switch-off confirmation postcontrast.

Another potential use of T2* maps beyond iron overload is in the investigation of microvascular obstruction and intramyocardial hemorrhage. Hemoglobin breakdown, especially in the acute phases of myocardial infarction, leads to areas of signal nulling within infarcted areas, which can be appreciated with T2* maps. In a comparison with T2 techniques, T2* proved more sensitive in detecting areas of hemorrhagic infarctions, with significant reductions in signal of 54% versus only marginal increases in remote areas.[70] Given the important prognostic role of both microvascular obstruction and intramyocardial hemorrhage in adverse events and negative left ventricle remodeling, accurate identification and quantification of these phenomena have been an important goal in treating patients with acute coronary artery disease.[71] Therefore, current evidence suggests that T2* mapping is recommended during the multiparametric evaluation of

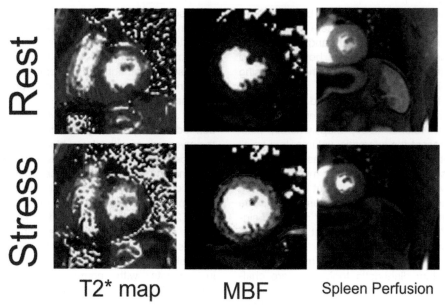

Fig. 8. Free-breathing motion-corrected 3 T T2* maps, myocardial blood flow (MBF) maps, and first-pass perfusion images of the heart/spleen at rest and stress. T2* at rest increased from 21.2 milliseconds to 24.4 milliseconds (+15.1%) in this patient with normal coronary arteries, with the correlated increase in MBF and splenic switch-off. The T2* maps were obtained before any contrast infusion, allowing accurate assessment of a positive vaso-dilatory induction of dipyridamole before injection.[72] (*Courtesy of* Peter Kellman, NIH, Bethesda, MD.)

patients with acute or recent myocardial infarction.[69] In addition, Bulluck and colleagues[73] have shown that patients with ST segment elevation myocardial infarction with intramyocardial hemorrhage had residual myocardial iron at follow-up and this may drive chronic inflammation (high T2 value in the surrounding infarct tissue), which is associated with adverse left ventricular remodeling.

ACKNOWLEDGMENTS

The authors thank Dr Peter Kellman (Medical Signal and Image Processing Program; National Heart, Lung, and Blood Institute; NIH, Bethesda, MD) for his valuable comments and suggestions to improve the article and overall support on implementing some of the sequences used in the figures.

REFERENCES

1. Messroghli DR, Moon JC, Ferreira VM, et al. Clinical recommendations for cardiovascular magnetic resonance mapping of T1, T2, T2* and extracellular volume: a consensus statement by the Society for Cardiovascular Magnetic Resonance (SCMR) endorsed by the European Association for Cardiovascular Imaging (EACVI). J Cardiovasc Magn Reson 2017;19(1):75.

2. Anderson LJ, Holden S, Davis B, et al. Cardiovascular T2-star (T2*) magnetic resonance for the early diagnosis of myocardial iron overload. Eur Heart J 2001;22(23):2171–9.

3. Chavhan GB, Babyn PS, Thomas B, et al. Principles, techniques, and applications of T2*-based MR imaging and its special applications. Radiographics 2009;29(5):1433–49.

4. Baksi AJ, Pennell DJ. T2* imaging of the heart: methods, applications, and outcomes. Top Magn Reson Imaging 2014;23(1):13–20.

5. Wood JC, Ghugre N. Magnetic resonance imaging assessment of excess iron in thalassemia, sickle cell disease and other iron overload diseases. Hemoglobin 2008;32(1–2):85–96.

6. Gossuin Y, Muller RN, Gillis P. Relaxation induced by ferritin: a better understanding for an improved MRI iron quantification. NMR Biomed 2004;17(7):427–32.

7. Ghugre NR, Enriquez CM, Coates TD, et al. Improved R2* measurements in myocardial iron overload. J Magn Reson Imaging 2006;23(1):9–16.

8. Westwood M, Anderson LJ, Firmin DN, et al. A single breath-hold multiecho T2* cardiovascular magnetic resonance technique for diagnosis of myocardial iron overload. J Magn Reson Imaging 2003;18(1):33–9.

9. Smith GC, Carpenter JP, He T, et al. Value of black blood T2* cardiovascular magnetic resonance. J Cardiovasc Magn Reson 2011;13(1):21.

10. Tanner MA, He T, Westwood MA, et al. Multi-center validation of the transferability of the magnetic resonance T2* technique for the quantification of tissue iron. Haematologica 2006;91(10):1388–91.

11. Carpenter JP, He T, Kirk P, et al. On T2* magnetic resonance and cardiac iron. Circulation 2011; 123(14):1519–28.

12. He T, Gatehouse PD, Smith GC, et al. Myocardial T2* measurements in iron-overloaded thalassemia: An in vivo study to investigate optimal methods of quantification. Magn Reson Med 2008;60(5):1082–9.

13. Westwood MA, Anderson LJ, Firmin DN, et al. Inter-scanner reproducibility of cardiovascular magnetic resonance T2* measurements of tissue iron in thalassemia. J Magn Reson Imaging 2003;18(5):616–20.

14. Feng Y, He T, Feng M, et al. Improved pixel-by-pixel MRI R2* relaxometry by nonlocal means. Magn Reson Med 2014;72(1):260–8.

15. Feng Y, He T, Gatehouse PD, et al. Improved MRI R2* relaxometry of iron-loaded liver with noise correction. Magn Reson Med 2013;70(6):1765–74.

16. www.cmrtools.com. 2010; Available at: http://www.cmrtools.com/cmrweb/Regulatory.htm. Accessed December 03, 2010.

17. www.circlecvi.com. 2010;Available at: http://www.circlecvi.com/site/regulatory.php. Accessed December 03, 2010.

18. Mavrogeni S, Bratis K, van Wijk K, et al. The reproducibility of cardiac and liver T2* measurement in thalassemia major using two different software packages. Int J Cardiovasc Imaging 2013;29:1511–6.

19. Bacigalupo L, Paparo F, Zefiro D, et al. Comparison between different software programs and post-processing techniques for the MRI quantification of liver iron concentration in thalassemia patients. Radiol Med 2016;121(10):751–62.

20. Fernandes JL, Sampaio EF, Verissimo M, et al. Heart and liver T2 assessment for iron overload using different software programs. Eur Radiol 2011; 21(12):2503–10.

21. Git KA, Fioravante LA, Fernandes JL. An online open-source tool for automated quantification of liver and myocardial iron concentrations by T2* magnetic resonance imaging. Br J Radiol 2015; 88(1053):20150269.

22. Messroghli DR, Rudolph A, Abdel-Aty H, et al. An open-source software tool for the generation of relaxation time maps in magnetic resonance imaging. BMC Med Imaging 2010;10:16.

23. Fernandes JL, Fioravante LAB, Verissimo MP, et al. A free software for the calculation of T2* values for iron overload assessment. Acta Radiol 2017;58(6):698–701.

24. Sandino CM, Kellman P, Arai AE, et al. Myocardial T2* mapping: influence of noise on accuracy and precision. J Cardiovasc Magn Reson 2015; 17(1):7.

25. House MJ, Fleming AJ, de Jonge MD, et al. Mapping iron in human heart tissue with synchrotron x-ray fluorescence microscopy and cardiovascular magnetic resonance. J Cardiovasc Magn Reson 2014;16(1):80.

26. Positano V, Meloni A, Santarelli MF, et al. Fast generation of T2* maps in the entire range of clinical interest: application to thalassemia major patients. Comput Biol Med 2015;56:200–10.

27. Kellman P, Xue H, Spottiswoode BS, et al. Free-breathing T2* mapping using respiratory motion corrected averaging. J Cardiovasc Magn Reson 2015; 17(1):3.

28. Saiviroonporn P, Viprakasit V, Boonyasirinant T, et al. Comparison of the region-based and pixel-wise methods for cardiac T2* analysis in 50 transfusion-dependent Thai thalassemia patients. J Comput Assist Tomogr 2011;35(3):375–81.

29. Jin N, da Silveira JS, Jolly MP, et al. Free-breathing myocardial T2* mapping using GRE-EPI and automatic non-rigid motion correction. J Cardiovasc Magn Reson 2015;17:113.

30. Modell B, Khan M, Darlison M, et al. Improved survival of thalassaemia major in the UK and relation to T2* cardiovascular magnetic resonance. J Cardiovasc Magn Reson 2008;10:42.

31. Chouliaras G, Berdoukas V, Ladis V, et al. Impact of magnetic resonance imaging on cardiac mortality in thalassemia major. J Magn Reson Imaging 2011; 34(1):56–9.

32. Angelucci E, Barosi G, Camaschella C, et al. Italian Society of Hematology practice guidelines for the management of iron overload in thalassemia major and related disorders. Haematologica 2008;93(5):741–52.

33. Musallam KM, Angastiniotis M, Eleftheriou A, et al. Cross-talk between available guidelines for the management of patients with beta-thalassemia major. Acta Haematol 2013;130(2):64–73.

34. Verissimo MP, Loggetto SR, Fabron Junior A, et al. Brazilian Thalassemia Association protocol for iron chelation therapy in patients under regular transfusion. Rev Bras Hematol Hemoter 2013;35(6):428–34.

35. Pennell DJ, Udelson JE, Arai AE, et al. Cardiovascular function and treatment in beta-thalassemia major: a consensus statement from the American Heart Association. Circulation 2013;128(3):281–308.

36. Wood JC, Origa R, Agus A, et al. Onset of cardiac iron loading in pediatric patients with thalassemia major. Haematologica 2008;93(6):917–20.

37. Fernandes JL, Fabron A Jr, Verissimo M. Early cardiac iron overload in children with transfusion-dependent anemias. Haematologica 2009;94(12):1776–7.

38. Cappellini MD, Cohen A, Eleftheriou A, et al. Iron overload. Guidelines for the clinical management

of thalassemia. 2nd rev edition. Nicosia (Cyprus): Thalassemia International Federation; 2008. p. 33–63.

39. Fernandes JL. MRI for iron overload in thalassemia. Hematol Oncol Clin North Am 2018;32(2):277–95.

40. He T, Gatehouse PD, Kirk P, et al. Black-blood T2* technique for myocardial iron measurement in thalassemia. J Magn Reson Imaging 2007;25(6): 1205–9.

41. Positano V, Pepe A, Santarelli MF, et al. Multislice multiecho T2* cardiac magnetic resonance for the detection of heterogeneous myocardial iron distribution in thalassaemia patients. NMR Biomed 2009; 22(7):707–15.

42. Positano V, Pepe A, Santarelli MF, et al. Standardized T2* map of normal human heart in vivo to correct T2* segmental artefacts. NMR Biomed 2007; 20(6):578–90.

43. Kirk P, Roughton M, Porter JB, et al. Cardiac T2* magnetic resonance for prediction of cardiac complications in thalassemia major. Circulation 2009; 120(20):1961–8.

44. Torlasco C, Cassinerio E, Roghi A, et al. Role of T1 mapping as a complementary tool to T2* for noninvasive cardiac iron overload assessment. PLoS One 2018;13(2):e0192890.

45. Garbowski MW, Carpenter JP, Smith G, et al. Biopsy-based calibration of T2* magnetic resonance for estimation of liver iron concentration and comparison with R2 Ferriscan. J Cardiovasc Magn Reson 2014;16:40.

46. Storey P, Thompson AA, Carqueville CL, et al. R2* imaging of transfusional iron burden at 3T and comparison with 1.5T. J Magn Reson Imaging 2007; 25(3):540–7.

47. Messroghli DR, Greiser A, Frohlich M, et al. Optimization and validation of a fully-integrated pulse sequence for modified look-locker inversion-recovery (MOLLI) T1 mapping of the heart. J Magn Reson Imaging 2007;26(4):1081–6.

48. Messroghli DR, Radjenovic A, Kozerke S, et al. Modified Look-Locker inversion recovery (MOLLI) for high-resolution T1 mapping of the heart. Magn Reson Med 2004;52(1):141–6.

49. Piechnik SK, Ferreira VM, Dall'Armellina E, et al. Shortened Modified Look-Locker Inversion recovery (ShMOLLI) for clinical myocardial T1-mapping at 1.5 and 3 T within a 9 heartbeat breathhold. J Cardiovasc Magn Reson 2010;12:69.

50. Chow K, Flewitt JA, Green JD, et al. Saturation recovery single-shot acquisition (SASHA) for myocardial T(1) mapping. Magn Reson Med 2014;71(6): 2082–95.

51. Abdel-Gadir A, Vorasettakarnkij Y, Ngamkasem H, et al. Ultrafast magnetic resonance imaging for iron quantification in thalassemia participants in the developing world: the TIC-TOC Study (Thailand and UK International Collaboration in Thalassaemia Optimising Ultrafast CMR). Circulation 2016;134(5): 432–4.

52. Abdel-Gadir A, Treibel T, Moon JC. Myocardial T1 mapping: where are we now and where are we going? Res Rep Clin Cardiol 2014;5:339–47.

53. Abdel-Gadir A, Berber R, Porter JB, et al. Detection of metallic cobalt and chromium liver deposition following failed hip replacement using T2* and R2 magnetic resonance. J Cardiovasc Magn Reson 2016;18(1):29.

54. Roujol S, Weingartner S, Foppa M, et al. Accuracy, precision, and reproducibility of four T1 mapping sequences: a head-to-head comparison of MOLLI, ShMOLLI, SASHA, and SAPPHIRE. Radiology 2014;272(3):683–9.

55. Wood JC, Otto-Duessel M, Aguilar M, et al. Cardiac iron determines cardiac T2*, T2, and T1 in the gerbil model of iron cardiomyopathy. Circulation 2005; 112(4):535–43.

56. Sado DM, Maestrini V, Piechnik SK, et al. Noncontrast myocardial T1 mapping using cardiovascular magnetic resonance for iron overload. J Magn Reson Imaging 2015;41(6):1505–11.

57. Abdel-Gadir A, Sado D, Murch S, et al. Myocardial iron quantification using T2* and native T1mapping - a 250 patient study. J Cardiovasc Magn Reson 2015;17(1):P312.

58. Alam MH, Auger D, Smith GC, et al. T1 at 1.5T and 3T compared with conventional T2* at 1.5T for cardiac siderosis. J Cardiovasc Magn Reson 2015;17:102.

59. Hanneman K, Nguyen ET, Thavendiranathan P, et al. Quantification of myocardial extracellular volume fraction with cardiac MR imaging in thalassemia major. Radiology 2016;279(3):720–30.

60. Radenkovic D, Weingartner S, Ricketts L, et al. T1 mapping in cardiac MRI. Heart Fail Rev 2017; 22(4):415–30.

61. Krittayaphong R, Zhang S, Saiviroonporn P, et al. Detection of cardiac iron overload with native magnetic resonance T1 and T2 mapping in patients with thalassemia. Int J Cardiol 2017;248: 421–6.

62. Guo H, Au WY, Cheung JS, et al. Myocardial T2 quantitation in patients with iron overload at 3 Tesla. J Magn Reson Imaging 2009;30(2):394–400.

63. Li D, Dhawale P, Rubin PJ, et al. Myocardial signal response to dipyridamole and dobutamine: demonstration of the BOLD effect using a double-echo gradient-echo sequence. Magn Reson Med 1996; 36(1):16–20.

64. Friedrich MG, Karamitsos TD. Oxygenation-sensitive cardiovascular magnetic resonance. J Cardiovasc Magn Reson 2013;15:43.

65. Wacker CM, Bock M, Hartlep AW, et al. Changes in myocardial oxygenation and perfusion under pharmacological stress with dipyridamole: assessment

using T*2 and T1 measurements. Magn Reson Med 1999;41(4):686–95.

66. Wacker CM, Hartlep AW, Pfleger S, et al. Susceptibility-sensitive magnetic resonance imaging detects human myocardium supplied by a stenotic coronary artery without a contrast agent. J Am Coll Cardiol 2003;41(5):834–40.

67. Friedrich MG, Niendorf T, Schulz-Menger J, et al. Blood oxygen level-dependent magnetic resonance imaging in patients with stress-induced angina. Circulation 2003;108(18):2219–23.

68. Jahnke C, Manka R, Kozerke S, et al. Cardiovascular magnetic resonance profiling of coronary atherosclerosis: vessel wall remodelling and related myocardial blood flow alterations. Eur Heart J Cardiovasc Imaging 2014;15(12):1400–10.

69. Manka R, Paetsch I, Schnackenburg B, et al. BOLD cardiovascular magnetic resonance at 3.0 tesla in myocardial ischemia. J Cardiovasc Magn Reson 2010;12:54.

70. Kali A, Tang RL, Kumar A, et al. Detection of acute reperfusion myocardial hemorrhage with cardiac MR imaging: T2 versus T2. Radiology 2013;269(2):387–95.

71. Hamirani YS, Wong A, Kramer CM, et al. Effect of microvascular obstruction and intramyocardial hemorrhage by CMR on LV remodeling and outcomes after myocardial infarction: a systematic review and meta-analysis. JACC Cardiovasc Imaging 2014;7(9):940–52.

72. Hansen MS, Sorensen TS. Gadgetron: an open source framework for medical image reconstruction. Magn Reson Med 2013;69(6):1768–76.

73. Bulluck H, Rosmini S, Abdel-Gadir A, et al. Residual myocardial iron following intramyocardial hemorrhage during the convalescent phase of reperfused ST-segment-elevation myocardial infarction and adverse left ventricular remodeling. Circ Cardiovasc Imaging 2016;9(10) [pii: e004940].

The Role of Cardiac MR Imaging in the Assessment of Patients with Cardiac Amyloidosis

Filipe Penna de Carvalho, MD[a], Fernanda Erthal, MD[a],
Clerio F. Azevedo, MD, PhD[a,b,*]

KEYWORDS

- Cardiac MR • Amyloidosis • Delayed enhancement • T1 mapping • Extracellular volume fraction

KEY POINTS

- Cardiac MR imaging provides detailed assessment of cardiac function, volumes, and tissue characterization, thus it is very useful in the diagnostic pathway of cardiac amyloidosis (CA).
- Delayed enhancement detects myocardial infiltration secondary to amyloid deposition in patients with CA, and has both diagnostic and prognostic utility.
- Native T1 and extracellular volume calculation are recent mapping techniques that indirectly measure amyloid burden. These not only have high diagnostic accuracy for CA but are also strong independent predictors of outcomes.

INTRODUCTION

Amyloidosis is a multiorgan, infiltrative disease caused by abnormal protein deposition of insoluble amyloid fibrils on the extracellular matrix. There are a variety of different subtypes of amyloid disease, either hereditary or nonhereditary, each associated with specific precursor proteins, organ involvement, and prognosis.

Cardiac involvement plays an important role in patient prognosis and therapy decision.[1–3] More than 95% of all cardiac amyloidoses (CAs) are related to immunoglobulin light-chain amyloidosis (AL) or transthyretin amyloidosis (ATTR).[2] In AL-CA, which is related to multiple myeloma in up to 15% of cases, amyloid fibrils are derived from monoclonal immunoglobulin light-chains. AL-CA is associated with a poor prognosis, with a median survival after diagnosis not longer than 1 year.[2] Transthyretin (TTR), the precursor protein in ATTR-CA, is a liver-derived plasma protein that acts as a transporter for thyroxine and retinol-binding protein. ATTR can occur either as a hereditary mutant (ATTRm) variant or as an acquired wild-type (ATTRwt) variant, the latter is also known as senile amyloidosis.[2,4] ATTR is associated with a better prognosis compared with the AL-CA type, with a mean survival of 3 to 5 years for ATTRwt and about 2 years for the most common form of ATTRm in the United States (V122I mutation).[2]

Despite recent efforts, both in terms of novel research and optimization of clinical management, and in the face of its increasingly recognized clinical relevance, amyloidosis remains an underdiagnosed disease for which the true incidence is still

Disclosure: The authors have no conflicts to disclose.
[a] Diagnósticos da America (DASA), Unidade CID Leblon, Av. Ataulfo de Paiva 669, CEP 22440-032, Rio de Janeiro, RJ, Brazil; [b] Division of Cardiology, Duke University Medical Center, Duke Medical Pavilion, 10 Medicine Circle, Room 1E63, DUMC 3934, Durham, NC 27710, USA
* Corresponding author. Duke Cardiovascular Magnetic Resonance Center, Duke Medical Pavilion, 10 Medicine Circle Room 1E63, DUMC 3934, Durham, NC 27710.
E-mail address: clerio.azevedo@duke.edu

Magn Reson Imaging Clin N Am 27 (2019) 453–463
https://doi.org/10.1016/j.mric.2019.04.005
1064-9689/19/© 2019 Elsevier Inc. All rights reserved.

unknown. According to the most recent estimates, AL occurs in 6 to 10 per million individuals in the United States,[5] whereas the most common variant of ATTRm (V122I mutation) is present in 3% to 4% of African Americans.[2,6] ATTRwt (senile amyloidosis) is reported to be present in up to 25% of the elderly population on autopsy studies[7] and in up to 13% of patients admitted with heart failure with preserved ejection fraction on a recent study using nuclear imaging techniques.[2,8]

Novel specific and effective treatments for AL-CA and ATTR-CA are being increasingly reported,[1,2] which has led to a growing interest in the early and accurate diagnosis of CA.[9] Despite advancements in noninvasive cardiac imaging, with the recent introduction of echocardiographic speckle tracking techniques[10] and nuclear imaging methods such as bone tracer scintigraphy,[11] diagnosing CA is still challenging. This is particularly true for early-stage CA, in which serum biomarkers and electrocardiographic and echocardiographic findings might not yet be evident or typical for CA. In this context, cardiac MR (CMR) imaging has emerged as a valuable technique that is playing an increasingly important role in the assessment of CA.[12]

The focus of this article is to summarize the state-of-the-art applications of CMR imaging for the diagnostic and prognostic assessment of patients with suspected or confirmed CA (Table 1).

MORPHOLOGIC FEATURES

Cardiac amyloidosis is characterized by the infiltration and deposition of amyloid fibrils in the interstitial space of the myocardial tissue, resulting in progressive cardiac wall thickening and diastolic dysfunction, and eventually leading to restrictive cardiomyopathy.[13]

Endomyocardial biopsy (EMB) is the gold standard for the diagnosis of CA.[14] However, EMB is an invasive technique, limited by local expertise, and not widely available. Therefore, current diagnostic strategies are frequently based on clinical, laboratory, and imaging findings, often associated with a noncardiac biopsy.[15]

In the past decade, CMR imaging has emerged as a powerful imaging technique that provides detailed assessment of the classic features present in the later stages of CA (Box 1), including left ventricular hypertrophy (LVH), disproportionate atria enlargement, and increased atrial wall thickness[16,17] (Fig. 1).

Left Ventricle Volumes and Systolic Function

Typically, the left ventricle (LV) is not dilated in up to 80% of patients with CA on autopsy studies.[13]

In vivo, LV end-diastolic volume (LVEDV) is usually reduced. This frequently leads to a reduced LV stroke volume (LVSV) despite preserved or only mildly reduced LV ejection fraction (LVEF).[12] This pattern has been reported in several prior studies, with the mean LVEDV ranging from 100 to 131 mL (58–69 mL/m^2), LVSV from 59 to 72 mL (32–38 mL/m^2), and LVEF from 56% to 60%.[17–19] However, importantly, LVEF can be severely compromised in cases of advanced CA.[12]

Left Ventricle Hypertrophy

Although concentric LVH is regarded as a hallmark of CA, several studies have shown that alternative remodeling patterns may be present.[16,17] Pozo and colleagues[16] reported that subjects with CA often have increased LV mass and wall thickness, with concentric LVH present in 58%, whereas alternative patterns are present in 42% (18% eccentric LVH, 16% concentric remodeling, and 8% normal geometry). Interestingly, in the same study, the investigators showed that the region of maximal LV wall thickness, which is located in the basal anteroseptum in 99% of patients without CA, was found in other LV wall locations in 33% of subjects with confirmed CA.[16]

Recently, Martinez-Naharro and colleagues[17] reported asymmetrical septal LVH to be the most common pattern of LV remodeling in ATTR-CA (79% of subjects), whereas concentric LVH was more common on AL-CA (68% of subjects). The 2 main subtypes of asymmetrical septal hypertrophy were seen in 55% (sigmoid septum) and 24% (reverse septal contour) of subjects with ATTR, the latter also being considered a typical finding in hypertrophic cardiomyopathy[17] (Figs. 2 and 3). Asymmetrical LVH was seen in only 14% of subjects with AL-CA and all of them had the sigmoid septal pattern.[17] No LVH was seen in 3% of subjects with AL-CA and in 18% of the subjects with ATTR-CA.[17]

These findings highlight the importance of clinicians and imaging experts to be aware that the morphologic phenotype of patients with CA may differ from the traditionally described concentric LVH, and that asymmetric septal LVH can be consistent with CA in the appropriate setting.[16,17]

Atrial Enlargement and Atrial Septal Thickness

Atrial structure, volume, and function can be reliably assessed by CMR imaging.[12] Virtually all patients with advanced CA present with biatrial enlargement and increased atrial septal thickness due to amyloid deposition within the atrial walls[13](see Fig. 1). Maceira and colleagues[18] described a significant increase in the atrial septal

Table 1
Summary of published literature on cardiac amyloidosis and cardiac MR imaging

Author, Year	Number of Subjects (amyloidosis)	Diagnostic Evaluation	Tissue Characterization Techniques Used	Prognostic Evaluation	Mean Follow-up (months)
Maceira et al,[18] 2005	30	—	DE	No	—
vanden Driesen et al,[20] 2006	8	—	DE	No	—
Perugini et al,[23] 2006	21 (AL = 9; ATTR = 12)	—	DE	No	—
Vogelsberg et al,[48] 2008	33	SENS = 80%; SPEC = 94%; PPV = 92%; NPV = 85%	DE	No	—
Ruberg et al,[27] 2009	28 (AL only)	SENS = 86%; SPEC = 86%; PPV = 95%; NPV = 67%	DE	Yes	29 (range 5–36)
Austin et al,[28] 2009	47	SENS = 88%; SPEC = 90%; PPV = 88%; NPV = 90%	DE	Yes	12
Syed et al,[19] 2010	120 (AL = 100, ATTR = 20)	—	DE	No	—
Banypersad et al,[34] 2013	60 (AL only)	—	DE, native T1, ECV	No	—
Karamitsos et al,[31] 2013	46	SENS = 92%; SPEC = 91%; ACC = 92%	DE, native T1	No	—
Dungu et al,[4] 2014	97 (AL = 46, ATTR = 51)	—	DE	No	—
Pozo et al,[16] 2014	130	SENS = 67%; SPEC = 86%; ACC = 88%	DE	No	—
White et al,[21] 2014	90	SENS = 93%; SPEC = 70%; ACC = 84%	DE, TI scout	Yes	29 (IQR: 12–44)
Fontana et al,[22] 2014	164 (AL = 79, ATTR = 85)	AUC = 0.85 (0.79–0.92)	DE, native T1	No	—
Banypersad et al,[30] 2015	100 (AL only)	—	DE, native T1, ECV	Yes	23 (IQR: 6–25)
Fontana et al,[26] 2015	250 (AL = 119, ATTR = 122)	—	DE, native T1, ECV	Yes	24 ± 13
Martinez-Naharro et al,[17] 2017	342 (AL = 50, ATTR = 292)	—	DE, native T1, ECV	Yes	19 ± 14
Martinez-Naharro et al,[35] 2018	227 (ATTR only)	AUC = 0.91 (0.87–0.94)	DE, native T1, ECV	Yes	32 ± 17

Abbreviations: ACC, accuracy; AUC, area under the receiver-operator curve; DE, delayed enhancement; ECV, extracellular volume; IQR, interquartile range; NPV, negative predictive value; PPV, predictive positive value; SENS, sensitivity; SPEC, specificity.

thickness in subjects with CA when compared with hypertensive controls (5.6 mm vs 3.9 mm, respectively). Similar findings were also reported by vanden Driesen and colleagues.[20]

Other Morphologic Findings

Amyloid infiltration is also present in other cardiac structures, such as the valves and small intramural coronary arteries.[13] Although not specific, thickening of at least 1 cardiac valve has been reported in 85% of autopsy subjects with CA, being the tricuspid valve the most frequently affected (83%), followed by the mitral valve (80%), and the pulmonic and aortic valves (54% each).[13] Thickening of all 4 cardiac valves was reported in approximately 50% of subjects.[13] Similar findings

have also been described in CMR imaging studies, often associated with mild to moderate regurgitation.[2,15]

Pericardial and pleural effusions may be present as a nonspecific finding in 39% to 52% and 41% to 47% of patients with CA, respectively.[16,19,21] Pericardial effusions are usually mild and secondary to amyloid infiltration of the pericardium, though rare cases of large effusions have also been described.[2] Pleural effusion, if present, is often due to heart failure. Large refractory effusion should raise the suspicion of concomitant pleural amyloidosis.[15]

Interestingly, amyloid infiltration of small intramural coronary arteries may lead to ischemic symptoms without associated obstructive epicardial coronary atherosclerotic disease, with angina pectoris being the presenting symptom in a subset of patients.[2]

DELAYED-ENHANCEMENT TECHNIQUE: DIAGNOSTIC ASSESSMENT

CMR imaging is not only able to precisely characterize heart morphology and function but also to reliably detect amyloid infiltration.[17,22] Tissue characterization using the delayed-enhancement (DE) technique has been shown to detect the myocardial infiltration secondary to amyloid deposition in 69% to 100% of patients with CA.[17–19,23]

Importantly, patients with CA demonstrate abnormal gadolinium kinetics (faster washout of gadolinium from the myocardium and blood pool when compared with controls),[18] which may increase the difficulty in finding the appropriate inversion time (TI) to null normal myocardium on magnitude DE images.[21,24] The increasing availability of the phase-sensitive inversion recovery (PSIR) technique for DE, which decreases the need for optimal TI setting and allows for lower operator-dependent variations in image quality,[24] has somewhat mitigated this problem. Regardless, a recent meta-analysis by Zhao and colleagues[25] (n = 257) found DE to be an effective

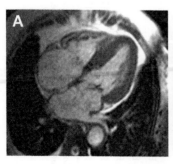
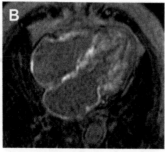

Fig. 1. A typical presentation of cardiac amyloidosis, with concentric LVH, biatrial enlargement, and increased atrial septal thickness, seen on cine 4-chamber image (*A*). Delayed enhancement shows an also typical diffuse transmural LV enhancement associated with enhancement of both atrial walls (*B*).

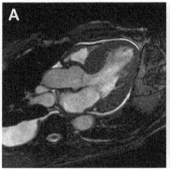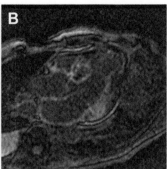

Fig. 2. A patient with ATTR amyloidosis. Asymmetric LVH with sigmoid septum pattern is seen on cine imaging (*A*). Delayed enhancement (*B*) reveals a typical diffuse transmural pattern with unusually black blood.

tool to diagnose patients with suspected CA, with a pooled sensitivity and specificity of 85% (95% confidence interval [CI] 77–91) and 92% (95% CI 83–97), respectively, and an area under the curve (AUC) of 0.9530.

Delayed-Enhancement Patterns

A few typical patterns of DE have been described as being present on different stages of CA[17–19,23] (**Fig. 4**). These patterns can be categorized into 3 main subtypes: (1) a diffuse transmural pattern, with transmural enhancement in at least 1 LV segment (reported in 60% to 71% of patients with CA); (2) a diffuse subendocardial pattern, with the enhancement involving the whole subendocardium without any segment with transmural involvement (present in 23%–29% of patients with CA); and (3) a patchy focal pattern, with regions of midwall enhancement permeated by normal myocardium (present in up to 6% of patients with CA).[17–19,23] Interestingly, both diffuse patterns (transmural and subendocardial) usually present with unusually dark blood pool, reflecting the abnormal gadolinium kinetics seen in advanced CA.[17–19,23]

In addition, different patterns of DE may suggest specific subtypes of CA and assist in the differentiation between ATTR-CA and AL-CA[4,26] (see later discussion).

Rapid Visual T1 Assessment (Inversion Time Scout)

White and colleagues[21] described an ingenious method that exploits the abnormal gadolinium kinetics typically present in patients with CA. They used an early postcontrast DE sequence with variable TI (commonly referred to as a TI scout sequence) to visually compare the signal intensity of the blood pool and myocardium. Normally, postcontrast blood pool has a shorter T1 than the myocardium, and thus crosses the null point earlier (becomes black at a lower TI).[21] However, in CA this relationship is inverted because there is an abnormal retention of gadolinium in the myocardium secondary to amyloid infiltration[21] (**Fig. 5**). The investigators found that greater than 50% of the myocardium nulling faster than the blood pool was a useful criterion for the diagnosis of CA, particularly with the diffuse enhancement pattern, and, more importantly, was associated with a worse prognosis.[21]

DIFFERENTIATING LIGHT-CHAIN CARDIAC AMYLOIDOSIS FROM TRANSTHYRETIN CARDIAC AMYLOIDOSIS WITH CARDIAC MR IMAGING

Morphologically, CA is frequently associated with LV volumes and ejection fraction within the normal

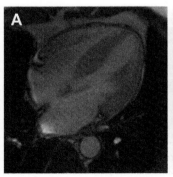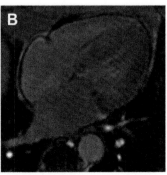

Fig. 3. A patient with ATTR amyloidosis. Asymmetric LVH with reverse septal contour pattern is seen on 4-chamber cine imaging (*A*). Delayed enhancement (*B*) reveals a typical diffuse subendocardial pattern.

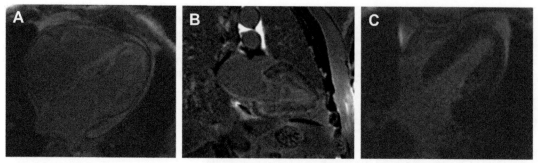

Fig. 4. Three main DE patterns in patients with histologically confirmed CA. Diffuse transmural (*A*), diffuse sub-endocardial (*B*), and patchy focal (*C*).

range regardless of subtype at presentation.[4] It has been reported, however, that ATTR-CA is associated with markedly higher LV mass index than AL-CA at presentation (122 vs 93 g/m^2 for men and 104 vs 83 g/m^2 for women, respectively).[4]

Although both AL-CA and ATTR-CA can present with any of the different patterns of DE, recent data have shown that diffuse transmural DE is more prevalent in AL-ATTR than in AL-CA, ranging from 63% to 71% versus 27% to 50% of patients, respectively.[17,26] Conversely, diffuse subendocardial DE was present more frequently in patients with AL-CA than in those with ATTR-CA (39% vs 12% to 24%, respectively).[26] Additionally, a higher prevalence of right ventricle (RV) free wall DE has been reported in ATTR-CA when compared with AL-CA (96% to 100% vs 72% to 77%, respectively).[4,17]

A DE scoring system (Query Amyloid Late Enhancement [QALE]) to assist differentiation between ATTR-CA and AL-CA has been proposed.[4] It is calculated using short-axis DE images of the LV and RV on 3 levels (basal, midventricular, and apical) with each level scored according to the degree of LV enhancement: no DE equals 0; noncircumferential or patchy DE equals 1; circumferential with no transmural DE equals 2; any transmural DE equals 3;

and circumferential transmural DE equals 4 (maximum total LV DE score = 12). The presence of any RV DE adds 6 to the total score (**Fig. 6**). Thus, the QALE score ranges from 0 (no DE on LV or RV) to 18 (global transmural LV DE on 3 levels plus RV involvement). ATTR-CA seems to be associated with higher scores than AL-CA. A cutoff point of greater than or equal to 13 has been reported to differentiate ATTR-CA from AL-CA with 82% sensitivity and 76% specificity.[4] Though promising, this score requires further external validation.

DELAYED-ENHANCEMENT: PROGNOSTIC ASSESSMENT

Although DE is the cornerstone of prognostic evaluation in most cardiomyopathies, the results reported in CA were somewhat conflicting.[24] It has been suggested that the presence of DE is strongly associated with other biomarkers of poor prognosis, including clinical, morphologic, functional, and biochemical features.[19] In a small series of 28 subjects with AL-CA, however, Ruberg and colleagues[27] have found that even though DE was strongly associated with heart failure severity it was not an independent predictor of survival. On the other hand, Austin and colleagues[28] demonstrated in a series of 47 subjects with suspected

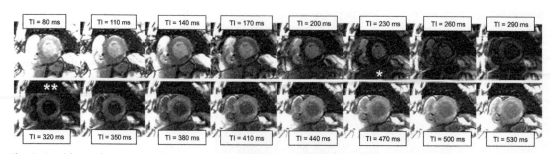

Fig. 5. Rapid visual T1 assessment (TI scout) in a patient with confirmed cardiac amyloidosis. In this case, the myocardium crosses the null point (*asterisk*) at a shorter TI when compared with the blood pool (*double asterisk*), a finding suggestive of diffuse amyloid infiltration.

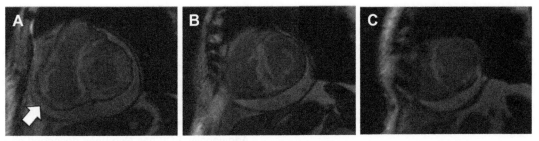

Fig. 6. QALE score calculation. Short-axis basal (*A*), midventricular (*B*), and apical (*C*) slices all present noncircumferential transmural DE (score = 3 each, total LV score = 9). RV DE is seen on basal slice (*A*, *arrow*), adding another 6 points, for a total QALE score equals 15 (suggestive of ATTR-CA).

CA that the presence of DE was the strongest predictor of 1-year mortality.

These conflicting results can be partially explained by the difficulty imposed by the abnormal gadolinium kinetics and lack of standardized DE parameters in earlier series, leading to suboptimal DE images and possible misclassification of patients.[24]

More recent data, derived from studies that included larger number of subjects, and using newer optimized and more standardized image acquisition and postprocessing protocols, demonstrated that DE does, indeed, provide valuable prognostic information in subjects with CA.[2,26] Fontana and colleagues[26] investigated the prognostic value of DE using PSIR in 250 subjects with ATTR-CA or AL-CA. The investigators found that diffuse transmural DE was independently associated with an overall 4.1-fold increase in mortality after adjustments for known prognostic factors (LVEF, LV mass index, N-terminal probrain natriuretic peptide, stroke volume index, E/E′). The median survival was 17 months for AL-CA and 38 months for ATTR-CA.[26]

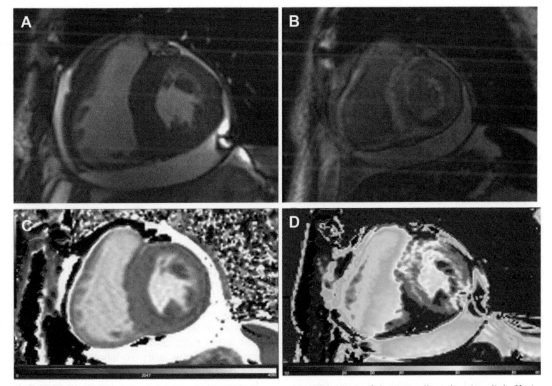

Fig. 7. A basal short-axis slice showing concentric hypertrophy, thickening of the RV wall, and pericardial effusion on cine steady-state free precession (*A*), with a typical diffuse transmural pattern of delayed enhancement (*B*). Mean native T1 (*C*) was elevated (T1 1442 ms; normal range 1165–1289 ms for this sequence at 3T), with a mean extracellular volume (*D*) of 77%.

T1 MAPPING TECHNIQUES

T1 mapping registers the course of longitudinal magnetization and enables the absolute quantification of tissue T1 values in a continuous fashion.[29] Myocardial T1 is directly related to the intrinsic myocardial tissue properties and, therefore, most pathologic conditions affecting the heart can result in abnormal myocardial T1 values.[29]

Current approaches for CA relies on precontrast T1 mapping (native T1) and postcontrast extracellular volume fraction (ECV) calculation, both demonstrated to correlate well with cardiac disease burden[30] (Fig. 7).

Native T1

Several studies have shown that native T1 is markedly increased in both ATTR and AL-CA and is associated with high diagnostic accuracy for both types of CA when compared with subjects with other causes of LVH.[22,30,31] This information is particularly useful in patients in whom contrast is contraindicated.

Moreover, increased native T1 also correlated well with known markers of systolic dysfunction, diastolic dysfunction, and cardiac biomarkers.[31] In AL-CA, elevated native T1 has been associated with a 5.39-fold increase of mortality.[30] Some investigators have also reported that the native T1 changes often precede the LV morphologic changes and thus seem to be a marker of early cardiac involvement.[22,30]

However, widespread native T1 reporting still presents some challenges, with recent efforts driven to standardize data acquisition and optimize workflows.[32] The normal range of native T1 varies depending on the CMR imaging system and sequence used, requiring that normal ranges need to be determined locally.[32,33] Thus, although many investigators reported different cutoff points for native T1, those cannot be easily translated into clinical practice.

Additionally, native T1 mapping represents a composite signal from cells and the interstitium, and not the interstitium alone.[30] Therefore, ECV has been suggested to be a better technique to measure the interstitial space and, thus, better quantify the amyloid burden.[24,34]

Extracellular Volume Fraction

ECV reflects the fraction of interstitial space on the myocardium and can be calculated using the patient hematocrit and the signal intensity change after gadolinium administration in blood and myocardium.[29,30]

Similar to native T1, ECV has also been found to be increased in ATTR and AL-CA, and to correlate well with known markers of worse prognosis.[17,30] It has been suggested that an ECV greater than 0.40 is highly specific for CA.[24] Moreover, ECV independently predicted mortality in both AL-CA (hazard ratio [HR] = 3.85 for ECV >0.45)[30] and in ATTR-AL (HR = 1.115 for each 3% increase in ECV),[35] even after adjustment for covariates.[17]

Additionally, ECV has also been described as a marker of early disease in both subtypes of CA, with modest increases (ECV = 0.30–0.40) reported in patients without any other evidence of cardiac involvement, suggesting subclinical low-grade cardiac disease and a potential target for early aggressive therapy to prevent disease progression.[17,30]

Because it is a T1 ratio, ECV does not suffer as much from the limitations regarding standardization of data acquisition as seen in native T1. Thus, ECV is believed to be a more reliable technique for the quantification of amyloid burden and identification of the full spectrum of different stages of CA evolution, possibly allowing the clinician to better diagnose and understand the prognostic implications of CA.[17,24,35]

OTHER IMAGING MODALITIES
Scintigraphy

Scintigraphy with bone-seeking tracers has high diagnostic accuracy and plays an important role in the diagnosis of CA.[2,11,36–40] Three technetium (Tc)-labeled radiotracers may be used: ^{99m}Tc-methylene diphosphonate, ^{99m}Tc-3,3-diphosphono-1,2-propanodicarboxylic acid, and ^{99m}Tc-pyrophosphate (PYP).[11,36,38] Cardiac uptake can be measured by semiquantitative visual score or by quantitative analysis.

In the visual score approach, the cardiac uptake is compared with the bone uptake, and results can range from no uptake (0) to diffuse uptake (3). When using the quantitative analysis, a region of interest is drawn over the heart and compared with the contralateral chest to account for background counts (a heart to contralateral chest [H/CL] ratio).[2,39,41,42] A meta-analysis by Treglia and colleagues,[36] with 6 studies and 529 subjects, found a sensitivity of 92.2% (95% CI 89–95), a specificity of 95.4% (95% CI 77–99), and a diagnostic odds ratio of 81.6 (95% CI 44–153) for bone scintigraphy with Tc-labeled radiotracers for diagnosing CA.

In particular, scintigraphy plays an important role in distinguishing and diagnosing ATTR. Gillmore and colleagues[11] studied 1217 subjects (857 with biopsy-proven CA and 360 with confirmed nonamyloid cardiomyopathy) and found myocardial uptake on bone scintigraphy to be greater than 99% specific and 86% sensitive for ATTR-CA. Moreover, when 2 findings were combined (absence of serum or urine monoclonal protein, and grades 2 or 3 of myocardial tracer uptake), the specificity and positive predictive value for ATTR were 100%.[11] The investigators suggested that the diagnosis of ATTR could be made using bone scintigraphy, with no need for biopsy, in patients without monoclonal gammopathy.[11]

Interestingly, ^{99m}Tc-PYP scintigraphy may also be used as a prognostic tool.[42] A multicenter study with 171 subjects reported worse survival in subjects with greater cardiac uptake.[42] Over a period of 5 years, survival was worse in those with an uptake H/CL ratio greater than or equal to 1.6.[42]

Echocardiography

Echocardiography is a noninvasive and widely available tool to assess cardiac function and morphology. The most common findings in CA, although not specific, are biatrial enlargement, thickened valves, small pericardial effusion, and biventricular and atrial septal thickening due to amyloid deposition. However, these findings may also be present in other infiltrative cardiomyopathies.[43,44] Moreover, CA may have asymmetric hypertrophy of the septum and mimic hypertrophic cardiomyopathy.[43]

Currently, strain imaging has gained importance in the differential diagnosis of CA and other causes of restrictive cardiomyopathy.[45–47] A study with 100 subjects (40 with biopsy-proven CA, 40 with hypertrophic cardiomyopathy, and 20 with hypertensive cardiomyopathy and myocardial remodeling) found the ejection fraction to longitudinal strain ratio to be the best parameter to discriminate CA (AUC = 0.95; 95% CI 0.89–0.98, $P<.00005$).[45] Strain imaging is also promising for the early diagnosis of patients with mild hypertrophy and normal EF.[45]

SUMMARY

Despite recent advancements in terms of newer biomarkers development and improved imaging techniques, the diagnosis of CA remains a frequent clinical challenge. Recent novel therapies have been shown to improve patient survival in randomized clinical trials, such as proteasome inhibitors (bortezomib) for AL and the TTR-stabilizing agent tafamidis for ATTR. This underscores the fundamental role of early diagnosis and correct phenotyping of patients with suspected or known CA.[1,2]

Current diagnostic pathways for CA usually rely on a combination of clinical features (eg, heart failure symptoms, autonomic dysfunction, macroglossia, carpal tunnel syndrome, or multiple myeloma), electrocardiographic manifestations (eg, low voltage, conduction abnormalities, and/or atrial fibrillation), and echocardiographic findings (eg, LVH, diastolic dysfunction, and impaired global longitudinal strain with typical apical sparing pattern[2,6]). In this context, CMR imaging not only provides further insight into cardiac function and morphology but also provides unique noninvasive tissue characterization, which offers additional prognostic and diagnostic information.[24]

Specifically, a comprehensive CMR imaging examination, including cine; DE; and, possibly, native T1 and/or ECV assessment, has been shown to provide high diagnostic accuracy for CA.[25] Importantly, the presence, extent, and pattern of myocardial hyperenhancement on DE images can help differentiate the 2 main subtypes of CA and, in addition, provide valuable prognostic information. Of note, native T1 and ECV, which also represent an indirect measure of amyloid burden, are significantly increased in both subtypes of CA and are also associated with worse outcomes.[17,22,30,31,35]

Given the aforementioned incremental diagnostic and prognostic value of CMR imaging, the authors believe that it should be an integral part of the diagnostic pathway of patients with suspected CA after an initial evaluation that includes clinical history, electrocardiogram, and echocardiography. The combined information obtained from this comprehensive assessment not only can help confirm or exclude the diagnosis of CA and determine its severity but it can also help guide further testing for AL (serum or urine immunofixation and serum free light-chain assay), ATTR (^{99m}Tc-PYP scintigraphy), or both (endomyocardial or extracardiac biopsies).

REFERENCES

1. Maurer MS, Schwartz JH, Gundapaneni B, et al. Tafamidis treatment for patients with transthyretin amyloid cardiomyopathy. N Engl J Med 2018; 379(11):1007–16.

2. Donnelly JP, Hanna M. Cardiac amyloidosis: an update on diagnosis and treatment. Cleve Clin J Med 2017;84(12 Suppl 3):12–26.

3. Gertz MA, Lacy MQ, Dispenzieri A, et al. Refinement in patient selection to reduce treatment-related mortality from autologous stem cell transplantation in amyloidosis. Bone Marrow Transplant 2013;48(4): 557–61.

4. Dungu JN, Valencia O, Pinney JH, et al. CMR-based differentiation of AL and ATTR cardiac amyloidosis. JACC Cardiovasc Imaging 2014;7(2):133–42.

5. Kyle RA, Linos A, Beard CM, et al. Incidence and natural history of primary systemic amyloidosis in Olmsted County, Minnesota, 1950 through 1989. Blood 1992;79(7):1817–22.

6. Bhogal S, Ladia V, Sitwala P, et al. Cardiac amyloidosis: an updated review with emphasis on diagnosis and future directions. Curr Probl Cardiol 2018;43(1):10–34.

7. Tanskanen M, Peuralinna T, Polvikoski T, et al. Senile systemic amyloidosis affects 25% of the very aged and associates with genetic variation in alpha2-macroglobulin and tau: a population-based autopsy study. Ann Med 2008;40(3):232–9.

8. González-López E, Gallego-Delgado M, Guzzo-Merello G, et al. Wild-type transthyretin amyloidosis as a cause of heart failure with preserved ejection fraction. Eur Heart J 2015;36(38):2585–94.

9. Pinney JH, Whelan CJ, Petrie A, et al. Senile systemic amyloidosis: clinical features at presentation and outcome. J Am Heart Assoc 2013;2(2):1–11.

10. Phelan D, Collier P, Thavendiranathan P, et al. Relative apical sparing of longitudinal strain using two-dimensional speckle-tracking echocardiography is both sensitive and specific for the diagnosis of cardiac amyloidosis. Heart 2012;98(19):1442–8.

11. Gillmore JD, Maurer MS, Falk RH, et al. Nonbiopsy diagnosis of cardiac transthyretin amyloidosis. Circulation 2016;133(24):2404–12.

12. Falk RH, Quarta CC, Dorbala S. How to image cardiac amyloidosis. Circ Cardiovasc Imaging 2014;7(3):552–62.

13. Roberts WC, Waller BF. Cardiac amyloidosis causing cardiac dysfunction: analysis of 54 necropsy patients. Am J Cardiol 1983;52(1):137–46.

14. Duston MA, Skinner M, Shirahama T, et al. Diagnosis of amyloidosis by abdominal fat aspiration. Analysis of four years' experience. Am J Med 1987;82(3):412–4.

15. Falk RH. Diagnosis and management of the cardiac amyloidoses. Circulation 2005;112(13):2047–60.

16. Pozo E, Kanwar A, Deochand R, et al. Cardiac magnetic resonance evaluation of left ventricular remodelling distribution in cardiac amyloidosis. Heart 2014;100(21):1688–95.

17. Martinez-Naharro A, Treibel TA, Abdel-Gadir A, et al. Magnetic resonance in transthyretin cardiac amyloidosis. J Am Coll Cardiol 2017;70(4):466–77.

18. Maceira AM, Joshi J, Prasad SK, et al. Cardiovascular magnetic resonance in cardiac amyloidosis. Circulation 2005;111(2):186–93.

19. Syed IS, Glockner JF, Feng D, et al. Role of cardiac magnetic resonance imaging in the detection of cardiac amyloidosis. JACC Cardiovasc Imaging 2010;3(2):155–64.

20. vanden Driesen RI, Slaughter RE, Strugnell WE. MR findings in cardiac amyloidosis. Am J Roentgenol 2006;186(6):1682–5.

21. White JA, Kim HW, Shah D, et al. CMR imaging with rapid visual T1 assessment predicts mortality in patients suspected of cardiac amyloidosis. JACC Cardiovasc Imaging 2014;7(2):143–56.

22. Fontana M, Banypersad SM, Treibel TA, et al. Native T1 mapping in transthyretin amyloidosis. JACC Cardiovasc Imaging 2014;7(2):157–65.

23. Perugini E, Rapezzi C, Piva T, et al. Non-invasive evaluation of the myocardial substrate of cardiac amyloidosis by gadolinium cardiac magnetic resonance. Heart 2006;92(3):343–9.

24. Fontana M, Chung R, Hawkins PN, et al. Cardiovascular magnetic resonance for amyloidosis. Heart Fail Rev 2015;20(2):133–44.

25. Zhao L, Tian Z, Fang Q. Diagnostic accuracy of cardiovascular magnetic resonance for patients with suspected cardiac amyloidosis: a systematic review and meta-analysis. BMC Cardiovasc Disord 2016;16(1):129.

26. Fontana M, Pica S, Reant P, et al. Prognostic value of late gadolinium enhancement cardiovascular magnetic resonance in cardiac amyloidosis. Circulation 2015;132(16):1570–9.

27. Ruberg FL, Appelbaum E, Davidoff R, et al. Diagnostic and prognostic utility of cardiovascular magnetic resonance imaging in light-chain cardiac amyloidosis. Am J Cardiol 2009;103(4):544–9.

28. Austin BA, Tang WHW, Rodriguez ER, et al. Delayed hyper-enhancement magnetic resonance imaging provides incremental diagnostic and prognostic utility in suspected cardiac amyloidosis. JACC Cardiovasc Imaging 2009;2(12):1369–77.

29. Puntmann VO, Peker E, Chandrashekhar Y, et al. T1 mapping in characterizing myocardial disease. Circ Res 2016;119(2):277–99.

30. Banypersad SM, Fontana M, Maestrini V, et al. T1 mapping and survival in systemic light-chain amyloidosis. Eur Heart J 2015;36(4):244–51.

31. Karamitsos TD, Piechnik SK, Banypersad SM, et al. Noncontrast T1 mapping for the diagnosis of cardiac amyloidosis. JACC Cardiovasc Imaging 2013;6(4):488–97.

32. Messroghli DR, Moon JC, Ferreira VM, et al. Clinical recommendations for cardiovascular magnetic resonance mapping of T1, T2, T2 and extracellular volume: a consensus statement by the Society for Cardiovascular Magnetic Resonance (SCMR) endorsed by the European Association for Cardiovascular Imagin. J Cardiovasc Magn Reson 2017;19(1):1–24.

33. Moon JC, Messroghli DR, Kellman P, et al. Myocardial T1 mapping and extracellular volume quantification: a Society for Cardiovascular Magnetic Resonance (SCMR) and CMR Working Group of

the European Society of Cardiology consensus statement. J Cardiovasc Magn Reson 2013;15(1):1.

34. Banypersad SM, Sado DM, Flett AS, et al. Quantification of myocardial extracellular volume fraction in systemic AL amyloidosis: an equilibrium contrast cardiovascular magnetic resonance study. Circ Cardiovasc Imaging 2013;6(1):34–9.

35. Martinez-Naharro A, Kotecha T, Norrington K, et al. Native T1 and extracellular volume in transthyretin amyloidosis. JACC Cardiovasc Imaging 2018. [Epub ahead of print].

36. Treglia G, Glaudemans AWJM, Bertagna F, et al. Diagnostic accuracy of bone scintigraphy in the assessment of cardiac transthyretin-related amyloidosis: a bivariate meta-analysis. Eur J Nucl Med Mol Imaging 2018;45(11):1945–55.

37. Chen W, Ton V-K, Dilsizian V. Clinical phenotyping of transthyretin cardiac amyloidosis with bone-seeking radiotracers in heart failure with preserved ejection fraction. Curr Cardiol Rep 2018;20(4):23.

38. Bokhari S, Shahzad R, Castaño A, et al. Nuclear imaging modalities for cardiac amyloidosis. J Nucl Cardiol 2014;21(1):175–84.

39. Bokhari S, Castaño A, Pozniakoff T, et al. 99m Tc-pyrophosphate scintigraphy for differentiating light-chain cardiac amyloidosis from the transthyretin-related familial and senile cardiac amyloidoses. Circ Cardiovasc Imaging 2013;6(2):195–201.

40. Yamamoto Y, Onoguchi M, Haramoto M, et al. Novel method for quantitative evaluation of cardiac amyloidosis using 201TlCl and 99mTc-PYP SPECT. Ann Nucl Med 2012;26(8):634–43.

41. Castaño A, DeLuca A, Weinberg R, et al. Serial scanning with technetium pyrophosphate (99mTc-PYP) in advanced ATTR cardiac amyloidosis. J Nucl Cardiol 2016;23(6):1355–63.

42. Castano A, Haq M, Narotsky DL, et al. Multicenter study of planar technetium 99m pyrophosphate cardiac imaging. JAMA Cardiol 2016;1(8):880.

43. Picano E, Pinamonti B, Ferdeghini EM, et al. Two-dimensional echocardiography in myocardial amyloidosis. Echocardiography 1991;8(2):253–9.

44. Falk RH, Quarta CC. Echocardiography in cardiac amyloidosis. Heart Fail Rev 2015;20(2):125–31.

45. Pagourelias ED, Mirea O, Duchenne J, et al. Echo parameters for differential diagnosis in cardiac amyloidosis: a head-to-head comparison of deformation and nondeformation parameters. Circ Cardiovasc Imaging 2017;10(3):e005588.

46. Roslan A, Kamsani SH, Nay TW, et al. Echocardiographic and electrocardiographic presentations of patients with endomyocardial biopsy-proven cardiac amyloidosis. Med J Malaysia 2018;73(6):388–92.

47. Pradel S, Magne J, Jaccard A, et al. Left ventricular assessment in patients with systemic light chain amyloidosis: a 3-dimensional speckle tracking transthoracic echocardiographic study. Int J Cardiovasc Imaging 2019;35(5):845–54.

48. Vogelsberg H, Mahrholdt H, Deluigi CC, et al. Cardiovascular magnetic resonance in clinically suspected cardiac amyloidosis. noninvasive imaging compared to endomyocardial biopsy. J Am Coll Cardiol 2008;51(10):1022–30.

Applications of Cardiac MR Imaging in Electrophysiology
Current Status and Future Needs

David R. Okada, MD[a], Katherine C. Wu, MD[b],*

KEYWORDS

- Arrhythmia risk prediction • Cardiac arrhythmias • Cardiac electrophysiology
- Cardiac implantable electrical devices • Cardiac MR imaging • Catheter ablation

KEY POINTS

- The role of cardiac MR imaging in the diagnosis, risk-stratification, and treatment of patients with cardiac arrhythmias is rapidly evolving.
- Beyond substrate identification and characterization, it is now feasible to perform MR imaging–based noninvasive virtual programmed stimulation to identify potential ablation targets.
- The next phase of MR imaging–guided electrophysiology may involve intraprocedural guidance of electrophysiologic interventions using real-time MR imaging.

INTRODUCTION

Cardiac MR imaging (CMR) has become a cornerstone of the diagnostic and prognostic evaluation of patients with cardiac arrhythmias. However, several limitations currently limit its wider applicability, including artifacts from cardiac implantable electronic devices (CIEDs), safety concerns in patients with CIEDs, and potential toxicities of gadolinium chelates. At the same time, there are many key unmet needs in electrophysiology that CMR is poised to address. These needs include a robust platform for coregistering anatomic and electrophysiologic data in the setting of catheter ablation, a means of distinguishing irreversible injury from edema in the setting of catheter ablation, and a real-time imaging modality that does not involve ionizing radiation to replace intraprocedural fluoroscopy. The aims in this review are, first, to provide an overview of established CMR applications in clinical electrophysiology, and second, to highlight emerging techniques that may be able to address both current limitations of CMR in practice and unmet needs in clinical electrophysiology.

ARRHYTHMOGENIC MYOCARDIAL SUBSTRATE CHARACTERIZATION

CMR offers a variety of tools for identifying and characterizing arrhythmogenic myocardial substrate in both atrial and ventricular arrhythmias. The most established of these is the late gadolinium enhancement (LGE) technique, which provides valuable diagnostic and prognostic information in a variety of substrates.[1–4] Intravenously administered gadolinium, a heavy metal with differential T1 shortening properties, leads to accumulation in the extracellular space and demonstrates delayed washout from regions with

Disclosures: The authors have nothing to disclose.
[a] Division of Cardiology, Department of Medicine, Johns Hopkins Hospital, Johns Hopkins Medicine, 1800 Orleans Street, Baltimore, MD 21287, USA; [b] Division of Cardiology, Department of Medicine, Johns Hopkins Hospital, Johns Hopkins Medicine, 600 North Wolfe Street, Blalock 536, Baltimore, MD 21287, USA
* Corresponding author.
E-mail address: kwu@jhmi.edu

Magn Reson Imaging Clin N Am 27 (2019) 465–473
https://doi.org/10.1016/j.mric.2019.04.006

increased interstitial fibrosis. This property facilitates identification, localization, and quantitation particularly of replacement fibrosis using T1-weighted imaging and segmented inversion recovery techniques.[1,2,4,5] These characteristics enable detailed 2- or 3-dimensional characterization of arrhythmogenic substrate in a variety of diseases, including ischemic cardiomyopathy,[6,7] nonischemic cardiomyopathy (NICM),[8–10] cardiac sarcoidosis (CS),[11–13] hypertrophic cardiomyopathy (HCM),[14–17] arrhythmogenic right ventricular cardiomyopathy,[18] and atrial fibrillation.[19–21]

In ischemic substrate, the presence, total volume, and transmural extent of LGE provide prognostic information about the risk of subsequent ventricular arrhythmias and death.[6,7,22] In NICM, the presence of LGE is a strong prognostic marker of adverse events.[7–9,23] A recent meta-analysis of 34 studies that encompassed 4554 patients with nonischemic dilated cardiomyopathy reported a 44.8% prevalence of LGE.[23] Compared with those without LGE, dilated cardiomyopathy patients with LGE had increased odds ratios (OR) for cardiovascular death (OR 3.4, 95% confidence interval [CI], 2.0–5.7), ventricular arrhythmic events (OR 4.5, 95% CI, 3.4–6.0), and recurrent hospitalization for heart failure (OR 2.7, 95% CI 1.7–4.2).[23] The absence of LGE predicted favorable left ventricular (LV) remodeling. A prior meta-analysis reported similar ORs for the predictive values of presence and extent of LGE in both ischemic and nonischemic causes.[7]

In other forms of cardiomyopathy, such as CS, the presence of LGE, especially right ventricular LGE, is associated with an increased risk of adverse events. Coleman and colleagues[13] performed a meta-analysis including 760 patients with CS undergoing LGE-CMR. The presence of LGE conferred an OR of 10.7 for the combined endpoint of ventricular arrhythmia, implantable cardioverter-defibrillator (ICD) shock, sudden cardiac death, or all-cause mortality. Similar relationships have been noted in HCM and acute and chronic myocarditis, which has been reviewed recently.[4]

An emerging technique for improving the prognostic utility of LGE imaging involves using varying signal intensities (SI) within the hyperenhanced area to distinguish regions of core infarct from the so-called border zone or gray zone, and thereby characterize scar heterogeneity. Heterogeneous tissue in the gray zone appears to represent the arrhythmogenic component of post-infarction substrate for ventricular arrhythmias. Specifically, gray zone may harbor critical components of circuitry for reentrant arrhythmias[24,25] (Fig. 1). Different methods have been described to define core infarct versus gray zone. For instance, core infarct or dense scar may be delineated as a region with SI greater than 3 standard deviations (SD) above that of the null myocardium and gray zone as a region with SI greater than 2 but less than 3 SD above that of the null

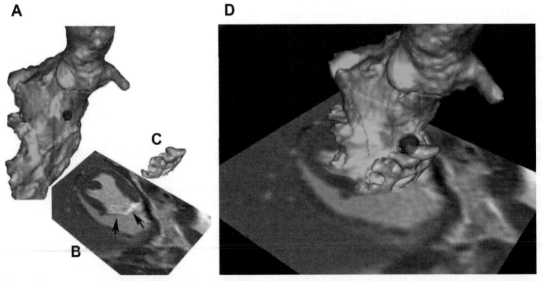

Fig. 1. Gray zone and critical isthmus colocalization in a swine model of scar-based reentrant VT. (*A*) Invasively determined critical isthmus (*red dot*). (*B, C*) The CMR-determined gray zone. Region of LGE (*arrows*). (*D*) The co-localization of the two. (*From* Estner HL, Zviman MM, Herzka D, et al. The critical isthmus sites of ischemic ventricular tachycardia are in zones of tissue heterogeneity, visualized by magnetic resonance imaging. Heart Rhythm 2011;8(12):1942–9; with permission.)

myocardium. Alternatively, core infarct may be delineated as a region with SI greater than 50% of the peak SI of the total hyperenhanced area, and gray zone is defined as a region with SI greater than peak normal SI or between 35% and 50% of the peak SI.[4] Several studies have shown that gray zone extent was a stronger predictor of subsequent ventricular arrhythmic events compared with core extent, with a recent meta-analysis reporting a pooled relative risk of 5.94 versus 3.82.[6]

Proof-of-concept studies show that by combining CMR imaging data with assumed information about myofiber orientation, myocyte biology, and tissue conduction properties, a personalized, image-based model of individual patient hearts can be developed[26–28] (Fig. 2). Such models can be used to perform virtual electrical programmed stimulation as a means of noninvasively identifying inducible substrate for risk stratification as well as for detecting potential targets for catheter ablation in both ventricular and atrial arrhythmias in addition to improving the understanding of mechanisms.[29–32] Arevalo and colleagues[29] studied patient-specific imaging-based noninvasive programmed stimulation in 41 patients with chronic myocardial infarction and LV ejection fraction ≤35% undergoing primary-prevention ICD placement. Noninvasive inducibility of ventricular arrhythmias conferred a hazard ratio of 4 for appropriate ICD firing or cardiac

death, whereas invasive electrophysiology testing conferred a lower hazard ratio of 2.6 for the same combined outcome.

Despite this proliferation of applications, the LGE technique has several important limitations. First, the use of intravenous gadolinium chelates is generally avoided in patients with significant renal dysfunction given concern for systemic nephrogenic fibrosis. Second, reliance on the differential kinetics of gadolinium in different tissues types requires precise timing of image acquisition with respect to contrast administration and precludes rapid serial imaging.[33] Third, because the LGE technique relies on differential SI between areas of fibrosis and normal myocardium, it is best suited to detect replacement fibrosis as opposed to diffuse interstitial myocardial fibrosis.[1,2,5,10] Emerging alternatives to LGE imaging may help to circumvent these challenges.

The native T1 mapping technique[34] is an endogenous contrast method that relies on measurement or estimation of T1 relaxation, which is the course of recovery of longitudinal magnetization. The T1 value depends on intrinsic tissue properties, which differ between normal and diffusely diseased tissue. Methods of estimating T1, rather than obtaining true T1 via turbo spin-echo sequences, enable more rapid image acquisition with fewer breath-holds. The technique appears to be most reproducible when the region of interest is taken from the septum. The technique is

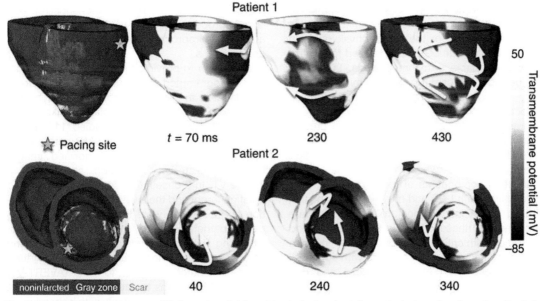

Patient 1

Pacing site $t = 70$ ms   230   430

Patient 2

noninfarcted Gray zone Scar   40   240   340

50

Transmembrane potential (mV)

−85

Fig. 2. Image-based patient-specific heart model for virtual electrophysiology study. Imaging from 2 patients in whom scar-based substrate enables initiation of reentrant tachycardia with noninvasive virtual pacing. (*From* Arevalo HJ, Vadakkumpadan F, Guallar E, et al. Arrhythmia risk stratification of patients after myocardial infarction using personalized heart models. Nat Commun. 2016;7:11437, with permission.)

less well suited for detecting regional differences in tissue characteristics, but rather for a global assessment of health versus disease in a diffusely altered substrate. The T1ρ technique is another endogenous contrast method that uses a spin-lock sequence to measure T1 relaxation in the rotating frame.[35] This technique appears to be comparable to the LGE technique in differentiating normal remote myocardium from replacement fibrosis.

CARDIAC MR IMAGING–GUIDED ELECTROPHYSIOLOGY INTERVENTION

CMR has become an increasingly important tool in the preprocedural, intraprocedural, and post-procedural assessment of patients undergoing catheter ablation for cardiac arrhythmias. Mapping systems that enable merging of imaging data with catheter position and intracardiac electrophysiologic data are now routinely used in clinical practice. Furthermore, the development of experimental MR imaging–compatible catheters that avoid issues with catheter heating, current induction, image distortion, and electromagnetic interference has made intraprocedural MR imaging feasible.[36–40] Such a platform would enable real-time assessment of anatomy, catheter position, and lesion formation and would limit or eliminate the need for ionizing radiation from fluoroscopy.

Preprocedural Applications

Preprocedural imaging with CMR in anticipation of catheter ablation for cardiac arrhythmias provides helpful information for the electrophysiologist. In routine practice, the LGE-CMR is used to localize areas of probable arrhythmogenesis. LGE-CMR may be especially useful in cases of midwall septal scar, which may not be apparent based on endocardial electroanatomical mapping. Several emerging techniques may provide more precise locations of potential ablation targets.

Conducting channels of viable tissue interdigitating with scar, which form critical slow-conduction components of reentry circuits, may be identified with LGE and may serve as ablation targets. Investigational postprocessing software that identifies these channels has shown good correlation with critical sites identified by invasive electrophysiology study in patients with structural heart disease[41–44] (Fig. 3). Berruezo and colleagues[45] studied 101 patients with LV scar-mediated ventricular tachycardia (VT). Using preprocedural LGE-CMR to identify potential conducting channels, electrophysiology operators first ablated putative channels and then performed

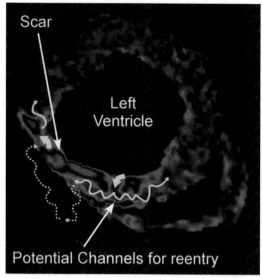

Fig. 3. LGE-CMR–based 3-dimensional imaging of scar-based substrate showing theoretic channels for reentry. (*From* Nazarian S, Bluemke D, and Halperin H. Applications of Cardiac Magnetic Resonance in Electrophysiology. Circ Arrhythmia Electrophysiol. 2009;2:63-71, with permission.)

programmed electrical stimulation. If there were residual inducible VTs, the operators proceeded to ablate these. Imaging-based channel identification and dechanneling with radiofrequency (RF) ablation rendered 54.4% of patients noninducible. Further electrogram-guided ablation rendered 78.2% of patients noninducible. Those who required only image-based dechanneling had shorter procedure time, fewer RF ablation lesions, and fewer intraprocedural external cardioversions/defibrillations.

In addition to providing prognostic information, virtual programmed stimulation, described above, may localize targets for catheter ablation in both ventricular and atrial arrhythmias. Ashikaga and colleagues[46] retrospectively studied 11 patients who underwent preprocedural CMR before catheter ablation for VT. They performed image-based simulated programmed stimulation to induce VT. In 9 cases, the simulation-determined ablation target and the invasively determined ablation target regions were the same. In 8 of these cases, catheter ablation was acutely successful, rendering the patient noninducible. An ongoing trial at the authors' institution, Ablation at VirtualhEart pRedicted Targets for VT (AVERT-VT; NCT03536052), aims to validate this technique in a prospective cohort of patients with ischemic cardiomyopathy who are undergoing catheter ablation for refractory VT. Similar techniques may be applicable in atypical atrial flutter and atrial fibrillation. Zahid and colleagues[47] retrospectively studied 10 patients who underwent preprocedural CMR followed by catheter ablation for left-sided atrial flutter. By use of in silico rapid pacing, left-sided atrial flutter was induced in 7 patients. Simulation-guided ablation targets were identified and compared with actual RF lesions, which were similar in size and location in all 7 patients. In a separate study, Zahid and colleagues[30] retrospectively assessed 20 patients with persistent atrial fibrillation undergoing LGE-CMR. Using 30 virtual pacing sites within the atria, atrial fibrillation was induced in 13 patients and enabled identification and localization of reentrant drivers. There were, on average, 2.7 reentrant drivers per patient. The investigators observed that these drivers were localized in tissue with high fibrosis density and high fibrosis entropy.

Intraprocedural Applications

Catheter ablation traditionally relies on the use of fluoroscopy to determine catheter position. However, fluoroscopy is 2-dimensional, provides limited anatomic detail, and involves administration of ionizing radiation. Limitations with fluoroscopy represent an unmet need in clinical electrophysiology that MR imaging may be poised to address.

At present, the use of intraprocedural MR imaging is limited to static images that are acquired preprocedurally. Preacquired imaging may be used to provide anatomic definition of the cardiac chambers, and associated structures can be used as a "shell" or scaffold with reference to which catheter position can be determined in real time and invasively acquired parameters like voltage can be mapped.[48] These scaffolds can also help operators to avoid potential missteps like ablation within a pulmonary vein. However, this application may be limited by translational shifts in the location of the heart or phasic cardiac motion that creates discordance between the actual locations of structures and their apparent locations on preacquired images.[49]

The development of experimental MR imaging–compatible catheters that circumvent problems with catheter heating, current induction, image distortion, and electromagnetic interference has made intraprocedural MR imaging feasible.[36–40] These catheters, coupled with emerging noncontrast MR imaging techniques for distinguishing irreversible injury from edema, may permit real-time intraprocedural information about catheter ablation lesions.

Catheter ablation relies on the creation of RF or cryoablation lesions to create controlled, well-defined areas of necrosis. Once ablations are formed, various assays may be performed to define success. For example, following catheter ablation for VT, programmed electrical stimulation may be performed to demonstrate lack of inducible ventricular arrhythmias, which is a common procedural endpoint.[50,51] Similarly, following pulmonary vein isolation for atrial fibrillation, the absence of pulmonary vein potentials during sinus rhythm or coronary sinus pacing demonstrates pulmonary vein entrance block and is a common procedural endpoint.[52] However, the electrophysiology captured by these assays may reflect the effects of both necrosis and edema from RF or cryoablation lesions. Over time, as edema resolves, the electrophysiologic properties of the lesion may change. Therefore, an intraprocedural means of delineating necrosis versus edema would be useful.

Several groups have shown the utility of combining both T1-weighted and T2-weighted imaging, the latter of which is more specific for edema, to track the time course of ablation lesions and distinguish between necrosis and edema.[53,54] Although the LGE technique is useful to characterize RF ablation lesions, differential kinetics of gadolinium in different tissues requires careful timing of image acquisition following contrast administration. The ability of noncontrast native T1 mapping approaches to characterize ablation lesions and track their evolution has been reported.[55] A novel, noncontrast T1-weighted technique with long inversion time (TI = 700 ms) permits differentiation of necrosis from edema and permits differentiation of acute from chronic lesions[33] (Fig. 4). With minimal postprocessing, this technique also enables 3-dimensional volume rendering. Finally, because native T1 mapping is a noncontrast technique and does not rely on wash-in and wash-out kinetics of gadolinium chelates, imaging may be performed serially, as needed. A separate technique, proton resonance frequency shift thermography, uses the sensitivity of the proton resonance frequency to temperature and may provide complementary intraprocedural information about RF ablation lesions.[56] Future work in this area could focus on the comparative utility of imaging-based and electrophysiologic assay-based endpoints for ablation procedures in predicting long-term procedural success.

CARDIAC IMPLANTABLE ELECTRICAL DEVICES

Historically, thoracic MR imaging has been avoided or approached with great caution in patients with CIEDs because of concern for patient

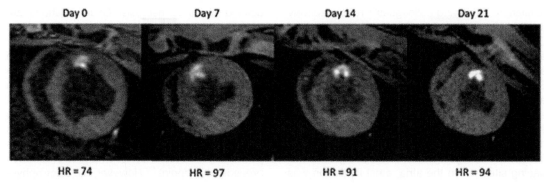

Fig. 4. RF ablation lesion imaging with T1 inversion recovery using a long inversion time. This technique differentiates necrosis from edema and demonstrates stable lesion appearance over time. (*From* Guttman MA, Tao S, Fink S, et al. Non-Contrast-Enhanced T1-Weighted MRI of Myocardial Radiofrequency Ablation Lesions. Magn Reson Med 2018. 79:879–889, with permission.)

safety and potentially prohibitive imaging artifacts. The magnetic field generated by an RF pulse may exert torque on ferromagnetic material, may cause heating of leads and potentially cause damage at the device-tissue interface, and may provide electromagnetic interference that could cause device malfunction or programming changes. Furthermore, CIEDs may cause large susceptibility artifacts using standard acquisition techniques that may preclude diagnostic visualization of a large segment of the myocardium.[57] However, emerging techniques for artifact suppression, such as wideband pulse sequences, as well as evolving institutional safety protocols, may enable high-quality CMR imaging in many patients with CIEDs.

Accumulating experience suggests that MR imaging is safe in most patients with CIEDs. Nazarian and colleagues[58] prospectively studied 1509 patients with non-MR imaging conditional CIEDs (58% with pacemakers and 42% with defibrillators) undergoing 1.5-T MR imaging at a single center. Patients were excluded if they had undergone lead implantation within the previous 4 weeks, had surgical epicardial leads or permanent abandoned, nonfunctional leads, had a subcutaneous ICD, or were pacing-dependent and had an ICD without the option for asynchronous pacing. The pacing mode was changed to asynchronous pacing for all pacemaker-dependent patients, and to demand mode for all other patients, and tachyarrhythmia therapies were disabled for all patients. Long term follow-up was available in 63% of patients. No clinically significant adverse events were reported. A decrease in p-wave amplitude was noted in 4% of patients; an increase in atrial capture threshold was noted in 4% of patients; an increased right ventricular capture threshold

was noted in 4% of patients; and an increase in LV capture threshold was noted in 5% of patients. The similarly sized MagnaSafe Registry, a prospective multicenter study, also showed no significant adverse events when patients are appropriately screened and undergo device reprogramming in keeping with prespecified safety protocols.[59] Hence, several professional cardiology societies are issuing updated guidelines to direct safe performance of imaging the presence of devices.[60]

Emerging techniques, such as wideband pulse sequences, may provide high-quality CMR imaging in patients with CIEDs at 1.5 T and 3 T[61,62] (**Fig. 5**). Do and colleagues[63] performed CMR at 1.5 T on 111 patients with non-MR imaging conditional CIEDs using a hyperbolic secant pulse. Among these, the investigators reported that 87% of images were free of device-related artifacts limiting clinical interpretation. Ranjan and colleagues[61] studied the wideband technique in a canine model of RF ablation at 3 T. Using a hyperbolic secant pulse, they assessed 97 experimental RF lesions in 7 dogs with ICD generators externally affixed to the left shoulder. They scored image quality on a 1 to 5 scale and showed that image quality was significantly higher using wideband imaging as compared with standard LGE-CMR.

Further advances in both patient safety protocols and artifact suppression techniques may enable not only routine clinical CMR in patients with CIEDs but also CMR-guided electrophysiology procedures, as described above, in patients with CIEDs. Future work could focus on both safety and image quality in patients with subcutaneous ICDs and permanent epicardial leads, and on imaging with field strengths higher than 1.5 T.

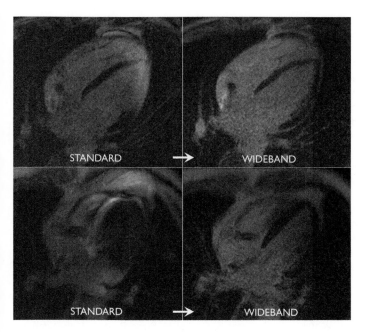

Fig. 5. Wideband LGE-CMR for artifact suppression in the presence of CIEDs. (*From* Stevens SM, Tung R, Rashid S, et al. Device artifact reduction for magnetic resonance imaging of patients with implantable cardioverter-defibrillators and ventricular tachycardia: late gadolinium enhancement correlation with electroanatomic mapping. Heart Rhythm. 2014;11(2):289-98, with permission.)

SUMMARY

There is an expanding range of tools offered by CMR that address both current limitations of CMR in practice and several key unmet needs in clinical electrophysiology. Endogenous contrast techniques for imaging myocardial fibrosis may limit the need for gadolinium chelates. Artifact suppression techniques and institutional safety protocols may enable diagnostic-quality imaging in many patients with CIEDs. Novel approaches to postprocessing enable identification of conducting channels that may provide targets for catheter ablation. The use of LGE-CMR in patient-specific heart models enables virtual noninvasive programmed stimulation that may help with risk stratification and localization of ablation targets. Finally, ablation catheters that are MR imaging–compatible have opened the door to real-time, intraprocedural MR imaging for guidance of electrophysiology interventions.

REFERENCES

1. Captur G, Manisty C, Moon J. Cardiac MRI evaluation of myocardial disease. Heart 2016;102: 1429–35.

2. Pattanayak P, Bleumke D. Tissue characterization of the myocardium: state of the art characterization by magnetic resonance and computed tomography imaging. Radiol Clin North Am 2015;53:413–23.

3. Motwani M, Kidambi A, Greenwood J, et al. Advances in cardiovascular magnetic resonance in ischaemic heart disease and non-ischaemic cardiomyopathies. Heart 2014;100:1722–33.

4. Wu K. Sudden cardiac death substrate imaged by magnetic resonance imaging: from investigational tool to clinical applications. Circ Cardiovasc Imaging 2017;10:e005461.

5. Kramer C. Role of cardiac MR imaging in cardiomyopathies. J Nucl Med 2015;56(Suppl 4): 39S–45S.

6. Scott P, Rosengarten J, Curzen N, et al. Late gadolinium enhancement cardiac magnetic resonance imaging for the prediction of ventricular tachyarrhythmic events: a meta-analysis. Eur J Heart Fail 2013;15:1019–27.

7. Disertori M, Rigoni M, Pace N, et al. Myocardial fibrosis assessment by LGE is a powerful predictor of ventricular tachyarrhythmias in ischemic and non-ischemic LV dysfunction: a meta-analysis. JACC Cardiovasc Imaging 2016;9:1046–55.

8. Kuruvilla S, Adenaw N, Katwal A, et al. Late gadolinium enhancement on cardiac magnetic resonance predicts adverse cardiovascular outcomes in nonischemic cardiomyopathy: a systematic review and meta-analysis. Circ Cardiovasc Imaging 2014;7: 250–8.

9. Di Marco A, Anguera I, Schmitt M, et al. Late gadolinium enhancement and the risk for ventricular arrhythmias or sudden death in dilated cardiomyopathy: systematic review and meta-analysis. JACC Heart Fail 2017;5:28–38.

10. Patel A, Kramer C. Role of cardiac magnetic resonance in the diagnosis and prognosis of nonischemic cardiomyopathy. JACC Cardiovasc Imaging 2017;10:1180–93.

11. Patel M, Cawley P, Heitner J, et al. Detection of myocardial damage in patients with sarcoidosis. Circulation 2009;120:1969–77.

12. Hulten E, Agarwal V, Cahill M, et al. Presence of late gadolinium enhancement by cardiac magnetic resonance among patients with suspected cardiac sarcoidosis is associated with adverse cardiovascular prognosis: a systematic review and meta-analysis. Circ Cardiovasc Imaging 2016;9:e005001.

13. Coleman G, Shaw P, Balfour PCJ, et al. Prognostic value of myocardial scarring on CMR in patients with cardiac sarcoidosis. JACC Cardiovasc Imaging 2017;10:411–20.

14. Weng Z, Yao J, Chan R, et al. Prognostic value of LGE-CMR in HCM a meta-analysis. JACC Cardiovasc Imaging 2016;9:1392–402.

15. Maron M. Clinical utility of cardiovascular magnetic resonance in hypertrophic cardiomyopathy. J Cardiovasc Magn Reson 2012;14:13.

16. Maron B, Maron M. LGE means better selection of HCM patients for primary prevention implantable defibrillators. JACC Cardiovasc Imaging 2016;9: 1403–6.

17. Green J, Berger J, Kramer C, et al. Prognostic value of late gadolinium enhancement in clinical outcomes for hypertrophic cardiomyopathy. JACC Cardiovasc Imaging 2012;5:370–7.

18. Te Riele A, Tandri H, Sanborn D, et al. Noninvasive multimodality imaging in ARVD/C. JACC Cardiovasc Imaging 2015;8:597–611.

19. Cochet H, Dubois R, Yamashita S, et al. Relationship between fibrosis detected on late gadolinium-enhanced cardiac magnetic resonance and re-entrant activity assessed with electrocardiographic imaging in human persistent atrial fibrillation. JACC Clin Electrophysiol 2018;4:17–29.

20. Zghaib T, Nazarian S. New insights into the use of cardiac magnetic resonance imaging to guide decision making in atrial fibrillation management. Can J Cardiol 2018;34(11):1461–70.

21. Schmidt E, Halperin H. MRI use for atrial tissue characterization in arrhythmias and for EP procedure guidance. Int J Cardiovasc Imaging 2018;34:81–95.

22. Stone G, Selker H, Thiele H, et al. Relationship between infarct size and outcomes following primary PCI: patient-level analysis from 10 randomized trials. J Am Coll Cardiol 2016;67:1674–83.

23. Becker M, Cornel J, van de Ven P, et al. The prognostic value of late gadolinium-enhanced cardiac magnetic resonance imaging in nonischemic dilated cardiomyopathy: a review and meta-analysis. JACC Cardiovasc Imaging 2018;11:1274–84.

24. Ashikaga H, Sasano T, Dong J, et al. Magnetic resonance-based anatomical analysis of scar-related ventricular tachycardia: implications for catheter ablation. Circ Res 2007;101:939–47.

25. Estner H, Zviman M, Herzka D, et al. The critical isthmus sites of ischemic ventricular tachycardia are in zones of tissue heterogeneity, visualized by magnetic resonance imaging. Heart Rhythm 2011; 8:1942–9.

26. Trayanova N, Pashakhanloo F, Wu K, et al. Imaging-based simulations for predicting sudden death and guiding ventricular tachycardia ablation. Circ Arrhythm Electrophysiol 2017;10:e004743.

27. Gray R, Pathmanathan P. Patient-specific cardiovascular computational modeling: diversity of personalization and challenges. J Cardiovasc Transl Res 2018;11:80–8.

28. Rodriguez B, Carusi A, Abi-Gerges N, et al. Human-based approaches to pharmacology and cardiology: an interdisciplinary and intersectorial workshop. Europace 2016;18:1287–98.

29. Arevalo H, Vadakkumpadan F, Guallar E, et al. Arrhythmia risk stratification of patients after myocardial infarction using personalized heart models. Nat Commun 2016;10:11437.

30. Zahid S, Cochet H, Boyle P, et al. Patient-derived models link re-entrant driver localization in atrial fibrillation to fibrosis spatial pattern. Cardiovasc Res 2016;110:443–54.

31. Vagos M, van Herck I, Sundnes J, et al. Computational modeling of electrophysiology and pharmacotherapy of atrial fibrillation: recent advances and future challenges. Front Physiol 2018;9:1221.

32. Chen Z, Niederer S, Shanmugam N, et al. Cardiac computational modeling of ventricular tachycardia and cardiac resynchronization therapy: a clinical perspective. Minerva Cardioangiol 2017;65:380–97.

33. Guttman M, Tao S, Fink S, et al. Non-contrast-enhanced T1 -weighted MRI of myocardial radiofrequency ablation lesions. Magn Reson Med 2018;79: 879–89.

34. Puntmann V, Peker E, Chandrashekhar Y, et al. T1 mapping in characterizing myocardial disease: a comprehensive review. Circ Res 2016;119:277–99.

35. Stoffers R, Madden M, Shahid M, et al. Assessment of myocardial injury after reperfused infarction by T1ρ cardiovascular magnetic resonance. J Cardiovasc Magn Reson 2017;19:17.

36. Rogers T, Lederman R, Interventional CMR. Clinical applications and future directions. Curr Cardiol Rep 2015;15:31.

37. Campbell-Washburn A, Tavallaei M, Pop M, et al. Real-time MRI guidance of cardiac interventions. J Magn Reson Imaging 2017;46:935–50.

38. Mukherjee R, Roujol S, Chubb H, et al. Epicardial electroanatomical mapping, radiofrequency ablation, and lesion imaging in the porcine left ventricle under real-time magnetic resonance imaging guidance-an in vivo feasibility study. Europace 2018;20:f254–62.

39. Vergara G, Vijayakumar S, Kholmovski E, et al. Real-time magnetic resonance imaging-guided radiofrequency atrial ablation and visualization of lesion formation at 3 Tesla. Heart Rhythm 2011;8:295–303.

40. Bhagirath P, van der Graaf M, Karim R, et al. Interventional cardiac magnetic resonance imaging in electrophysiology: advances toward clinical translation. Circ Arrhythm Electrophysiol 2015;8:203–11.

41. Fernández-Armenta J, Berruezo A, Andreu D, et al. Three-dimensional architecture of scar and conducting channels based on high resolution ce-CMR: insights for ventricular tachycardia ablation. Circ Arrhythm Electrophysiol 2013;6:528–37.

42. Andreu D, Berruezo A, Ortiz-Pérez J, et al. Integration of 3D electroanatomic maps and magnetic resonance scar characterization into the navigation system to guide ventricular tachycardia ablation. Circ Arrhythm Electrophysiol 2011;4:674–83.

43. Andreu D, Ortiz-Pérez J, Fernández-Armenta J, et al. 3D delayed-enhanced magnetic resonance sequences improve conducting channel delineation prior to ventricular tachycardia ablation. Europace 2015;17:938–45.

44. Andreu D, Penela D, Acosta J, et al. Cardiac magnetic resonance-aided scar dechanneling: influence on acute and long-term outcomes. Heart Rhythm 2017;14:1121–8.

45. Berruezo A, Fernández-Armenta J, Andreu D, et al. Scar dechanneling: new method for scar-related left ventricular tachycardia substrate ablation. Circ Arrhythm Electrophysiol 2015;8:326–36.

46. Ashikaga H, Arevalo H, Vadakkumpadan F, et al. Feasibility of image-based simulation to estimate ablation target in human ventricular arrhythmia. Heart Rhythm 2013;10:1109–16.

47. Zahid S, Whyte K, Schwarz E, et al. Feasibility of using patient-specific models and the "minimum cut" algorithm to predict optimal ablation targets for left atrial flutter. Heart Rhythm 2016;13:1687–98.

48. Dickfeld T, Calkins H, Zviman M, et al. Anatomic stereotactic catheter ablation on three-dimensional magnetic resonance images in real time. Circulation 2003;108:2407–13.

49. Muthalaly R, Nerlekar N, Ge Y, et al. MRI in patients with cardiac implantable electronic devices. Radiology 2018;289:281–92.

50. Piers S, Leong D, van Huls van Taxis C, et al. Outcome of ventricular tachycardia ablation in patients with nonischemic cardiomyopathy: the impact of noninducibility. Circ Arrhythm Electrophysiol 2013;6:513–21.

51. Della Bella P, De Ponti R, Uriarte J, et al. Catheter ablation and antiarrhythmic drugs for haemodynamically tolerated post-infarction ventricular tachycardia; long-term outcome in relation to acute electrophysiological findings. Eur Heart J 2002;23: 414–24.

52. Verma A, Marrouche N, Natale A. Pulmonary vein antrum isolation: intracardiac echocardiography-guided technique. J Cardiovasc Electrophysiol 2004;15:1335–40.

53. Ghafoori E, Kholmovski E, Thomas S, et al. Characterization of gadolinium contrast enhancement of radiofrequency ablation lesions in predicting edema and chronic lesion size. Circ Arrhythm Electrophysiol 2017;10:e005599.

54. Krahn P, Singh S, Ramanan V, et al. Cardiovascular magnetic resonance guided ablation and intra-procedural visualization of evolving radiofrequency lesions in the left ventricle. J Cardiovasc Magn Reson 2018;20:20.

55. Kholmovski E, Silvernagel J, Angel N, et al. Acute noncontrast T1-weighted magnetic resonance imaging predicts chronic radiofrequency ablation lesions. J Cardiovasc Electrophysiol 2018;29(11):1556–62.

56. Kolandaivelu A, Zviman M, Castro V, et al. Noninvasive assessment of tissue heating during cardiac radiofrequency ablation using MRI thermography. Circ Arrhythm Electrophysiol 2010;3:521–9.

57. Mesubi O, Ahmad G, Jeudy J, et al. Impact of ICD artifact burden on late gadolinium enhancement cardiac MR imaging in patients undergoing ventricular tachycardia ablation. Pacing Clin Electrophysiol 2014;37:1274–83.

58. Nazarian S, Hansford R, Rahsepar A, et al. Safety of magnetic resonance imaging in patients with cardiac devices. N Engl J Med 2017;377:2555–64.

59. Russo R, Costa H, Silva P, et al. Assessing the risks associated with MRI in patients with a pacemaker or defibrillator. N Engl J Med 2017;376:755–64.

60. Shulman R, Hunt B. Cardiac implanted electronic devices and MRI safety in 2018—the state of play. Eur Radiol 2018;28:4062–5.

61. Ranjan R, McGann C, Jeong E, et al. Wideband late gadolinium enhanced magnetic resonance imaging for imaging myocardial scar without image artefacts induced by implantable cardioverter-defibrillator: a feasibility study at 3 T. Europace 2015;17:483–8.

62. Rashid S, Rapacchi S, Vaseghi M, et al. Improved late gadolinium enhancement MR imaging for patients with implanted cardiac devices. Radiology 2014;270:269–74.

63. Do D, Eyvazian V, Bayoneta A, et al. Cardiac magnetic resonance imaging using wideband sequences in patients with nonconditional cardiac implantable electronic devices. Heart Rhythm 2018; 15:218–25.

The Role of Contrast-Enhanced Cardiac Magnetic Resonance in the Assessment of Patients with Malignant Ventricular Arrhythmias

Dahlia Banerji, MD[a], Dexter Mendoza, MD[b],
Brian B. Ghoshhajra, MD, MBA[a], Sandeep S. Hedgire, MD[a],*

KEYWORDS

- Ventricular arrhythmia • Cardiac arrest • Scar mapping • Electrophysiology
- Cardiac magnetic resonance imaging • Sudden cardiac death • Risk stratification

KEY POINTS

- Myocardial fibrosis often results in tissue heterogeneity resulting in re-entry circuits and thereby predisposing individuals to malignant ventricular arrhythmias and sudden cardiac death.
- Cardiac magnetic resonance (CMR) imaging can provide valuable information to facilitate the management of patients presenting with malignant ventricular arrhythmias of ischemic and nonischemic origins.
- By virtue of its strength in tissue characterization sequences such as late gadolinium enhancement imaging, CMR can provide additional information in a myriad of diseases in relation to prognostication and risk stratification.

INTRODUCTION

Ventricular arrhythmias are common in patients with cardiomyopathy and heart failure of ischemic and nonischemic origin. These include premature ventricular contractions (PVC), nonsustained ventricular tachycardia (NSVT), accelerated idioventricular rhythm, sustained ventricular tachycardia (VT), and ventricular fibrillation (VF).[1] PVCs are frequently seen in individuals with heart failure, often in up to 70% to 95% of such individuals. They may vary in frequency (such as ventricular bigeminy and trigeminy) or complexity (multifocal or couplets). Complex PVCs may predict more malignant arrhythmias and sudden cardiac death (SCD). PVCs in individuals with previous myocardial infarctions (MIs) are associated with increased risk of death.[2,3] Malignant ventricular arrhythmias include sustained VT, torsades de pointes (a form of polymorphic VT), and VF. Patients with

Funding/Support: Dr D. Banerji was supported by National Institutes of Health (NIH)/National Heart, Lung and Blood Institute (NHLBI) (5T32HL076136).

[a] Cardiac MR PET CT Program, Department of Radiology (Cardiovascular Imaging), Division of Cardiology, Massachusetts General Hospital, Harvard Medical School, 165 Cambridge Street, Suite 400, Boston, MA 02114, USA;
[b] Thoracic Imaging and Intervention, Department of Radiology, Massachusetts General Hospital, Harvard Medical School, 55 Fruit Street, Founders 202, Boston, MA 02114, USA
* Corresponding author. Department of Radiology, Massachusetts General Hospital, 55 Fruit Street, Boston, MA 02114.
E-mail address: hedgire.sandeep@mgh.harvard.edu

Magn Reson Imaging Clin N Am 27 (2019) 475–490
https://doi.org/10.1016/j.mric.2019.04.011

spontaneous, sustained VT or VF have a much higher risk of SCD.

Cardiac fibroblasts comprise approximately 90% of the noncardiomyocyte cells of the heart and are the primary component responsible for many of the extracellular matrix components, including collagens I, III, IV, laminin, and fibronectin. Histologically, a signature feature of worsening heart failure is progressive accumulation of collagen in the heart, resulting in myocardial fibrosis. This scarring or replacement fibrosis is a compensatory mechanism of the heart to substitute for normal parenchyma. Myocardial fibrosis and the resultant heterogeneity often provide the structural substrate for malignant ventricular arrhythmias, which often culminate in SCD.[4]

Cardiac magnetic resonance (CMR) imaging is an advanced, multifaceted noninvasive imaging modality that can accurately assess myocardial structure and physiology. Specifically, the usefulness of gadolinium-based contrast and late gadolinium enhancement (LGE) makes it a powerful tool to assess the presence of scar, as it disperses in the extracellular space, with excellent histologic correlation.[5–7] Gadolinium is injected intravenously and can diffuse across the intravascular space but does not cross an intact myocardial cell membrane. Areas of myocardial injury, however, are associated with higher distribution/unit volume, and appear bright on LGE images. The distribution of LGE assists in determination of the various causes of cardiomyopathies, and serves as a prognostic marker for SCD.[8]

Compared with other imaging modalities, CMR has a distinct advantage of its high spatial resolution, allowing for clear scar delineation and quantification, which has prognostic value in determination of SCD. In addition, CMR is not limited by poor acoustic windows and provides more accurate detection of left ventricular ejection fraction (LVEF) compared with transthoracic echocardiography, which is seminal in further management as primary prevention of individuals with malignant arrhythmias and the decision of implantable cardiac defibrillators (ICDs) implantation relies on this.[9–11]

CARDIAC CONDUCTION SYSTEM AND INTRODUCTION TO CARDIAC MAGNETIC RESONANCE IMAGING

Coordinated contraction of the heart relies on the cardiac conduction system, which consists of specialized cardiomyocytes that generate and propagate electrical impulse. In a normal heart, electrical impulses arise from the sinoatrial junction, which is located near the superior cavoatrial junction. The impulse then travels to and is delayed at the atrioventricular node, near the interatrial septum. This delay allows for atrial contraction and ventricular filling before ventricular contraction. Electrical passage from the atrium to the ventricular myocardium is through the atrioventricular bundle (of His). This bundle conducts the electrical impulse to the left and right bundles and ultimately to the Purkinje fiber network, which activates the ventricular myocardium. Injury or pathology along this pathway can lead to arrhythmias.

A basic CMR imaging protocol for the investigation of ventricular arrhythmias requires assessment of cardiac anatomy and function. Functional assessment relies on cine cardiac imaging through the different cardiac planes (short and long axes), which typically uses steady-state free precession (SSFP) sequences. SSFP sequences are modified gradient echo sequences, which provide excellent contrast between the bright blood and the myocardium with high temporal resolution, making it indispensable in the evaluation of wall motion and in volumetric measurement necessary in the assessment of ventricular function. Detection of myocardial pathology relies on late gadolinium-enhanced mages following intravenous contrast administration and myocardial nulling. Myocardial nulling is achieved although inversion recovery pulses, which result in a dark appearance of the normal myocardium. Myocardial fibrosis or scarring is characterized by LGE, and the pattern and extent of LGE may be indicative of specific diagnoses.[12] Depending on clinical suspicion, additional sequences may be added to the protocol to answer specific diagnostic questions. These sequences are discussed as they pertain to specific pathologies below.

IMAGING FINDINGS/PATHOLOGY
Ischemic

- Ischemic heart disease is often associated with LGE, typically in a subendocardial or transmural distribution in myocardial segments, following a coronary artery territory[13] (Fig. 1).
- Often, the pattern involves a central core of dense fibrosis within a heterogenous peri-infarct (gray) zone, suggestive of the presence of viable and nonviable myocardium.[14] The extent of LGE is a reliable marker for the likelihood of functional recovery with

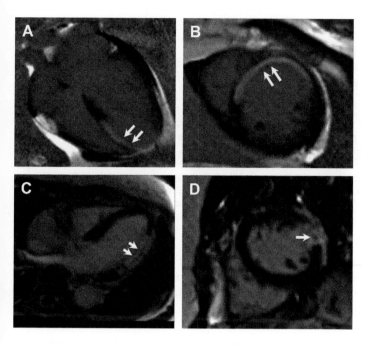

Fig. 1. Ischemic cardiomyopathy. Typical subendocardial LGE in the left anterior descending territory including the septal and anterior walls (*arrows, A, B*). Involvement of greater than 50% of the wall thickness portends low likelihood of recovery after revascularization. Transmural LGE of the lateral wall (*C, D*) seen on a different patient found to have spontaneous coronary arterial dissection and occlusion of the first and second obtuse marginal branches. Central focus of nonenhancement (*arrows, C, D*) is suggestive of microvascular obstruction, which is a poor prognostic indicator.

revascularization, taking a threshold of 50% to determine viability.

- Microvascular obstruction (MVO) is seen in a proportion of individuals with acute MI after reperfusion of a previously occluded coronary artery. Typically, it appears as a central dark focus within an area of early enhancing myocardium. This signifies a focal area of absent contrast enhancement within a site of MI. It may be seen on first-pass perfusion, early gadolinium enhancement (EGE) as well as LGE images, but the presence of MVO on LGE is a more accurate prognostic marker than when seen on first-pass perfusion or EGE, in determining risk of adverse left ventricular remodeling and future major adverse cardiovascular events.[15]
- The presence and extent of LGE are significant prognostic markers in the setting of coronary artery disease (CAD). According to 1 study, any LGE is associated with a hazard ratio of 10.9 for cardiac mortality.[16]
- A group from Duke demonstrated that the extent of total scar (threshold >5% left ventricular [LV] mass) was the most important prognostic parameter in ischemic as well as nonischemic cardiomyopathy.[17]

Nonischemic Cardiomyopathy

Dilated cardiomyopathy

- Dilated cardiomyopathy (DCM) is typically associated with no or minimal obstructive

CAD. Up to 71% of such patients have been seen to have LGE, often in a midwall distribution, less often in a subepicardial pattern (**Fig. 2**).

- Subendocardial injury is seen in approximately 17% of individuals and may be reflective of embolic phenomena.
- The extent of LGE and percentage of LV mass affected are related to the occurrence of inducible VT, SCD, or ICD therapy.[18]
- A previous pooled cohort analysis of 7 studies of patients with DCM and ischemic cardiomyopathy demonstrated that, although the presence of scar was an independent predictor of endpoints, the extent of scar (either

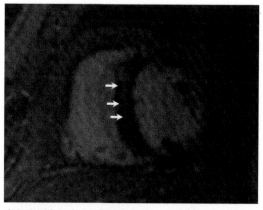

Fig. 2. Dilated cardiomyopathy. Although not specific, linear midwall LGE in the basal septum is commonly seen with dilated cardiomyopathy.

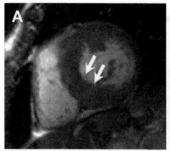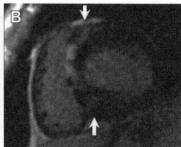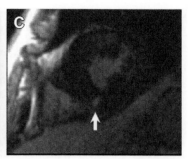

Fig. 3. Hypertrophic cardiomyopathy. Short axis SSFP image (*A*) shows asymmetric septal wall thickening measuring 25 mm in diastole (*arrows, A*). Post-contrast images (*B, C*) show subepicardial and midwall LGE predominantly in the septal and anterior walls with additional nodular LGE at the right ventricular insertion points (*B, C, arrows*).

transmurality or percentage of LV mass) was most predictive of outcomes, including inducible VT on electrophysiology studies, ventricular arrhythmias or ICD therapy, or a composite endpoint of ICD therapy or SCD.[19]

Hypertrophic cardiomyopathy

- Hypertrophic cardiomyopathy (HCM) is the most common genetic cardiomyopathy with many genes encoding for cardiac sarcomere. It is characterized by a heterogenic phenotypic expression.[20]
- SCD is a catastrophic disease consequence seen in a small subset of patients. It may be unpredictable and often arises in youth or middle-age.[21]
- ICD therapy has been instrumental in decreasing rates of SCD in patients with HCM to approximately 0.5%/year.[22]
- LGE on CMR has immense potential to identify areas of myocardial fibrosis, which is postulated to be the arrhythmogenic substrate in this cohort, as previous studies have demonstrated that individuals with LGE have higher rates of NSVT on Holter monitoring, compared with those without LGE (**Fig. 3**).
- Extensive LGE, comprising greater than 15% LV mass involvement is associated with a 2-fold increased risk of SCD, regardless of the presence of other risk factors (left ventricular wall thickness >30 mm, family history of SCD, presence of NSVT, unexplained syncope, or abnormal blood pressure response).[20]
- The most common locations for LGE involve the hypertrophic segments and the right ventricular (RV) insertion points; however, it may be diffuse and follow a non-territorial pattern.[23]

- A threshold of 6SD has been established as a reliable and reproducible metric to determine the extent of LGE in patients with HCM.[24]

Sarcoidosis

- Sarcoidosis is a multisystem granulomatous disease of unclear origin with characteristic noncaseating granulomas. Cardiac involvement is clinically evident in about 5% of affected individuals and may result in LV dysfunction, scar, and significant arrhythmias, but autopsy findings demonstrate myocardial lesions in about 20% to 60%.[25–27] Sarcoidosis is suspected when there is unexplained LV systolic dysfunction with an LVEF less than 40% or if there is unexplained spontaneous or induced sustained VT.[28] The principal manifestations are conduction abnormalities, ventricular arrhythmias including SCD, and heart failure.[29]
- Although there is no specific diagnostic pattern of LGE on CMR for cardiac sarcoidosis (CS), it often presents as a patchy or multifocal distribution with sparing of the endocardial border. It is more often seen in the basal segments, especially in the septal and lateral walls, and more often in a midmyocardial to subepicardial distribution.[30] Occasionally, a transmural pattern may also be seen with rare involvement of the RV free wall.[31] Occasionally, one may notice a prominent involvement of the insertion points with direct and contiguous extension across the septum into the RV, and this has been termed the "hook sign." The presence of this on CMR increases the probability of CS to greater than 90%[32] (**Fig. 4**).
- A multimodality imaging assessment of 29 patients with CS and VT demonstrated a higher tendency of abnormal electrograms

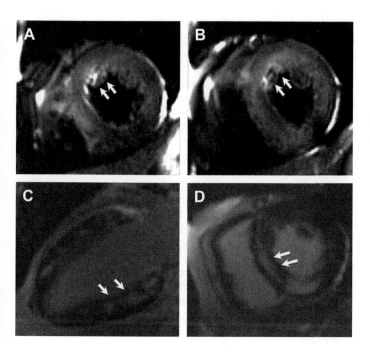

Fig. 4. Cardiac sarcoid. Short-axis T2-weighted image (*A, B*) show near diffuse increased signal particularly of the anterior and septal walls, consistent with myocardial edema (*arrows, A, B*). Two-chamber and short axis post contrast images show patchy and nodular areas of mid-wall myocardial LGE with relative sparing of the subendocardial border (*C, D, arrows*).

on electroanatomical mapping to correlate with scar on CMR and less so with inflammation on PET, suggesting the dominant role of scar in ventricular arrhythmogenesis.[33]

Myocarditis

- The most recent update on the expert consensus recommendations for the CMR diagnosis of acute myocarditis[34] (the "Lake Louse Criteria") proposes 2 main criteria:
  1. The presence of myocardial edema;
  2. Evidence of nonischemic myocardial injury.
- Myocardial edema is indicated by increased myocardial signal on T2-weighted sequences. T2 mapping allows for quantitative

assessment of the myocardium, which may increase the accuracy of detecting edema and may have prognostic value.[35,36]
- Myocardial injury is indicated by nonischemic pattern LGE. Classically, although neither sensitive nor specific, LGE in myocarditis has been described to be in subepicardial in the basal-to-mid LV inferolateral segments (**Fig. 5**).
- Myocardial injury may also be indicated by abnormally increased signal on T1-weighted images or increased extracellular volume, which can be determined using T1 mapping techniques.[37]
- Practically speaking, however, in routine clinical practice, the presence of evidence of nonischemic myocardial injury on CMR (ie,

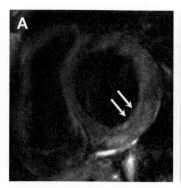
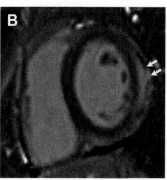

Fig. 5. Acute myocarditis. Short axis dual echo T2-weighted sequence image (*A*) myocardial edema in the basal inferolateral, lateral, and anterolateral segments (*arrows, A*). There is corresponding subepicardial LGE (*arrows, B*) in the same distribution.

nonischemic pattern of LGE) in the appropriate clinical setting would be adequate for the diagnosis of acute myocarditis.

Chagas cardiomyopathy

- Chagas disease is an infectious myocarditis caused by the protozoan, *Trypanosoma cruzi*, which is endemic to Central and South America.
- Most patients have a self-limited course, but approximately 30% develop persistent parasitemia and latent infection that manifests years later as a DCM, and subsequently chronic Chagas cardiomyopathy (CCC) may manifest as myocardial damage, characterized by marked fibrosis often associated with ventricular arrhythmias and apical aneurysms.
- Scar in patients with CCC has been determined to be a strong predictor of a combination of death and sustained VT.[38]
- The distribution of LGE scar is more often seen along the inferolateral wall of the left ventricle, but no specific distribution of fibrosis was noted to correlated with pathogenesis or outcomes. Varying observed LGE patterns included apical, transmural, focal and diffuse[39] (Fig. 6).

Left ventricular noncompaction

- Left ventricular noncompaction (LVNC) is an uncommon cardiomyopathy associated with prominent and deep LV trabeculations and

intertrabecular recesses, altering the myocardial framework, and thought to be associated with a developmental arrest in the embryogenic period causing lack of compaction of the myocardium.[40]

- LGE has been observed in approximately 40% of individuals who meet diagnostic criteria for LVNC. The underlying mechanisms have been postulated to be related to coronary microcirculatory dysfunction, resulting in ischemia and fibrosis in noncompacted and compacted myocardial segments, in a variegated fashion. The distribution has been observed to be heterogeneous as well, and may involve subendocardial, midmyocardial, subepicardial, or transmural segments (Fig. 7). Although some studies have demonstrated a predilection for LGE involvement of the interventricular septum, LGE involvement of the noncompacted segments is often less common.[41] As the presence of LGE in LVNC is infrequent, its presence is specific, but not sensitive enough to make the diagnosis.[42]
- Hyper-enhancement within the trabeculations of the noncompacted segment may also suggest fibrosis, which may serve as a marker for high-risk patient delineation because this may serve as a focus for malignant ventricular arrhythmias.[43] Another study of 113 patients demonstrated LGE in only 11 patients, but this was predictive of cardiac events, suggestive of a prognostic benefit.[44]

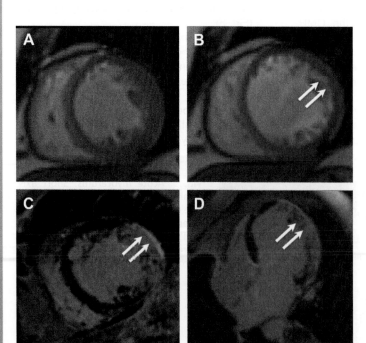

Fig. 6. Chagas cardiomyopathy. Representative still frames demonstrating systolic (*A*) and diastolic (*B*) mid-ventricular short axis slices showing thinning of the lateral wall (*arrows, B*), which was dyskinetic on cine imaging (not shown here). Short axis (*C*) and 4-chamber (*D*) post contrast images show transmural LGE (*arrows, C, D*) in the lateral and inferior walls consistent with acute myocarditis with a differential diagnosis of chronic infarct, subsequently proven to be secondary to Chagas cardiomyopathy based on serology.

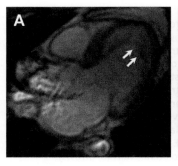
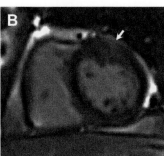

Fig. 7. Left ventricular noncompaction. Three chamber view SSFP image (A) shows prominent and deep intertrabecular recesses with greater than 2.3 ratio of noncompacted to compacted myocardium, particularly of the mid to apical segments (arrows, A). There is also patchy subepicardial LGE noted in the anterior wall on post contrast imaging (B, arrow).

Valvular Diseases

Arrhythmogenic mitral valve prolapse

- Similar to findings in echocardiography, mitral valve prolapse (MVP) is characterized by at least 2 mm excursion of the valve leaflet into the left atrium in LV outflow tract views (**Fig. 8**).
- Presence of LGE in the papillary muscles is suggestive of underlying fibrosis and has been associated with increased risk for complex VTs.[45]

Mitral annular disjunction

- On imaging, up to approximately 20% of patients with mitral annular disjunction (MAD) do not have associated MVP, and arrhythmias can be present irrespective of the presence or absence of MVP.[46]

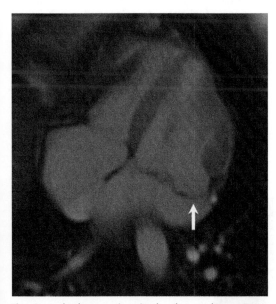

Fig. 8. Arrhythmogenic mitral valve prolapse. Four-chamber SSFP sequence shows ballooning and excursion of the mitral valve leaflet greater than 2 mm into the left atrium (arrow).

- On CMR, MAD is characterized by increased distance of the mitral annular roots to the ventricular myocardium, mainly affecting the posterior leaflet. The finding is best demonstrated in systole, in which there is a typical "curling motion" of the basal posterolateral wall, accentuating the disjunction. Although variable, MAD has been reported to affect up to two-thirds of the mitral annular circumference[46] (**Fig. 9**).

Other Cardiomyopathies

Infiltrative diseases
Anderson-Fabry

- Fabry disease (FD) is an X-linked lysosomal storage disorder caused by deficiency of the enzyme, α-galactosidase A. SCD is a common cause of mortality in FD. According to a recent meta-analysis, factors associated with SCD in FD included age, male sex, LVH, LGE, and NSVT.[47]
- Characteristically, LGE is seen in the basal inferolateral wall, often seen in a midwall or subepicardial distribution[48] (**Fig. 10**).

Danon disease

- Danon disease (DD) is a rare X-linked dominant lysosomal storage disease, caused by defects in the lysosome-associated membrane protein 2 gene and leads to accumulation of intracellular vacuoles. The age of onset varies from infancy to adulthood and classically presents as a triad of cardiomyopathy, skeletal myopathy, and intellectual disability in teenage boys. Cardiovascular sequelae may result in severe ventricular hypertrophy and heart failure and SCD at a young age.
- LGE often involves the subendocardium with occasional transmural extent, but not generally following a coronary territorial distribution.[49]
- Other LGE patterns described in DD include transmural involvement of the anterior and lateral walls with midmyocardial LGE in the septum.[50]

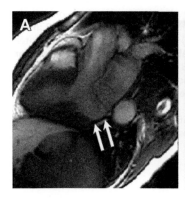
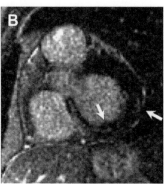

Fig. 9. Mitral annular disjunction. Three – chamber (*A*) SSFP image showing increased distance of the mitral annular root to the ventricular myocardium (*A, arrows*) involving the posterior leaflet. There is associated mitral valve prolapse with greater than 2 mm excursion of the mitral valve leaflets in the left atrium. Delayed post contrast images show LGE along the basal inferior and inferolateral walls (*B, arrows*).

Iron overload

- Cardiac siderosis, or myocardial iron overload, is a rare condition that may be associated with thalassemia or hemochromatosis. SCD may be a manifestation, if left untreated, from progression of heart failure.[51]
- T_2^* relaxation time is well poised to determine iron deposition, as it linearly falls with increasing iron overload.[52] Severe reduction of T_2^* relaxation time of less than 10 ms is associated with poor prognosis, associated with increased risk for VT despite normal LVEF and diastolic function, and requires initiation of iron chelation therapy. T_2^* relaxation time less than 20 ms is a proposed threshold to diagnose cardiac siderosis.[53]
- T2* imaging with 1.5-T has been validated, and is the current gold standard for noninvasive diagnosis of cardiac siderosis. Current studies also are in progress to demonstrate validity on 3-T machines.[54]

Athletes

- Athlete's heart refers to the structural and functional cardiac adaptation changes that occur with long-term exercise. Cardiomyopathy and arrhythmias often predispose to death in athletes, thus emphasizing the role of CMR in improving diagnosis.

- LGE/fibrosis has been associated with exercise-induced hypertension and race distances, particularly among triathletes.[55] Another study demonstrated that 14% of male athletes, but no controls, had LGE, half of whom had a pattern consistent with previous MI.[56] Similarly, another study among lifelong veteran male endurance athletes with age-matched controls demonstrated LGE in a pattern consistent with myocardial fibrosis, suggestive of previous acute myocarditis, in 50% of the veteran athletes[57] (**Fig. 11**).

Duchenne and Becker muscular dystrophies

- Duchenne muscular dystrophy (DMD) and Becker muscular dystrophy (BMD) are characterized by progressive wasting and weakness of skeletal muscles and are X-linked disorders caused by mutations in the dystrophin gene.
- Cardiac complications remain an important prognostic marker in DMD and BMD and is seen in about 70% of patients with BMD by the fourth decade. The most common manifestation in both is DCM.[58]
- Cardiomyopathy in DMD is rarely a diagnostic dilemma. The role of CMR in these patients is early detection and surveillance. Consensus guidelines recommend baseline

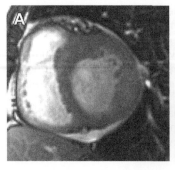
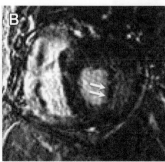

Fig. 10. Anderson Fabry Disease: Myocardial involvement of Fabry disease can present as circumferential left ventricular hypertrophy (*A*). LGE can vary, but characteristically involve the basal inferior and lateral wall (*B, arrow*).

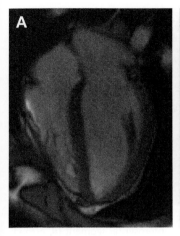
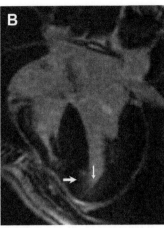

Fig. 11. Athlete's heart. CMR of a 20-year-old female, marathon runner shows normal circumferential left ventricular wall thickness (A) with subendocardial LGE involving the apical segments and apex (B, arrows). The biventricular function (not shown) was preserved.

assessment of cardiac function at the time of diagnosis, including noninvasive cardiac imaging using echocardiography or CMR.[59]

- Echocardiogram may be preferred in younger children who may otherwise require sedation for CMR, but CMR is recommended in older children.
- The cardiomyopathy associated with DMD is characterized by extensive fibrosis of the posterobasal wall (Fig. 12).
- As the disease progresses, fibrosis may extend to the lateral free wall.
- Mitral regurgitation may also occur secondary to posterior papillary muscle involvement.
- BMD cardiomyopathy is often associated with extensive midmyocardial LGE—mostly involving the septum and inferolateral segments of the LV—although reports of subendocardial LGE patterns due to underlying MIs, have also been reported.[60,61]

Friedrich ataxia

- Friedrich ataxia is an autosomal recessive disorder with significant neurologic and myocardial involvement. Cardiomyopathy is common

and characterized by LV hypertrophy with subsequent SCD arising from arrhythmias or congestive heart failure.[62]

- Typically, LGE demonstrates mild midmyocardial fibrosis of the interventricular septum, particularly in proximity to the inferior RV insertion point.[63]

Transplant cardiomyopathy

- Acute cellular allograft rejection remains a leading cause of early mortality among cardiac transplant patients, despite advances in antirejection therapy. Beyond the first year, transplant CAD is a common cause of death, following malignancy.
- Steen and colleagues[64] demonstrated 50% of patients to have a nonischemic pattern of LGE, 30% of whom, with unobstructed coronaries, had a typical infarction pattern associated with worse LV function and higher BNP values (Fig. 13).

Arrhythmogenic right ventricular dysplasia

- Historically, the diagnosis of arrhythmogenic right ventricular cardiomyopathy/dysplasia

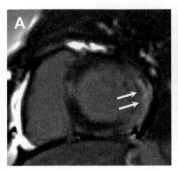
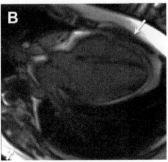

Fig. 12. Duchenne muscular dystrophy-related cardiomyopathy. Short-axis (A) and 4-chamber (B) late postcontrast images show extensive near transmural LGE involving the basal lateral wall and patchy midwall LGE in basal-to-mid ventricular septum. Note the atrophy of the thoracic musculature (B, arrows) in this patient with known Duchenne muscular dystrophy.

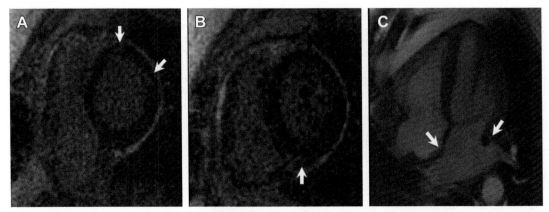

Fig. 13. Cardiac transplant rejection. CMR of a patient 2-years post orthotopic transplant shows small foci of LGE in the basal-to-mid anterior and anterolateral segments (*A, B*) and in the mid inferoseptal segment (*B, arrow*). Note the characteristic post-surgical "waisting" of the left atrium resulting from the anastomosis of the transplanted heart into the recipient's residual left atrium (*C, arrows*).

(ARVC/D) by MR imaging relied on assessment for RV wall thinning, wall motion abnormalities, and fibro-fatty infiltration of the myocardium, which can be relatively subjective and has been found to be unreliable and prone to misdiagnosis[65,66] **(Fig. 14)**

- In the most recent iteration of the CMR criteria for the diagnosis of ARVC/D, diagnosis requires the presence of "regional RV akinesia or dyskinesia or dyssynchronous RV contraction" and either:
  1. an increased RV end diastolic volume index ($\geq$100 mL/m^2 in men or 110 mL/m^2 in women) or
  2. a reduced RV ejection fraction ($\leq$40%).[67]

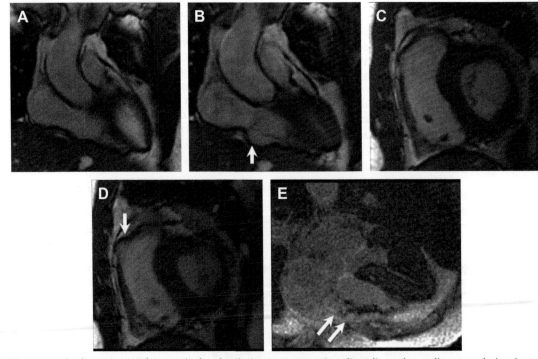

Fig. 14. Arrhythmogenic right ventricular dysplasia. Representative diastolic and systolic coronal cine images (*A, B, respectively*) show regional dyskinesia at the base of the right ventricle inferiorly during systole (*B, arrow*). Short axis diastolic (*C*) and systolic images (*D*) show a small focal aneurysm at the level of the right ventricular outflow tract (*D, arrow*) in the same patient. Although not a required criterion for the diagnosis of ARVD, post-contrast 4-chamber sequence shows LGE along the same distribution as the dyskinetic RV segments (*E*). CMR also demonstrated decreased RV function (not shown).

Uhl anomaly

- Uhl anomaly is defined by congenital absence of the RV myocardium and is a differential diagnosis of ARVC in young children with severely dilated RV volumes, presenting with ventricular arrhythmia.
- LGE on CMR in such cases may be limited to enhancement only of the RV, indicating a primary RV lesion.[68]

Naxos disease

- Naxos disease is an autosomal recessive disorder associated with ARVD and a cutaneous manifestation of palmo-plantar keratoderma and is associated with mutation of the desmoplakin gene.
- A variant seen in Ecuador and India is associated with predominantly LV involvement or Carvajal syndrome.[69]
- SSFP imaging on CMR often presents as RV dilatation. T1-weighted spin-echo images may demonstrate aneurysmal RV free wall without necessarily involving fibro-fatty replacement of the myocardium.
- LGE may demonstrate transmural enhancement of the RV wall, due to underlying fibrosis, usually extending from the subepicardial layers toward the endocardium.[70]

Systemic Diseases, and Autoimmune and Immune-Mediated Diseases

Thyrotoxicosis

- Thyrotoxicosis can often present with arrhythmias—more commonly atrial fibrillation, sinus tachycardia, and atrial flutter. However, malignant ventricular arrhythmias are an extremely unusual but important manifestation of this entity.
- Kobayashi and colleagues[71] demonstrated the usefulness of CMR in a patient with thyrotoxicosis who presented with VF, as the LGE pattern in the posteroseptal wall was suggestive of acute myocardial damage, distinguishing it from an ischemic pattern, and determining a cause other than vasospasm or coronary occlusion in that case.

Catastrophic antiphospholipid syndrome

- Catastrophic antiphospholipid syndrome is a rare subset of antiphospholipid antibody syndrome characterized by clotting in multiple vascular beds over a short time frame, leading to multiorgan failure and a high mortality rate—typically involving ≥3 organ systems with manifestations in less than 1 week.[72]

- Cardiac MR imaging may demonstrate a diffuse necrotic process with generalized myocardial involvement. However, differentiation between myocarditis and a diffuse microvascular ischemic process becomes more difficult. Another differential diagnosis for this is a diffuse vasculitis process.[73] However, CMR may prove useful in assessment of cardiac thrombi as well, using delayed enhancement CMR tissue characterization.[74]

Systemic lupus erythematosus

- SCD in patients with systemic lupus erythematosus (SLE) is most commonly due to CAD or myocarditis.[75]
- Varma and colleagues[76] demonstrated a novel method of postcontrast high-resolution T1-W inversion recovery pulse sequence in SLE patients to evaluate the pattern and burden of coronary wall contrast enhancement. Those with SLE had a diffuse pattern of coronary wall contrast enhancement, compared with traditional CAD, suggesting the mechanism of diffuse and not focal coronary inflammation in these subjects.
- Lupus myocarditis may also be detected on CMR.[77] Often those with SLE have a small amount of LGE, primarily found in the interventricular septum.[78] There may be an incremental role of quantifying the burden of myocarditis on CMR to guide therapy[79] (**Fig. 15**).

Systemic sclerosis

- Although the most common arrhythmias seen with systemic sclerosis (SSc) are PVCs, SCD

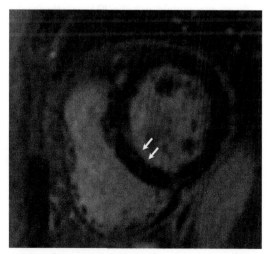

Fig. 15. Lupus myocarditis. Small punctate foci of LGE in the interventricular septum are a distinct finding in lupus myocarditis (*arrows*).

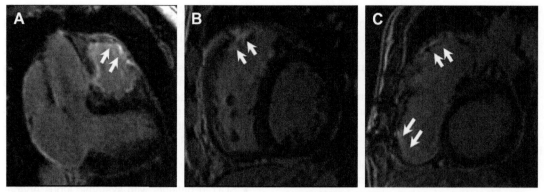

Fig. 16. Post tetralogy of Fallot (TOF) repair. Post contrast images show subendocardial of the right ventricle (RV), including of the trabeculation and moderator band and more patchy late gadolinium enhancement (LGE) at the base and at the level of the RV outflow tract (*arrows, A*). LGE involving the right ventricle particularly of outflow tract is commonly seen in patients who had undergone TOF repair (*arrow, B*). Extent of LGE can increase over time (*arrows, C*).

has been reported in 5% to 21% or unselected patients with SSc. SCD is more common in patients with skeletal and myocardial involvement.[75]

- Hachulla and colleagues[80] demonstrated contrast enhancement in 21% of their 52 study subjects with patterns ranging from linear to nodular. Most patients had midwall LGE, followed more rarely by a subendocardial or a subepicardial distribution. The main segments involved were midanterior, midanteroseptal, and midinferoseptal, and there was no correlation with coronary artery territorial distribution.

Rheumatoid arthritis

- The most common cause of SCD in patients with rheumatoid arthritis (RA) is atherosclerotic CAD, which may have sequelae of acute coronary syndrome and VT.[75] However, patients with RA are twice as likely to experience SCD, even after adjusting for a history of MI and this is thought to be due to systemic inflammation and autonomic dysfunction.[81]

Congenital Heart Diseases

Tetralogy of Fallot

- Congenital heart diseases are often associated with ventricular arrhythmias, particularly in individuals under 30 years of age.[82] Factors that have been associated with VT prediction in this cohort include prolonged QRS duration, decreased exercise capacity as well as ventricular fibrosis, as determined by LGE on CMR.[83]

- Tetralogy of Fallot (TOF) repair is associated with development of downstream pulmonary regurgitation and subsequently RV dilatation and subsequently, VT.[84]

- LV, RV, and RV outflow tract dysfunction, as determined by CMR, are predictors of major adverse clinical events.[85] The presence of LGE near the infundibular patch and RV anterior wall prove in agreement with low voltage areas, as determined by electroanatomical mapping, after TOF repair. These areas represent fibrofatty replacement due to infundibulotomy and ventriculotomy. The heterogeneous coexistence of scarred areas among normal myocardium predisposes to VT formation as a result of electrical re-entry[86] (**Fig. 16**).

SUMMARY

Cardiac MR imaging offers the ability to characterize the substrate for arrhythmia in the myocardium, chiefly by depicting myocardial fibrosis, but also by morphologic features such as thickening, dysplasia, and edema. Fibrosis often results in tissue heterogeneity resulting in re-entry circuits, which predispose to malignant ventricular arrhythmias and SCD. CMR plays a vital role in distinguishing ischemic from nonischemic causes of fibrosis, and can provide valuable information to differentiate among various causes of nonischemic insults. Once the diagnosis is established, CMR also offers the ability to quantify disease features such as scar burden, which can facilitate the management of patients presenting with malignant ventricular arrhythmias of ischemic and nonischemic causes.

REFERENCES

1. Hynes BJ, Luck JC, Wolbrette DL, et al. Arrhythmias in patients with heart failure. Curr Treat Options Cardiovasc Med 2002;4(6):467–85.

2. Lin CY, Chang SL, Lin YJ, et al. Long-term outcome of multiform premature ventricular complexes in structurally normal heart. Int J Cardiol 2015;180:80–5.

3. Ruberman W, Weinblatt E, Goldberg JD, et al. Ventricular premature beats and mortality after myocardial infarction. N Engl J Med 1977;297(14):750–7.

4. Wu TJ, Ong JJ, Hwang C, et al. Characteristics of wave fronts during ventricular fibrillation in human hearts with dilated cardiomyopathy: role of increased fibrosis in the generation of reentry. J Am Coll Cardiol 1998;32(1):187–96.

5. Moon JC, Reed E, Sheppard MN, et al. The histologic basis of late gadolinium enhancement cardiovascular magnetic resonance in hypertrophic cardiomyopathy. J Am Coll Cardiol 2004;43(12):2260–4.

6. Wagner A, Mahrholdt H, Holly TA, et al. Contrast-enhanced MRI and routine single photon emission computed tomography (SPECT) perfusion imaging for detection of subendocardial myocardial infarcts: an imaging study. Lancet 2003;361(9355):374–9.

7. Kim RJ, Fieno DS, Parrish TB, et al. Relationship of MRI delayed contrast enhancement to irreversible injury, infarct age, and contractile function. Circulation 1999;100(19):1992–2002.

8. Parsai C, O'Hanlon R, Prasad SK, et al. Diagnostic and prognostic value of cardiovascular magnetic resonance in non-ischaemic cardiomyopathies. J Cardiovasc Magn Reson 2012;14:54.

9. Gardner BI, Bingham SE, Allen MR, et al. Cardiac magnetic resonance versus transthoracic echocardiography for the assessment of cardiac volumes and regional function after myocardial infarction: an intrasubject comparison using simultaneous intrasubject recordings. Cardiovasc Ultrasound 2009;7:38.

10. Gouda S, Abdelwahab A, Salem M, et al. Scar characteristics for prediction of ventricular arrhythmia in ischemic cardiomyopathy. Pacing Clin Electrophysiol 2015;38(3):311–8.

11. Pontone G, Guaricci AI, Andreini D, et al. Prognostic benefit of cardiac magnetic resonance over transthoracic echocardiography for the assessment of ischemic and nonischemic dilated cardiomyopathy patients referred for the evaluation of primary prevention implantable cardioverter-defibrillator therapy. Circ Cardiovasc Imaging 2016;9(10).

12. Satoh H, Sano M, Suwa K, et al. Distribution of late gadolinium enhancement in various types of cardiomyopathies: significance in differential diagnosis, clinical features and prognosis. World J Cardiol 2014;6(7):585–601.

13. Schelbert EB, Cao JJ, Sigurdsson S, et al. Prevalence and prognosis of unrecognized myocardial infarction determined by cardiac magnetic resonance in older adults. JAMA 2012;308(9):890–6.

14. Disertori M, Gulizia MM, Casolo G, et al. Improving the appropriateness of sudden arrhythmic death primary prevention by implantable cardioverter-defibrillator therapy in patients with low left ventricular ejection fraction. Point of view. J Cardiovasc Med (Hagerstown) 2016;17(4):245–55.

15. Abbas A, Matthews GH, Brown IW, et al. Cardiac MR assessment of microvascular obstruction. Br J Radiol 2015;88(1047):20140470.

16. Kwong RY, Chan AK, Brown KA, et al. Impact of unrecognized myocardial scar detected by cardiac magnetic resonance imaging on event-free survival in patients presenting with signs or symptoms of coronary artery disease. Circulation 2006;113(23):2733–43.

17. Klem I, Weinsaft JW, Bahnson TD, et al. Assessment of myocardial scarring improves risk stratification in patients evaluated for cardiac defibrillator implantation. J Am Coll Cardiol 2012;60(5):408–20.

18. Assomull RG, Prasad SK, Lyne J, et al. Cardiovascular magnetic resonance, fibrosis, and prognosis in dilated cardiomyopathy. J Am Coll Cardiol 2006;48(10):1977–85.

19. Aljaroudi WA, Flamm SD, Saliba W, et al. Role of CMR imaging in risk stratification for sudden cardiac death. JACC Cardiovasc Imaging 2013;6(3):392–406.

20. Maron MS, Maron BJ. Clinical impact of contemporary cardiovascular magnetic resonance imaging in hypertrophic cardiomyopathy. Circulation 2015;132(4):292–8.

21. Gersh BJ, Maron BJ, Bonow RO, et al. 2011 ACCF/AHA guideline for the diagnosis and treatment of hypertrophic cardiomyopathy: a report of the American College of Cardiology Foundation/American Heart Association Task Force on Practice Guidelines. Circulation 2011;124(24):e783–831.

22. Maron BJ, Rowin EJ, Casey SA, et al. Hypertrophic cardiomyopathy in adulthood associated with low cardiovascular mortality with contemporary management strategies. J Am Coll Cardiol 2015;65(18):1915–28.

23. Maron MS, Appelbaum E, Harrigan CJ, et al. Clinical profile and significance of delayed enhancement in hypertrophic cardiomyopathy. Circ Heart Fail 2008;1(3):184–91.

24. Harrigan CJ, Peters DC, Gibson CM, et al. Hypertrophic cardiomyopathy: quantification of late gadolinium enhancement with contrast-enhanced

cardiovascular MR imaging. Radiology 2011;258(1): 128–33.

25. Hunninghake GW, Costabel U, Ando M, et al. ATS/ERS/WASOG statement on sarcoidosis. American Thoracic Society/European Respiratory Society/World Association of Sarcoidosis and other Granulomatous Disorders. Sarcoidosis Vasc Diffuse Lung Dis 1999;16(2):149–73.

26. Longcope WT, Freiman DG. A study of sarcoidosis; based on a combined investigation of 160 cases including 30 autopsies from The Johns Hopkins Hospital and Massachusetts General Hospital. Medicine (Baltimore) 1952;31(1):1–132.

27. Perry A, Vuitch F. Causes of death in patients with sarcoidosis. A morphologic study of 38 autopsies with clinicopathologic correlations. Arch Pathol Lab Med 1995;119(2):167–72.

28. Birnie DH, Sauer WH, Bogun F, et al. HRS expert consensus statement on the diagnosis and management of arrhythmias associated with cardiac sarcoidosis. Heart Rhythm 2014;11(7):1305–23.

29. Birnie DH, Nery PB, Ha AC, et al. Cardiac sarcoidosis. J Am Coll Cardiol 2016;68(4):411–21.

30. Ichinose A, Otani H, Oikawa M, et al. MRI of cardiac sarcoidosis: basal and subepicardial localization of myocardial lesions and their effect on left ventricular function. AJR Am J Roentgenol 2008;191(3):862–9.

31. Patel MR, Cawley PJ, Heitner JF, et al. Detection of myocardial damage in patients with sarcoidosis. Circulation 2009;120(20):1969–77.

32. Vita T, Okada DR, Veillet-Chowdhury M, et al. Complementary value of cardiac magnetic resonance imaging and positron emission tomography/computed tomography in the assessment of cardiac sarcoidosis. Circ Cardiovasc Imaging 2018;11(1):e007030.

33. Muser D, Santangeli P, Liang JJ, et al. Characterization of the electroanatomic substrate in cardiac sarcoidosis: correlation with imaging findings of scar and inflammation. JACC Clin Electrophysiol 2018;4(3):291–303.

34. Ferreira VM, Schulz-Menger J, Holmvang G, et al. Cardiovascular magnetic resonance in nonischemic myocardial inflammation: expert recommendations. J Am Coll Cardiol 2018;72(24):3158–76.

35. Giri S, Chung YC, Merchant A, et al. T2 quantification for improved detection of myocardial edema. J Cardiovasc Magn Reson 2009;11:56.

36. Spieker M, Haberkorn S, Gastl M, et al. Abnormal T2 mapping cardiovascular magnetic resonance correlates with adverse clinical outcome in patients with suspected acute myocarditis. J Cardiovasc Magn Reson 2017;19(1):38.

37. Haaf P, Garg P, Messroghli DR, et al. Cardiac T1 mapping and extracellular volume (ECV) in clinical practice: a comprehensive review. J Cardiovasc Magn Reson 2016;18(1):89.

38. Senra T, Ianni BM, Costa ACP, et al. Long-term prognostic value of myocardial fibrosis in patients with Chagas cardiomyopathy. J Am Coll Cardiol 2018;72(21):2577–87.

39. Volpe GJ, Moreira HT, Trad HS, et al. Left ventricular scar and prognosis in chronic Chagas cardiomyopathy. J Am Coll Cardiol 2018;72(21):2567–76.

40. Grothoff M, Pachowsky M, Hoffmann J, et al. Value of cardiovascular MR in diagnosing left ventricular non-compaction cardiomyopathy and in discriminating between other cardiomyopathies. Eur Radiol 2012;22(12):2699–709.

41. Wan J, Zhao S, Cheng H, et al. Varied distributions of late gadolinium enhancement found among patients meeting cardiovascular magnetic resonance criteria for isolated left ventricular non-compaction. J Cardiovasc Magn Reson 2013;15:20.

42. Nucifora G, Aquaro GD, Pingitore A, et al. Myocardial fibrosis in isolated left ventricular non-compaction and its relation to disease severity. Eur J Heart Fail 2011;13(2):170–6.

43. Jassal DS, Nomura CH, Neilan TG, et al. Delayed enhancement cardiac MR imaging in noncompaction of left ventricular myocardium. J Cardiovasc Magn Reson 2006;8(3):489–91.

44. Andreini D, Pontone G, Bogaert J, et al. Long-term prognostic value of cardiac magnetic resonance in left ventricle noncompaction: a prospective multicenter study. J Am Coll Cardiol 2016;68(20):2166–81.

45. Han Y, Peters DC, Salton CJ, et al. Cardiovascular magnetic resonance characterization of mitral valve prolapse. JACC Cardiovasc Imaging 2008;1(3):294–303.

46. Dejgaard LA, Skjolsvik ET, Lie OH, et al. The mitral annulus disjunction arrhythmic syndrome. J Am Coll Cardiol 2018;72(14):1600–9.

47. Baig S, Edward NC, Kotecha D, et al. Ventricular arrhythmia and sudden cardiac death in Fabry disease: a systematic review of risk factors in clinical practice. Europace 2018;20(FI2):f153–61.

48. Moon JC, Sachdev B, Elkington AG, et al. Gadolinium enhanced cardiovascular magnetic resonance in Anderson-Fabry disease. Evidence for a disease specific abnormality of the myocardial interstitium. Eur Heart J 2003;24(23):2151–5.

49. Piotrowska-Kownacka D, Kownacki L, Kuch M, et al. Cardiovascular magnetic resonance findings in a case of Danon disease. J Cardiovasc Magn Reson 2009;11:12.

50. Rowin EJ, Maron MS. The role of cardiac MRI in the diagnosis and risk stratification of hypertrophic cardiomyopathy. Arrhythm Electrophysiol Rev 2016;5(3):197–202.

51. Klintschar M, Stiller D. Sudden cardiac death in hereditary hemochromatosis: an underestimated cause of death? Int J Legal Med 2004;118(3):174–7.

52. Anderson LJ, Holden S, Davis B, et al. Cardiovascular T2-star (T2*) magnetic resonance for the early diagnosis of myocardial iron overload. Eur Heart J 2001;22(23):2171–9.

53. Kirk P, Roughton M, Porter JB, et al. Cardiac T2* magnetic resonance for prediction of cardiac complications in thalassemia major. Circulation 2009; 120(20):1961–8.

54. Krittayaphong R, Zhang S, Saiviroonporn P, et al. Assessment of cardiac iron overload in thalassemia with MRI on 3.0-T: high-field T1, T2, and T2* quantitative parametric mapping in comparison to T2* on 1.5-T. JACC Cardiovasc Imaging 2019;12(4):752–4.

55. Tahir E, Starekova J, Muellerleile K, et al. Myocardial fibrosis in competitive triathletes detected by contrast-enhanced CMR correlates with exercise-induced hypertension and competition history. JACC Cardiovasc Imaging 2018;11(9):1260–70.

56. Merghani A, Maestrini V, Rosmini S, et al. Prevalence of subclinical coronary artery disease in masters endurance athletes with a low atherosclerotic risk profile. Circulation 2017;136(2):126–37.

57. Wilson M, O'Hanlon R, Prasad S, et al. Diverse patterns of myocardial fibrosis in lifelong, veteran endurance athletes. J Appl Physiol (1985) 2011; 110(6):1622–6.

58. Aikawa T, Takeda A, Oyama-Manabe N, et al. Progressive left ventricular dysfunction and myocardial fibrosis in Duchenne and Becker muscular dystrophy: a longitudinal cardiovascular magnetic resonance study. Pediatr Cardiol 2019;40(2): 384–92.

59. Birnkrant DJ, Bushby K, Bann CM, et al. Diagnosis and management of Duchenne muscular dystrophy, part 2: respiratory, cardiac, bone health, and orthopaedic management. Lancet Neurol 2018;17(4): 347–61.

60. Petrie CJ, Mark PB, Dargie HJ. Cardiomyopathy in Becker muscular dystrophy – does regional fibrosis mimic infarction? J Cardiovasc Magn Reson 2005; 7(5):823–5.

61. Mavrogeni S, Markousis-Mavrogenis G, Papavasiliou A, et al. Cardiac involvement in Duchenne and Becker muscular dystrophy. World J Cardiol 2015;7(7):410–4.

62. Pandolfo M. Friedreich ataxia. Arch Neurol 2008; 65(10):1296–303.

63. Raman SV, Phatak K, Hoyle JC, et al. Impaired myocardial perfusion reserve and fibrosis in Friedreich ataxia: a mitochondrial cardiomyopathy with metabolic syndrome. Eur Heart J 2011;32(5):561–7.

64. Steen H, Merten C, Refle S, et al. Prevalence of different gadolinium enhancement patterns in patients after heart transplantation. J Am Coll Cardiol 2008;52(14):1160–7.

65. Bluemke DA, Krupinski EA, Ovitt T, et al. MR Imaging of arrhythmogenic right ventricular cardiomyopathy: morphologic findings and interobserver reliability. Cardiology 2003;99(3):153–62.

66. Bomma C, Rutberg J, Tandri H, et al. Misdiagnosis of arrhythmogenic right ventricular dysplasia/cardiomyopathy. J Cardiovasc Electrophysiol 2004;15(3): 300–6.

67. Marcus FI, McKenna WJ, Sherrill D, et al. Diagnosis of arrhythmogenic right ventricular cardiomyopathy/dysplasia: proposed modification of the task force criteria. Circulation 2010;121(13):1533–41.

68. Rizk J, Shehu N, Wolf C, et al. A case of Uhl's anomaly presenting with ventricular tachycardia. Eur Heart J Cardiovasc Imaging 2018;19(11):1312.

69. Noain JA, Golet AC, Calzada JN, et al. Living after sudden death: a case report of Naxos disease. Indian J Crit Care Med 2012;16(4):207–9.

70. Mavrogeni S, Bratis K, Protonotarios N, et al. Cardiac magnetic resonance can early assess the presence and severity of heart involvement in Naxos disease. Int J Cardiol 2012;154(1):e19–20.

71. Kobayashi H, Haketa A, Abe M, et al. Unusual manifestation of Graves' disease: ventricular fibrillation. Eur Thyroid J 2015;4(3):207–12.

72. Sciascia S, Lopez-Pedrera C, Roccatello D, et al. Catastrophic antiphospholipid syndrome (CAPS). Best Pract Res Clin Rheumatol 2012;26(4):535–41.

73. Hucker WJ, Chatzizisis YS, Steigner ML, et al. Myocardial catastrophe: a case of sudden, severe myocardial dysfunction. Circulation 2014;130(10): 854–62.

74. Goyal P, Weinsaft JW. Cardiovascular magnetic resonance imaging for assessment of cardiac thrombus. Methodist Debakey Cardiovasc J 2013; 9(3):132–6.

75. Seferovic PM, Ristic AD, Maksimovic R, et al. Cardiac arrhythmias and conduction disturbances in autoimmune rheumatic diseases. Rheumatology (Oxford) 2006;45(Suppl 4):iv39–42.

76. Varma N, Hinojar R, D'Cruz D, et al. Coronary vessel wall contrast enhancement imaging as a potential direct marker of coronary involvement: integration of findings from CAD and SLE patients. JACC Cardiovasc Imaging 2014;7(8):762–70.

77. Mavrogeni S, Karabela G, Stavropoulos E, et al. Heart failure imaging patterns in systemic lupus erythematosus. Evaluation using cardiovascular magnetic resonance. Int J Cardiol 2014;176(2):559–61.

78. Prochaska MT, Bergl PA, Patel AR, et al. Atrioventricular heart block and syncope coincident with diagnosis of systemic lupus erythematosus. Can J Cardiol 2013;29(10):1330.e5–7.

79. Saremi F, Ashikyan O, Saggar R, et al. Utility of cardiac MRI for diagnosis and post-treatment follow-up of lupus myocarditis. Int J Cardiovasc Imaging 2007;23(3):347–52.

80. Hachulla AL, Launay D, Gaxotte V, et al. Cardiac magnetic resonance imaging in systemic sclerosis:

a cross-sectional observational study of 52 patients. Ann Rheum Dis 2009;68(12):1878–84.

81. Lazzerini PE, Capecchi PL, Acampa M, et al. Arrhythmic risk in rheumatoid arthritis: the driving role of systemic inflammation. Autoimmun Rev 2014;13(9):936–44.

82. European Heart Rhythm A, Heart Rhythm S, Zipes DP, et al. ACC/AHA/ESC 2006 guidelines for management of patients with ventricular arrhythmias and the prevention of sudden cardiac death: a report of the American College of Cardiology/American Heart Association Task Force and the European Society of Cardiology Committee for practice guidelines (writing committee to develop guidelines for management of patients with ventricular arrhythmias and the prevention of sudden cardiac death). J Am Coll Cardiol 2006;48(5):e247–346.

83. Tsai SF, Chan DP, Ro PS, et al. Rate of inducible ventricular arrhythmia in adults with congenital heart disease. Am J Cardiol 2010; 106(5):730–6.

84. Van Aerschot I, Iserin L. Follow-up of tetralogy of Fallot after repair. Presse Med 2011;40(7–8):740–7 [in French].

85. Therrien J, Siu SC, Harris L, et al. Impact of pulmonary valve replacement on arrhythmia propensity late after repair of tetralogy of Fallot. Circulation 2001;103(20):2489–94.

86. Babu-Narayan SV, Kilner PJ, Li W, et al. Ventricular fibrosis suggested by cardiovascular magnetic resonance in adults with repaired tetralogy of Fallot and its relationship to adverse markers of clinical outcome. Circulation 2006;113(3): 405–13.

State-of-the-Art Quantitative Assessment of Myocardial Ischemia by Stress Perfusion Cardiac Magnetic Resonance

Thiago Quinaglia, MD, PhD[a], Michael Jerosch-Herold, PhD[b],
Otávio R. Coelho-Filho, MD, PhD, MPH[a,c],*

KEYWORDS

- Myocardial ischemia • Cardiac magnetic resonance and stress perfusion
- Cardiovascular magnetic resonance • Myocardial perfusion • Quantitative ischemia assessment

KEY POINTS

- Cardiac magnetic resonance (CMR) provides excellent temporal and spatial resolution without the limitations associated with unfavorable echocardiographic windows, and low temporal and spatial resolution in nuclear medicine studies, nor does it involve ionizing radiation.
- Myocardial perfusion by CMR can be integrated with a spatially registered interrogation of regional function (wall thickening, segmental contractility, and myocardial deformation image), edema, fibrosis, and viability.
- These simultaneous faculties are not present in other imaging modalities.

INTRODUCTION

Cardiac magnetic resonance (CMR) has arisen as a method of choice for myocardial ischemia assessment. CMR is endowed with a series of advantageous characteristics, which are only in part present with other modalities. Although arguably still not the gold-standard method, stress perfusion CMR permits excellent spatial and temporal resolution, evaluation of contractile function (wall motility and thickening) and myocardial perfusion quantification, in addition to assessment of myocardial viability and scar with late gadolinium enhancement (LGE) technique.[1] Moreover, multicenter studies[2–5] have demonstrated outstanding sensitivity and specificity in the detection of significant coronary artery disease (CAD) in patients submitted to perfusion imaging during pharmacologic stress by CMR. A compilation of 26 studies,[6] comprising more than 11,000 patients, predicted sensitivity of 89% and specificity of 80% in the detection of CAD by the stress perfusion of CMR (**Fig. 1**).

Disclosures: The authors have nothing to disclose.
[a] Faculdade de Ciências Médicas, Universidade Estadual de Campinas, Rua Tessália Viera de Camargo, 126 - Cidade Universitária "Zeferino Vaz", Campinas, São Paulo 13083-887, Brazil; [b] Noninvasive Cardiovascular Imaging Program, Department of Radiology, Brigham and Women's Hospital, 75 Francis Street, Room L1-RA050, Mailbox #22, Boston, MA 02115, USA; [c] Department of Internal Medicine, Hospital das Clínicas, State University of Campinas, UNICAMP, Rua Vital Brasil, 251- Cidade Universitária "Zeferino Vaz", Campinas, São Paulo 13083-888, Brazil
* Corresponding author. Department of Internal Medicine, Hospital das Clínicas, State University of Campinas, UNICAMP, Rua Vital Brasil, 251- Cidade Universitária "Zeferino Vaz", Campinas, São Paulo 13083-888, Brazil.
E-mail addresses: orcfilho@unicamp.br; tavicocoelho@gmail.com

Magn Reson Imaging Clin N Am 27 (2019) 491–505
https://doi.org/10.1016/j.mric.2019.04.002
1064-9689/19/© 2019 Elsevier Inc. All rights reserved.

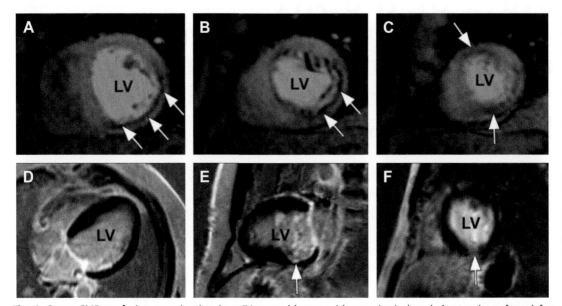

Fig. 1. Stress CMR perfusion examination in a 54-year-old man with exercise-induced chest pain, referred for ischemia assessment. (*A-C*) Stress first-pass perfusion images acquired during vasodilator pharmacologic stress, demonstrating a large subendocardial perfusion defect within the basal to mid-inferior and lateral LV walls as well as the apical anterior LV segment. (*D–F*) LGE images showing a small subendocardial myocardial infarction in the inferolateral wall (*arrows*). The stress perfusion first-pass defect was significantly larger than the areas with documented scar by LGE.

Compared with single photon emission computed tomography (SPECT),[5] multivendor studies demonstrated noninferior performance of stress perfusion CMR in the presence of at least one-vessel disease and a better performance in multivessel disease. More recently, the CE-MARC study reported superiority of CMR, even in patients with single-vessel coronary disease.[4,7] Compared with SPECT, PET offers a better spatial resolution (5–7 mm vs 12–15 mm of SPECT) and the promise not to misdiagnose microvascular or balanced multivessel disease. Also, PET provides absolute quantitative measures of radiotracer concentration, thus facilitating estimation of absolute myocardial perfusion in mL/min per g of myocardial tissue. However, radioisotopes have very a short half-life, requiring on-site production of tracers, which impedes more widespread use. Some other important limitations of nuclear perfusion imaging are the presence of attenuation artifacts, in the anterior wall for female patients with large breasts, and the inferior wall in male patients with large abdominal circumference, use of radiation, and relatively long examination duration.

In this scenario, CMR imaging could have growing importance because it has widespread availability, allows imaging with high temporal and spatial resolution, and does not involve ionizing radiation. However, some shortcomings still prevent CMR from reaching its full potential.

The most important of them is the lack of a dependable quantitative analysis because signal intensities on CMR images do not provide a direct measure of contrast concentration and require careful "calibration" of the contrast concentration estimation in the arterial input. Quantitative analyses are not routinely endorsed by current guidelines, despite their potential clinical utility, because of the lack of clinical studies demonstrating a positive difference in outcomes or even studies confirming a better accuracy compared with nonquantitative visual analysis.[8,9] In the present review, we aim to gather and appraise pivotal studies related to stress perfusion CMR and present the current state-of-the-art myocardial ischemia assessment by this promising method. The review has a special focus on quantitative analysis of ischemic myocardium.

NORMAL CORONARY FLOW DURING REST AND HYPEREMIA

The established physiologic rationale for stress perfusion imaging is based on the concept of coronary flow reserve.[10] The myocardium extracts virtually all oxygen delivered. Because of the high energy costs for the cardiac cycle, myocardial perfusion depends almost exclusively on coronary blood flow. Coronary flow reserve (**Fig. 2**) refers to the capacity of the coronary circulation to increase

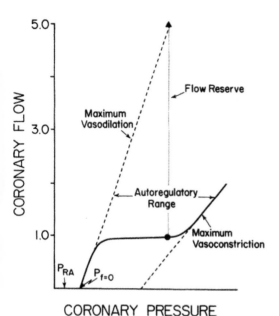

Fig. 2. Association of coronary flow with coronary arterial pressure in the LV. Normal relationship is seen in the solid line. At rest, coronary flow is conserved constant regardless of coronary pressure, between the limits of maximum coronary vasodilation and constriction (*dashed lines*). The solid circle represents basal conditions; the solid triangle represents flow at the same pressure during maximum vasodilation. Flow reserve is the ratio of flow during vasodilation to that measured before vasodilation, and in this example is 5.0. P_{RA}, right atrial pressure; $P_{f=0}$, back pressure opposing coronary flow. (*From* Klocke FJ. Measurements of coronary flow reserve: defining pathophysiology versus making decisions about patient care. Circulation. 1987;76(6):1183–1189. https://doi.org/10.1161/01.cir.76.6.1183; with permission).

the blood flow through the coronary tree until its microcirculation, when in maximum dilation. As for perfusion, it is expressed as the volume of blood flow (eg, in milliliters) through the microcirculation in a unit of myocardial mass (eg, gram), per unit of time (eg, minute). During CMR, coronary artery vasodilation is typically obtained with a pharmacologic vasodilator agent, such as adenosine or dipyridamole, and more recently with regadenoson,[11,12] an A2A adenosine receptor agonist with fewer side effects than adenosine. In healthy young adults, these drugs increase coronary flow up to 4 times and are particularly effective in minimizing resistance within distal coronary artery bed.

At rest, a coronary epicardial lesion will limit flow only when luminal narrowing reaches 85% or more, whereas with vasodilation this threshold is reduced to approximately 50%.[13,14] The response of coronary flow to vigorous exercise has the same magnitude as the increase observed during the

vasodilation with an adenosine receptor agonist agent.[15] Presuming that myocardial perfusion can be independently quantified at rest and during maximal vasodilatation, the perfusion reserve can be calculated as the flow rate during hyperemia (maximal vasodilatation) divided by the resting flow. (Sometimes the resting flow in the denominator is normalized by the rate-pressure product to achieve greater independence from the baseline cardiac workload, which can be elevated in hypertension and other pathologies.) In the healthy coronary circulation, the coronary flow reserve and myocardial perfusion reserve agree in magnitude, but the presence of a coronary epicardial obstruction can result in an epicardial reserve inferior to the myocardial perfusion reserve measured downstream of the lesion[16] due to the presence of coronary collaterals. The poststenosis vasodilatory response occurs at the prearteriolar level and depends on individual microvascular function, which, in turn, is determined by clinical factors, such as smoking status, diabetes, hypertension, and other conditions, known to impair microvascular function and induce endothelial dysfunction. Therefore, perfusion of the microcirculation may vary across individuals for a similar epicardial stenosis.

A compromised myocardial perfusion reserve is considered a useful substitute marker for ischemia, although the threshold below which myocardial perfusion reserve should fall to cause clinically relevant ischemia is not well defined. A coronary flow reserve of 2.5:1.0 has frequently been used as a cutoff point, as it results in a significant association with risk factors, presence of CAD, and with clinical outcomes after revascularization.[17] For CMR perfusion imaging with absolute myocardial blood flow (MBF) quantification a similar threshold may be appropriate.

DIAGNOSIS OF CORONARY ARTERY DISEASE
Myocardial Perfusion Imaging

Myocardial perfusion images are acquired for approximately 60 beats to cover a precontrast phase, the first pass of contrast in myocardium after injection, and recirculation of the contrast agent. Total time of acquisition is too long for a single breath-hold, although patients are usually asked to hold their breath for the initial phase of the study and resume breathing when necessary, but without having to take a deep breath, which would result in slice position misregistration. Breathing movement is sufficiently slow to not cause motion artifacts in individual images (acquisition time per image ~120–200 ms), but during postprocessing it is necessary to adjust for respiration-related cardiac motion. However, total correction for cardiac motion can probably only be solved with 3-dimensional (3D) acquisitions rather than 2D multislice imaging.

A substantial number of single-center[18–21] and multicenter[2,3] studies demonstrated favorable sensitivity and specificity of myocardial perfusion imaging with coronary vasodilation for the detection of CAD versus coronary angiography. Stress testing with adenosine yielded better sensitivity for diagnosis of CAD than dipyridamole (0.90, 95% confidence interval [CI]: 0.88–0.92 vs 0.86; 95% CI: 0.80–0.90; $P = .022$) and a trend toward a better specificity (0.81, 95% CI: 0.78–0.84 vs 0.77, 95% CI: 0.71–0.82, $P = .065$). In one multicenter study, Schwitter and colleagues[22] compared the diagnostic accuracy of myocardial perfusion stress by CMR with SPECT for the detection of significant CAD, defined as luminal narrowing $\geq$50% in at least 1 vessel. The investigators demonstrated noninferiority of myocardial perfusion stress CMR (area under the receiver operating characteristic curve [AUC], 0.86 + 0.06 vs 0.75 + 0.09; $P = .12$). Recent meta-analyses[6,23] confirmed this diagnostic accuracy.

The MR IMPACT II trial (n = 533) showed that CMR is a safe alternative to SPECT, revealing greater sensitivity (0.67 vs 0.59, $P = .024$), although lower specificity (0.61 vs 0.72, $P = .038$).[5] However, in another prospective study (n = 752), CE-MARC, Greenwood and colleagues[4] demonstrated greater sensitivity (86.5% vs 66.5%, $P<.0001$) and negative predictive value (90.5% vs 79.1%, $P<.0001$) of CMR compared with SPECT, whereas specificity (83.4% vs 82.6%, $P = .916$; respectively) and positive predictive value (77.2% vs 71.4%, $P = .061$, respectively) were similar. In addition, stress CMR was superior to SPECT flow limiting CAD across all CAD definitions (**Fig. 3**). Comparisons with invasive physiologic measures as fractional flow reserve (FFR) also yielded favorable results. Rieber and colleagues[24] demonstrated that the calculation of myocardial perfusion reserve index, with a cutoff value of 1.5:1.0 for a semiquantitative perfusion reserve index, allowed the detection of stenosis hemodynamically important, as determined by FFR less than 0.75.

MYOCARDIAL PERFUSION QUANTIFICATION
Semiquantitative Analysis

Semiquantitative techniques assess the signal intensity versus time curves across myocardial segments by determining simple curve properties, rather than estimating MBF.[9] Briefly, a segmentation model of 17 segments, as recommend by the American Heart Association,[25] divides the left ventricle (LV) in regions to be analyzed in parallel with wall motion and LGE. Myocardial segments are defined on short-axis views of the heart (and possibly 1 long-axis view for apical cap) by contouring the LV along the endocardial and epicardial borders, defining a reference point like the anterior LV–right ventricle junction, and subdividing the LV wall into 6 segments at the basal and mid-level, and 4 segments at the apical level. This form of segmentation of the LV allows tracking of the same portions of the LV wall, compensates for respiratory movements, and excludes epicardial fat and signal from the blood pool as potential sources of error. Images acquired during ectopic heartbeats are excluded. The rate of increase of the signal intensity during the first pass ("upslope" of signal-intensity curve) has been identified as useful parameter for a semiquantitative analyses and shown to yield good diagnostic accuracy.[3,20,21,26] Frequently evaluated parameters by postprocessing packages include maximal upslope of the myocardial signal intensity, AUC from start of contrast enhancement to first-pass peak in the blood pool,[9] and time to peak signal intensity (from start of contrast enhancement).

Estimating the spatial extent of ischemia provides important diagnostic and prognostic information. A recent prospective study with 1024 consecutive patients in referred to stress perfusion CMR suggests that simple quantification of the number of ischemic segments has a prognostic value and helps identify patients at risk.[27] Based on the 16-segment model (17-segment model excluding the apical cap), the investigators demonstrated that patients with $\geq$1.5 ischemic segments presented a worse prognosis, owing to more frequent cardiac death, nonfatal myocardial infarction, and myocardial revascularization within 90 days of the examination. The mean follow-up time of the study was 2.5 years. In the 17-segment model, ischemia in 2 or more segments corresponds to approximately a 12.0% ischemic burden mirroring nuclear medicine studies in which an ischemic load greater than 10.0% to 12.5% should be used to indicate coronary revascularization because myocardium would be at risk.

Full Quantification of Myocardial Perfusion

Fully automated quantitative analyses are still not established in clinical practice but have evolved and may help discriminate diagnosis in particular cases such as multivessel coronary disease, microvascular dysfunction, or suspicion of inadequate vasodilator response. Quantitative

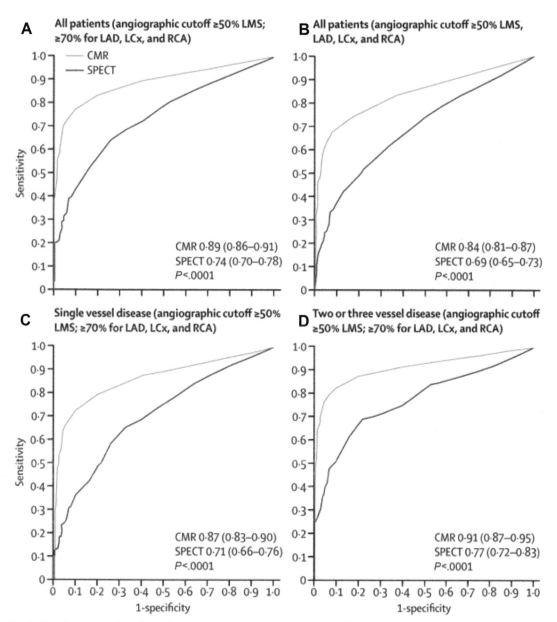

Fig. 3. Receiver operating characteristic curves comparing stress CMR (*blue line*) and SPECT (*pink line*) for detecting flow limiting CAD according to coronary heart disease definition (*A*) all patients with angiographic cutoff >/=50% for LMS or >/=70% for LAD, LCx and RCA; (*B*) all patients with angiographic cutoff>/=50% for LMS, LAD, LCx and RCA; (*C*) single vessel disease with angiographic cutoff >/=50% for LMS or >/=70% for LAD, LCx and RCA and (*D*) two or three vessel disease with angiographic cutoff >/=50% for LMS or >/=70% for LAD, LCx and RCA). LAD, left anterior descending; LCx, left circumflex; LMS, left main stenosis; RCA, right coronary artery. (*Reprinted with permission from* Elsevier [Greenwood JP, Maredia N, Younger JF, et al. Cardiovascular magnetic resonance and single-photo emission computed tomography for diagnosis of coronary heart disease (CE-MARC): a prospective trial. Lancet 2012;379(9814):453–60]).

CMR has been validated against microspheres in experimental models,[28] coronary sinus flow,[29] and PET in healthy volunteers.[30]

In patients undergoing coronary angiography, Morton and colleagues[31] applied a double bolus injection and Fermi deconvolution analysis to

fully quantitative stress perfusion by CMR and compare it with ^{13}N-ammonia PET, the current noninvasive reference standard. They demonstrated that myocardial perfusion reserve is highly correlated between the 2 methods (r = 0.75, P<.0001). When analyzing coronary territories with the lowest reserve scores, correlation remained significant (r = 0.79, P<.0001). However, absolute perfusion values, at rest and during stress, had only a modest association (r = 0.32, P<.002 and r = 0.37, P<.0001, respectively). These data may be explained by different properties of the tracers and model assumptions, but the relative stress/rest ratios are less affected by absolute disparities. The same study established cutoff values for MBF reserve that predicted significant coronary disease determined by angiography: ≤1.44 for PET and ≤1.45 for CMR (with 82% sensitivity and 87% specificity; and 82% sensitivity and 81% specificity, respectively). Different approaches have been proposed for MBF quantification, are frequently applied and appear to have similar diagnostic performance.[32] They are Fermi model, uptake model, 1-compartment model, model-independent deconvolution methods, and 2 model-independent methods.

Gadolinium Enhancement and Myocardial Blood Flow

These fully quantitative methods derive estimates of MBF from signal intensity versus time curves of myocardial contrast enhancement. Yet, signal intensity is only approximately proportional to gadolinium concentration in T1-weighted images and at higher concentrations this relation becomes nonlinear, giving rise to what is often referred to as signal saturation. Signal saturation in particular affects the signal intensity in the blood pool, where contrast concentrations are highest during the first pass compared with myocardium. Several options are available to avoid or minimize this problem: the contrast dose and delivery must be chosen to minimize saturation effects and doses are often lower than those applied in routine practice for visual interpretation of studies. A dual bolus of contrast with a dosage (or dilution) ratio of approximately 1:10 may help minimize saturation effects in the arterial input during the first pass of the lower-dosage bolus. The second larger bolus is used for measuring myocardial contrast enhancement, although it should be pointed out that saturation may still affect the vascular component of the signal in the myocardium, but there are no visual cues of saturation like in the case of the arterial input. For a quantitative analysis, the arterial input measured with the small bolus is scaled up to the dosage used for the measurement of the myocardial enhancement, and aligned with the start of blood pool enhancement from the second bolus. As can be surmised from the signal intensity curves measured with a dual-bolus technique, postprocessing requires selecting portions of signal-intensity curves for arterial input and myocardial enhancement, respectively, matching them up along the time axis, all requiring user input (**Fig. 4**).[28,33] A so-called dual-sequence approach may be an alternative to the dual bolus because it is based on the combined measurement of the blood pool input function and myocardial signals with different T1 weighting. For the arterial input images, one acquires low-resolution images within less than ~40 ms with a T1 weighting that is less sensitive to T1 changes but offers a wider linear range (for the relationship between signal intensity and R1 = 1/T1), followed by myocardial images with a stronger T1 weighting of the signal intensity, but smaller linear range. The dual-sequence approach avoids variation between bolus injections,[34] and ensures almost perfect temporal alignment for the signal intensity curves depicting contrast enhancement in the arterial input and myocardial segments.

Two approaches have been applied for the quantification of MBF from regional signal intensity curves: one is based on a tracer-kinetic model for the blood-tissue exchange (BTEX)[35,36] of contrast, representing the vascular and interstitial compartments as functional spaces between which contrast is exchanged via a (capillary) barrier, after contrast enters the tissue through its arterial input. This BTEX type of model was first applied for quantification of myocardial perfusion with an intravascular contrast agent by Kroll and colleagues[35] and later used also for studies with extravascular agents. It required careful adjustment of some fixed parameters of the model, as one can generally only leave blood flow and 1 volume parameter as variable fitting parameters to ensure reproducible results. (Alternatively, one can use an intravascular contrast agent, which allows simplification of the model.) A second approach for quantification is based on the central volume theorem of Meier and Zierler,[37] which states that the amplitude of the myocardial impulse response equals blood flow. It is illustrated in **Fig. 5**. Furthermore, the myocardial impulse response, when convolved with a measured arterial input, predicts the myocardial contrast enhancement. To be of practical value, this relationship between the myocardial impulse response and myocardial enhancement has to be inverted to estimate blood flow: the impulse response is estimated by deconvolving the measured myocardial contrast enhancement curve, with the measured arterial contrast enhancement curve. Deconvolution falls into a category of mathematical problems that are termed "ill-posed," as there is no mathematically unique solution, and one has to effectively apply constraints based on physiologic or empirical

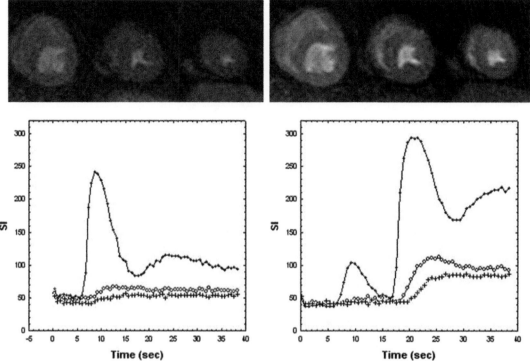

Fig. 4. Compared with single-bolus low-contrast injection (upper and lower left panels), high-contrast dual-bolus injection (upper and lower right panels), has less variability and better image quality. SI, signal intensity. (*From* Christian TF, Aletras AH, Arai AE. Estimation of absolute myocardial blood flow during first-pass MR perfusion imaging using a dual-bolus injection technique: Comparison to single-bolus injection method. J Magn Reson Imaging. 2008;27(6):1271–1277; with permission).

insights to recover a solution that represents a good "physiologic" approximation.[38] One approach is to constrain the impulse response to a certain class of shapes, based on observations from simulations with tracer-kinetic problems. A Fermi function has proven to be a reasonable approximation for the tissue impulse response,[39] at least during first pass of the contrast agent, and used as a parametrized representation of the impulse response for deconvolution of the measured myocardial contrast enhancement.[40] An advantage of the "deconvolution" approach is that it obviates the need a model of the BTEX, that may include parameters with poor sensitivity to the measurement conditions, and therefore may require some user adjustment. For further details the reader is referred to earlier reviews on blood flow quantification by CMR.[40,41]

High Spatial Resolution

A variety of recent techniques have provided a more than 10-fold reduction in image acquisition time from undersampling of the image data by taking advantage of spatial, temporal, or spatio-temporal redundancy in the image data.[42–44] Spatial redundancy follows from use of parallel receive coils/channels, and gave rise to parallel-imaging acceleration techniques. Temporal redundancy is due to the serial acquisition of images for a single time point in cardiac cycle, and because contrast enhancement proceeds at a slower rate than the image acquisition rate. These forms of data-redundancy in a "conventional" perfusion scan (ie, without use of undersampling) imply that undersampling in both the spatial and time domains (k-t) can be performed to reduce the image acquisition time within bounds deemed acceptable for signal-to-noise, image quality, artifact absence, and so forth. Various k-t undersampling/acceleration techniques have been used for myocardial perfusion CMR, such as TSENSE,[45,46] k-t BLAST,[47] and more recently k-t principal component analysis (PCA).[48,49] Other, arguably more esoteric methods relate to the highly constrained back-projection reconstruction (HYPR),[50] in which k-space data are obtained by undersampled radial projections, possibly combined with an overall rotation of the sampling pattern during the course of dynamic imaging.

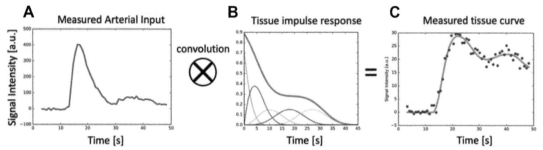

Fig. 5. The central volume principle of Meier and Zierler[37] states that the convolution of arterial input, shown in (A), with the myocardial impulse response in (B), predicts the myocardial response that would be observed, shown as solid red line in (C). Meier and Zierler[37] deduced from first principles that the amplitude of the impulse response equals MBF. In this example from a rest perfusion study, the arterial input and the myocardial contrast enhancement (*circles* in C) were extracted from CMR perfusion images. To estimate the impulse response from these measured curves, one must invert the relationship depicted in the figure and apply a *deconvolution* operation. Convolution can be thought of as a complex form of multiplication. Deconvolution would then be akin to division and is susceptible to producing spurious results from noise in the data. For a stable deconvolution, we required the impulse response to be smooth and monotonically decaying; contrast can only leave a region after an initial impulse input. Smoothness was enforced by representing the impulse response as a sum of smooth "basis" splines, shown as individual components under the blue curve in (B). MBF in this example was estimated to be 0.9 mL/min per g; the initial amplitude of the impulse response.

Missing data due to undersampling is restored from neighboring time frames.[50,51] This technique also presents a greater signal-to-noise ratio adjusted for pixel size.[52] The gains from imaging acceleration have been put to use to allow an in-plane spatial resolution of below 1.5 to 2.0 mm and still acquire 3 to 4 images per heartbeat, whereas traditional studies achieved an in-plane resolution of 2.5 to 3.0 mm for a similar number of slices per heartbeat.[4,5,22]

In CMR perfusion imaging, higher spatial resolution significantly reduces dark-rim artifacts because they are proportional to voxel size.[53] Application of k-t techniques in 3.0 T may reach up to eightfold acceleration and a resolution of 1.1 mm. This combination improved diagnostic performance of the method in CAD-suspected patients undergoing angiography (AUC, 0.93 vs 0.83; P<.001), which can be attributed to a better detection of subendocardial ischemia.[54] Quantitative analyses based on high-resolution perfusion stress imaging seems to be feasible and may even allow assessment of transmural gradients. However, temporal filtering effects inherent to k-t acceleration techniques may introduce a bias of underestimating blood flows and further optimization may still be needed to define the clinically acceptable limits for imaging acceleration.[55]

Three-Dimensional Whole-Heart Coverage

Faster image acquisition also paved the way for the development of whole-heart 3D myocardial perfusion CMR imaging. Three-dimensional perfusion CMR conceivably addresses an important limitation

of the multislice 2D imaging, which is the lack of complete myocardial coverage (in 2D, only 3–4 noncontiguous slices are obtained). Also, in 2D CMR sequences, slices correspond to different phases of the cardiac, whereas in 3D, acquisition is made in a diastolic phase and can be matched with other data obtained, for instance, of LGE.[55] A drawback of 3D perfusion imaging is that one can use only a relatively short fraction of the cardiac cycle for the acquisition of image data in order to minimize artifacts from cardiac motion. With 2D perfusion imaging, the acquisition of image data for each slice is self-contained, and avoidance of motion-induced artifacts or blurring involves minimizing this acquisition time per slice rather than the total acquisition time during each cardiac cycle.

Visually interpreted 3D-CMR perfusion examinations have achieved promising results, although superiority of 3D compared with 2D perfusion imaging remains to be shown in head-to-head comparisons. Manka and colleagues[56] assessed 146 patients at suspicion for CAD with a k-t imaging acceleration technique achieving 2.3-mm spatial resolution, and found sensitivity of 92%, specificity of 74%, and accuracy of 83% compared with quantitative coronary angiography ≥50%. At 3.0 T, diagnosis accuracy reaches 91% (sensitivity of 90% and specificity of 90%) when the standard comparison is a physiology method such as FFR by angiography.[57]

As for quantitative analyses, multicenter data demonstrate accuracy of 3D CMR perfusion imaging and accurate quantification of the ischemic volume relative to the entire myocardium.[56,58–60] Newly developed protocols have been released and promising results published. Fully 3D quantitative evaluations of MBF would eliminate the necessity to identify a "normally" perfused region of myocardium as reference, and could match up with the standard quantitative method PET but with the advantage of widespread availability, better spatial resolution, and absence of harmful radiation. Notwithstanding, some of the drawbacks related to the method must be addressed, such as the requirement for accurate arterial input sampling. A dual-sequence/dual-contrast using k-t PCA for spatially and temporally undersampled data yielded 3D perfusion images with higher signal-to-noise ratio (at contrast doses of 0.1 mmol/kg, and compared with 2D perfusion imaging), and addressed the issue of nonlinear (in relation to contrast concentration) contrast enhancement.[61] Acquisition of data for k-t PCA 3D perfusion imaging may take place either in diastole or systole,[62] but with a possible preference for systole because the LV wall is thicker, thereby facilitating an analysis of subendocardial perfusion. Also, during systole, dark-rim artifacts, which tend to have a constant width independent of cardiac phase, tend to be less of a nuisance than for diastolic images with a thinner LV wall. Other shortcomings of 3D fully quantitative analyses still need further research, such as a lack of standardized contrast-dosing, imaging acquisition and postprocessing protocols. More importantly, large clinical trials need to validate the current findings.

Microvascular Perfusion

Microvascular disease may appear as a subendocardial concentric perfusion defect. As it may not respect coronary territories its diagnosis may be difficult. It frequently coincides with the presence of LV hypertrophy and in individuals with diseases that lead to capillary rarefaction or dysfunction of the microcirculation, such as diabetes and hypertension. The appearance of a diffuse subendocardial perfusion defect may also take place in the presence of balanced multivessel coronary disease and a differential diagnosis may be challenging. In addition, although coronary angiography may differentiate microvascular disease and multivessel epicardial (macrovascular) disease, it may lead to inappropriate exclusion of microvascular disease when it is in fact present if accurate tools to rule out the diagnosis are not applied during angiography.[63–66]

Assessment of Wall Motion Segmental Contractility

Exercise has already been used in CMR to induce ischemia,[67] but the logistics to reach a sufficient

level of exercise is difficult to impossible within the confines of a magnet bore and pharmacologic stress remains the method of choice for clinical CMR studies. As the heterogeneity of the flow does not lead directly to ischemic abnormalities of wall motion except in cases of more severe perfusion reduction, it is not surprising that the assessment of wall motion during vasodilator stress results in a lower sensitivity[68] and higher specificity for the detection of coronary disease than the use of inotropic drugs. Therefore, stress-related contractility assessment should be preferably carried out with inotropes.

Nagel and colleagues[69] compared the segmental abnormalities of the LV wall induced by ischemia during dobutamine infusion by CMR with stress echocardiography in 208 consecutive patients with suspected CAD before cardiac catheterization. In this study, dobutamine CMR provided better sensitivity (89% vs 74%) and specificity (86% vs 70%) than stress echocardiography with dobutamine to detect coronary artery stenosis greater than 50%. Likewise, Hundley and colleagues,[70] using dobutamine in 163 patients with unfavorable echocardiographic windows, demonstrated sensitivity and specificity of 83% in the detection of coronary stenosis greater than 50% per coronary angiography. Various studies of CMR using dobutamine to induce of ischemia suggest that the presence of segmental contractile dysfunction in only 1 segment (6% of ischemic load) is already a predictor of worse outcome.[71,72] Any difference between the number of segments with reduced perfusion and the number of segments with wall motion abnormalities could be explained by the sequence of events in the ischemic cascade. As hypoperfusion precedes contraction abnormalities, it is possible that the extent of hypoperfusion exceeds the hypokinetic segments.

Myocardial Viability

Assessment of contractile reserve, as in stress echocardiography, was the first approach to assessing myocardial viability by CMR, but the technique has evolved considerably with the introduction of LGE images.[73] Viability can be estimated by wall thickness ratio (rest/stress), contractile reserve, and LGE currently considered gold-standard method for viability.[74,75]

Myocardial Contractile Reserve and Relative Wall Thickness

In line with echocardiographic data,[71] the presence of thinned myocardium can indicate lack of viability. Baer and colleagues[72] demonstrated that a diastolic wall thickness of 5.5 mm could be used to delimit myocardial segments with preserved metabolic function from those without, as evaluated by FDG PET. In a later study, the same group demonstrated that was almost never a recovery of regional function when the thickness of diastolic wall was less than 5.5 mm[76]; however, the reverse was not always true, that is, functional recovery did not occur universally in regions with wall thickness greater than 5.5 mm. Thus, the evaluation of diastolic wall thickness, although sensitive, offers poor specificity for predicting functional recovery.

Thickening of the ventricular wall of 2 mm during low-dose dobutamine greatly improves the specificity of technique. In the study by Baer and colleagues,[76] dobutamine increased specificity to 92% with sensitivity remaining at 86% to predict post-revascularization functional recovery. A consistent finding in dobutamine stress, however, is the high specificity of the technique, similar to the stress echocardiogram.[77] To achieve higher observer-independence techniques, such as tissue "tagging" and feature tracking for the analysis of myocardial deformation ("strain") offer the potential to further improve on the reported results, although the additional postprocessing required by these techniques has been a persistent deterrent to their clinical application.

Late Gadolinium Enhancement

Excellent tissue characterization is one of the main advantages of CMR and the exploitation of this through the use of T1-weighted contrast images to define infarcted and irreversibly damaged myocardium has been one of the most significant advances in CMR.[73] Although the exact reasons for the hypersignal in replacement (or interstitial) fibrosis continue to be a subject of intense scrutiny, the likely mechanism is a combination of arrival and output kinetics of the gadolinium within the myocardium and different volumes of distribution of gadolinium in viable cells and nonviable regions. The injected extracellular gadolinium contrast agent distributes within the entire tissue volume after myocardial infarction, whereas in normal myocardium, gadolinium is excluded from the intracellular space, that is, from approximately two-thirds of the tissue volume.

In acute myocardial ischemia the integrity of the membrane of the sarcolemma is lost, effectively a marker of cell death, allowing gadolinium to get into cardiomyocytes and resulting in signal hyperintensity. In chronic disease, the tissue transforms into a dense collagen matrix with a greatly expanded interstitial space accessible to

gadolinium contrast. Although some animal studies have demonstrated that the size and transmural depth of the infarction may be slightly overestimated (9%–12%) in the immediate postinfarction phase, these indicators are stable and reflect the actual extension of the scar after 1 week.

Late Gadolinium Enhancement in Clinical Practice

Experimental and clinical studies indicate that the extent of LGE is reproducible and closely correlates with the size of the myocardial necrosis or scar of infarction as determined by in vitro and in vivo methods established.[78–80] Subendocardial LGE is highly specific for the detection of myocardial infarction.[78] In addition, the detection of myocardial infarction is associated with a significantly increased risk of death subsequent to adverse cardiac events, adding incremental prognostic information to the evaluation of ventricular function.[81,82] Finally, the extent of myocardial LGE is emerging as a tool to determine the response to new medical and interventional therapies. The probability of functional recovery by segment is inversely related to the transmural extension of the infarct.[75] Zero percent to 25% transmural extension is associated with 82% probability of contractile function recovery, a 26% to 50% transmural extension, with 45% probability of recovery, and among segments with 51% to 75% transmural extension only 7% recovered. None of the segments presented recovery when the transmural extent of LGE was 75% or larger. Subsequent studies by other groups corroborated these results.[83–85] In addition to the response to revascularization, the extent of viable myocardium in ischemic cardiomyopathy also appears be a predictor of response to betablockade[86] and myocardial scar may be useful in the selection of patients who will benefit from resynchronization therapy.[87]

Clinical Prognosis Assessment

Coelho-Filho and colleagues[88] demonstrated in a relatively large number of women and men, that there were no significant differences between men and women regarding the diagnosis of CAD or for risk stratification of major adverse cardiovascular events using CMR stress perfusion imaging. But the method can shed light on the pathophysiology of chest pain with normal epicardial coronary arteries ("syndrome X"), a clinically not uncommon distressing condition in postmenopausal women. Quantitative myocardial perfusion CMR[89] has been validated against invasive measurements of coronary flow reserve in patients with microvascular dysfunction; it was found to provide excellent correlation with the catheter-based measurements. Panting and colleagues[65] identified myocardial subendocardial hypoperfusion during adenosine infusion in this set of patients (X syndrome), and Doyle and colleagues[90] reported reduction in coronary flow reserve in similar patients. Coronary flow reserve is also reduced in hypertension, myocardial hypertrophy,[91,92] and in some cardiomyopathies.[93]

Acute Chest Pain

Stress perfusion CMR can provide prognostic information in various clinical settings.[94–96] In the acute chest pain scenario, Ingkanisorn and colleagues[94] have shown that adenosine stress CMR may determine the prognosis in patients with inconclusive electrocardiogram for CAD and negative biomarkers for acute coronary syndrome. In such patients, a negative perfusion stress CMR virtually excluded CAD or unfavorable clinical outcomes: no patient with normal examination had an adverse cardiac event. In a population with chest pain presenting to the emergency department, perfusion stress CMR was shown to have a sensitivity of 100% and a 93% specificity in the prediction of subsequent myocardial infarction or detection of coronary stenosis during 1 year of follow-up.[95]

Chronic Chest Pain

Results are similar for patients with suspected CAD. In a cohort of 513 patients, Jahnke and colleagues[97] examined the value of adenosine stress CMR perfusion and dobutamine stress CMR to help predict cardiac death and nonfatal myocardial infarction. At 3 years of follow-up, event-free survival reached 99.2% for patients with normal CMR and 83.5% for those with an abnormal perfusion. Abnormal CMR yielded a probability of death or nonfatal infarction beyond estimated risk from the presence of clinical risk factors (likelihood ratio, χ^2 = 16.0–34.3, P = .001). In this study, stress CMR, either by perfusion or by wall motility, contributed with incremental value regarding traditional factors such as age, sex, smoking and diabetes, although the combination of both techniques did not increase stratification power. A normal perfusion was associated with an event rate extremely low, 0.7% at 2 years, 2.3% at 3 years, and an abnormal perfusion study with corresponding rates of 6.2%, 12.2%, and 16.3%. In the multivariate analysis, adjusting for other risks, the detection of an abnormality of perfusion was associated with a 10-fold increase in risk of cardiovascular events (death or myocardial infarction). In another study of 218 patients with negative perfusion studies followed for more than 2 years, there were no deaths or infarction, percutaneous coronary intervention or coronary revascularization surgery.[98]

SUMMARY

CMR provides excellent temporal and spatial resolution without the limitations associated with unfavorable echocardiographic windows, and low temporal and spatial resolution in nuclear medicine studies, nor does it involve ionizing radiation. Myocardial perfusion by CMR can be integrated with a spatially registered interrogation of regional function (wall thickening, segmental contractility, and myocardial deformation image), edema, fibrosis, and viability. These simultaneous faculties are not present in other imaging modalities. Quantitative analysis of myocardial perfusion is an evolving tool for stress perfusion CMR and may be incorporated into clinical practice within the next few years. Larger clinical studies are expected to pave the way for wider adoption. Although every other cardiac imaging modality may offer one equivalent or possibly superior match for assessing stress perfusion or function, fibrosis, or viability, the key to the success of CMR may lie in the power of an integrated cardiac examination in which each of these components provides an incremental benefit for diagnosis and prognosis. In that context, stress perfusion CMR will undoubtedly play a pivotal role for improving the diagnosis of myocardial ischemia and add to the already outstanding capabilities of CMR for assessing ventricular function and myocardial viability.

REFERENCES

1. Coelho-Filho OR, Rickers C, Kwong RY, et al. MR myocardial perfusion imaging. Radiology 2013; 266(3):701–15.
2. Wolff SD, Schwitter J, Coulden R, et al. Myocardial first-pass perfusion magnetic resonance imaging: a multicenter dose-ranging study. Circulation 2004; 110(6):732–7.
3. Giang TH, Nanz D, Coulden R, et al. Detection of coronary artery disease by magnetic resonance myocardial perfusion imaging with various contrast medium doses: first European multi-centre experience. Eur Heart J 2004;25(18):1657–65.
4. Greenwood JP, Maredia N, Younger JF, et al. Cardiovascular magnetic resonance and single-photon emission computed tomography for diagnosis of

coronary heart disease (CE-MARC): a prospective trial. Lancet 2012;379(9814):453–60.

5. Schwitter J, Wacker CM, Wilke N, et al. MR-IMPACT II: Magnetic Resonance Imaging for Myocardial Perfusion Assessment in Coronary artery disease Trial: perfusion-cardiac magnetic resonance vs. single-photon emission computed tomography for the detection of coronary artery disease: a comparative multicentre, multivendor trial. Eur Heart J 2013; 34(10):775–81.

6. Hamon M, Fau G, Nee G, et al. Meta-analysis of the diagnostic performance of stress perfusion cardiovascular magnetic resonance for detection of coronary artery disease. J Cardiovasc Magn Reson 2010;12(1):29.

7. Greenwood JP, Motwani M, Maredia N, et al. Comparison of cardiovascular magnetic resonance and single-photon emission computed tomography in women with suspected coronary artery disease from the Clinical Evaluation of Magnetic Resonance Imaging in Coronary Heart Disease (CE-MARC) Trial. Circulation 2014;129(10):1129–38.

8. Puntmann VO, Valbuena S, Hinojar R, et al. Society for Cardiovascular Magnetic Resonance (SCMR) expert consensus for CMR imaging endpoints in clinical research: part I - analytical validation and clinical qualification. J Cardiovasc Magn Reson 2018;20(1):67.

9. Schulz-Menger J, Bluemke DA, Bremerich J, et al. Standardized image interpretation and post processing in cardiovascular magnetic resonance: Society for Cardiovascular Magnetic Resonance (SCMR) board of trustees task force on standardized post processing. J Cardiovasc Magn Reson 2013;15:35.

10. Klocke FJ. Measurements of coronary flow reserve: defining pathophysiology versus making decisions about patient care. Circulation 1987; 76(6):1183–9.

11. Farzaneh-Far A, Shaw LK, Dunning A, et al. Comparison of the prognostic value of regadenoson and adenosine myocardial perfusion imaging. J Nucl Cardiol 2015;22(4):600–7.

12. Iqbal FM, Hage FG, Ahmed A, et al. Comparison of the prognostic value of normal regadenoson with normal adenosine myocardial perfusion imaging with propensity score matching. JACC Cardiovasc Imaging 2012;5(10):1014–21.

13. Gould KL, Kirkeeide RL, Buchi M. Coronary flow reserve as a physiologic measure of stenosis severity. J Am Coll Cardiol 1990;15(2):459–74.

14. Gould KL, Lipscomb K. Effects of coronary stenoses on coronary flow reserve and resistance. Am J Cardiol 1974;34(1):48–55.

15. Duncker DJ, Bache RJ. Regulation of coronary blood flow during exercise. Physiol Rev 2008; 88(3):1009–86.

16. Geldof MJ, Schalij MJ, Manger Cats V, et al. Comparison between regional myocardial perfusion reserve and coronary flow reserve in the canine heart. Eur Heart J 1995;16(12):1860–71.

17. Serruys PW, di Mario C, Piek J, et al. Prognostic value of intracoronary flow velocity and diameter stenosis in assessing the short- and long-term outcomes of coronary balloon angioplasty: the DEBATE Study (Doppler Endpoints Balloon Angioplasty Trial Europe). Circulation 1997;96(10):3369–77.

18. Panting JR, Gatehouse PD, Yang GZ, et al. Echo-planar magnetic resonance myocardial perfusion imaging: parametric map analysis and comparison with thallium SPECT. J Magn Reson Imaging 2001; 13(2):192–200.

19. Klem I, Heitner JF, Shah DJ, et al. Improved detection of coronary artery disease by stress perfusion cardiovascular magnetic resonance with the use of delayed enhancement infarction imaging. J Am Coll Cardiol 2006;47(8):1630–8.

20. Schwitter J, Nanz D, Kneifel S, et al. Assessment of myocardial perfusion in coronary artery disease by magnetic resonance: a comparison with positron emission tomography and coronary angiography. Circulation 2001;103(18):2230–5.

21. Al-Saadi N, Nagel E, Gross M, et al. Noninvasive detection of myocardial ischemia from perfusion reserve based on cardiovascular magnetic resonance. Circulation 2000;101(12):1379–83.

22. Schwitter J, Wacker CM, van Rossum AC, et al. MR-IMPACT: comparison of perfusion-cardiac magnetic resonance with single-photon emission computed tomography for the detection of coronary artery disease in a multicentre, multivendor, randomized trial. Eur Heart J 2008;29(4):480–9.

23. Nandalur KR, Dwamena BA, Choudhri AF, et al. Diagnostic performance of stress cardiac magnetic resonance imaging in the detection of coronary artery disease: a meta-analysis. J Am Coll Cardiol 2007;50(14):1343–53.

24. Rieber J, Jung P, Schiele TM, et al. Safety of FFR-based treatment strategies: the Munich experience. Z Kardiol 2002;91(Suppl 3):115–9.

25. Cerqueira MD, Weissman NJ, Dilsizian V, et al. Standardized myocardial segmentation and nomenclature for tomographic imaging of the heart. A statement for healthcare professionals from the Cardiac Imaging Committee of the Council on Clinical Cardiology of the American Heart Association. Circulation 2002;105(4):539–42.

26. Nagel E, Klein C, Paetsch I, et al. Magnetic resonance perfusion measurements for the noninvasive detection of coronary artery disease. Circulation 2003;108(4):432–7.

27. Vincenti G, Masci PG, Monney P, et al. Stress perfusion CMR in patients with known and suspected CAD: prognostic value and optimal ischemic

threshold for revascularization. JACC Cardiovasc Imaging 2017;10(5):526–37.

28. Christian TF, Rettmann DW, Aletras AH, et al. Absolute myocardial perfusion in canines measured by using dual-bolus first-pass MR imaging. Radiology 2004;232(3):677–84.

29. Ichihara T, Ishida M, Kitagawa K, et al. Quantitative analysis of first-pass contrast-enhanced myocardial perfusion MRI using a Patlak plot method and blood saturation correction. Magn Reson Med 2009;62(2): 373–83.

30. Fritz-Hansen T, Hove JD, Kofoed KF, et al. Quantification of MRI measured myocardial perfusion reserve in healthy humans: a comparison with positron emission tomography. J Magn Reson Imaging 2008;27(4):818–24.

31. Morton G, Chiribiri A, Ishida M, et al. Quantification of absolute myocardial perfusion in patients with coronary artery disease: comparison between cardiovascular magnetic resonance and positron emission tomography. J Am Coll Cardiol 2012;60(16): 1546–55.

32. Biglands JD, Magee DR, Sourbron SP, et al. Comparison of the diagnostic performance of four quantitative myocardial perfusion estimation methods used in cardiac MR imaging: CE-MARC Substudy. Radiology 2015;275(2):393–402.

33. Christian TF, Aletras AH, Arai AE. Estimation of absolute myocardial blood flow during first-pass MR perfusion imaging using a dual-bolus injection technique: comparison to single-bolus injection method. J Magn Reson Imaging 2008;27(6): 1271–7.

34. Kellman P, Hansen MS, Nielles-Vallespin S, et al. Myocardial perfusion cardiovascular magnetic resonance: optimized dual sequence and reconstruction for quantification. J Cardiovasc Magn Reson 2017; 19(1):43.

35. Kroll K, Wilke N, Jerosch-Herold M, et al. Modeling regional myocardial flows from residue functions of an intravascular indicator. Am J Physiol 1996; 271(4 Pt 2):H1643–55.

36. Jerosch-Herold M, Wilke N, Wang Y, et al. Direct comparison of an intravascular and an extracellular contrast agent for quantification of myocardial perfusion. Cardiac MRI Group. Int J Card Imaging 1999; 15(6):453–64.

37. Meier P, Zierler KL. On the theory of the indicator-dilution method for measurement of blood flow and volume. J Appl Physiol 1954;6(12):731–44.

38. Jerosch-Herold M, Swingen C, Seethamraju RT. Myocardial blood flow quantification with MRI by model-independent deconvolution. Med Phys 2002;29(5):886–97.

39. Jerosch-Herold M, Wilke N, Stillman AE. Magnetic resonance quantification of the myocardial perfusion reserve with a Fermi function model for constrained deconvolution. Med Phys 1998;25(1): 73–84.

40. Jerosch-Herold M. Quantification of myocardial perfusion by cardiovascular magnetic resonance. J Cardiovasc Magn Reson 2010;12:57.

41. Chung S, Shah B, Storey P, et al. Quantitative perfusion analysis of first-pass contrast enhancement kinetics: application to MRI of myocardial perfusion in coronary artery disease. PLoS One 2016;11(9): e0162067.

42. Kozerke S, Plein S. Accelerated CMR using zonal, parallel and prior knowledge driven imaging methods. J Cardiovasc Magn Reson 2008;10:29.

43. Motwani M, Lockie T, Greenwood JP, et al. Accelerated, high spatial resolution cardiovascular magnetic resonance myocardial perfusion imaging. J Nucl Cardiol 2011;18(5):952–8.

44. Tsao J, Kozerke S. MRI temporal acceleration techniques. J Magn Reson Imaging 2012;36(3):543–60.

45. Weber S, Kronfeld A, Kunz RP, et al. Comparison of three accelerated pulse sequences for semiquantitative myocardial perfusion imaging using sensitivity encoding incorporating temporal filtering (TSENSE). J Magn Reson Imaging 2007;26(3):569–79.

46. Kellman P, Derbyshire JA, Agyeman KO, et al. Extended coverage first-pass perfusion imaging using slice-interleaved TSENSE. Magn Reson Med 2004;51(1):200–4.

47. Gebker R, Jahnke C, Paetsch I, et al. MR myocardial perfusion imaging with k-space and time broad-use linear acquisition speed-up technique: feasibility study. Radiology 2007;245(3):863–71.

48. Pedersen H, Kozerke S, Ringgaard S, et al. k-t PCA: temporally constrained k-t BLAST reconstruction using principal component analysis. Magn Reson Med 2009;62(3):706–16.

49. Schmidt JF, Wissmann L, Manka R, et al. Iterative k-t principal component analysis with nonrigid motion correction for dynamic three-dimensional cardiac perfusion imaging. Magn Reson Med 2014;72(1): 68–79.

50. Ge L, Kino A, Griswold M, et al. Myocardial perfusion MRI with sliding-window conjugate-gradient HYPR. Magn Reson Med 2009;62(4):835–9.

51. Ma H, Yang J, Liu J, et al. Myocardial perfusion magnetic resonance imaging using sliding-window conjugate-gradient highly constrained back-projection reconstruction for detection of coronary artery disease. Am J Cardiol 2012;109(8):1137–41.

52. Plein S, Ryf S, Schwitter J, et al. Dynamic contrast-enhanced myocardial perfusion MRI accelerated with k-t sense. Magn Reson Med 2007;58(4): 777–85.

53. Maredia N, Radjenovic A, Kozerke S, et al. Effect of improving spatial or temporal resolution on image quality and quantitative perfusion assessment with k-t SENSE acceleration in first-pass CMR myocardial

perfusion imaging. Magn Reson Med 2010;64(6): 1616–24.

54. Motwani M, Maredia N, Fairbairn TA, et al. High-resolution versus standard-resolution cardiovascular MR myocardial perfusion imaging for the detection of coronary artery disease. Circ Cardiovasc Imaging 2012;5(3):306–13.

55. Motwani M, Jogiya R, Kozerke S, et al. Advanced cardiovascular magnetic resonance myocardial perfusion imaging: high-spatial resolution versus 3-dimensional whole-heart coverage. Circ Cardiovasc Imaging 2013;6(2):339–48.

56. Manka R, Jahnke C, Kozerke S, et al. Dynamic 3-dimensional stress cardiac magnetic resonance perfusion imaging: detection of coronary artery disease and volumetry of myocardial hypoenhancement before and after coronary stenting. J Am Coll Cardiol 2011;57(4):437–44.

57. Jogiya R, Kozerke S, Morton G, et al. Validation of dynamic 3-dimensional whole heart magnetic resonance myocardial perfusion imaging against fractional flow reserve for the detection of significant coronary artery disease. J Am Coll Cardiol 2012; 60(8):756–65.

58. Manka R, Paetsch I, Kozerke S, et al. Whole-heart dynamic three-dimensional magnetic resonance perfusion imaging for the detection of coronary artery disease defined by fractional flow reserve: determination of volumetric myocardial ischaemic burden and coronary lesion location. Eur Heart J 2012;33(16):2016–24.

59. Manka R, Wissmann L, Gebker R, et al. Multicenter evaluation of dynamic three-dimensional magnetic resonance myocardial perfusion imaging for the detection of coronary artery disease defined by fractional flow reserve. Circ Cardiovasc Imaging 2015; 8(5) [pii:e003061].

60. Jogiya R, Morton G, De Silva K, et al. Ischemic burden by 3-dimensional myocardial perfusion cardiovascular magnetic resonance: comparison with myocardial perfusion scintigraphy. Circ Cardiovasc Imaging 2014;7(4):647–54.

61. Wissmann L, Niemann M, Gotschy A, et al. Quantitative three-dimensional myocardial perfusion cardiovascular magnetic resonance with accurate two-dimensional arterial input function assessment. J Cardiovasc Magn Reson 2015;17:108.

62. Motwani M, Kidambi A, Sourbron S, et al. Quantitative three-dimensional cardiovascular magnetic resonance myocardial perfusion imaging in systole and diastole. J Cardiovasc Magn Reson 2014;16:19.

63. Pilz G, Klos M, Ali E, et al. Angiographic correlations of patients with small vessel disease diagnosed by adenosine-stress cardiac magnetic resonance imaging. J Cardiovasc Magn Reson 2008;10:8.

64. Kawecka-Jaszcz K, Czarnecka D, Olszanecka A, et al. Myocardial perfusion in hypertensive patients with normal coronary angiograms. J Hypertens 2008;26(8):1686–94.

65. Panting JR, Gatehouse PD, Yang GZ, et al. Abnormal subendocardial perfusion in cardiac syndrome X detected by cardiovascular magnetic resonance imaging. N Engl J Med 2002;346(25): 1948–53.

66. Stanton T, Marwick TH. Assessment of subendocardial structure and function. JACC Cardiovasc Imaging 2010;3(8):867–75.

67. Rerkpattanapipat P, Gandhi SK, Darty SN, et al. Feasibility to detect severe coronary artery stenoses with upright treadmill exercise magnetic resonance imaging. Am J Cardiol 2003;92(5):603–6.

68. Pennell DJ, Underwood SR, Ell PJ, et al. Dipyridamole magnetic resonance imaging: a comparison with thallium-201 emission tomography. Br Heart J 1990;64(6):362–9.

69. Nagel E, Lehmkuhl HB, Bocksch W, et al. Noninvasive diagnosis of ischemia-induced wall motion abnormalities with the use of high-dose dobutamine stress MRI: comparison with dobutamine stress echocardiography. Circulation 1999;99(6): 763–70.

70. Hundley WG, Hamilton CA, Thomas MS, et al. Utility of fast cine magnetic resonance imaging and display for the detection of myocardial ischemia in patients not well suited for second harmonic stress echocardiography. Circulation 1999;100(16): 1697–702.

71. Schinkel AF, Bax JJ, Boersma E, et al. Assessment of residual myocardial viability in regions with chronic electrocardiographic Q-wave infarction. Am Heart J 2002;144(5):865–9.

72. Baer FM, Voth E, Schneider CA, et al. Comparison of low-dose dobutamine-gradient-echo magnetic resonance imaging and positron emission tomography with [18F]fluorodeoxyglucose in patients with chronic coronary artery disease. A functional and morphological approach to the detection of residual myocardial viability. Circulation 1995;91(4):1006–15.

73. Kim RJ, Fieno DS, Parrish TB, et al. Relationship of MRI delayed contrast enhancement to irreversible injury, infarct age, and contractile function. Circulation 1999;100(19):1992–2002.

74. Schinkel AF, Poldermans D, Elhendy A, et al. Assessment of myocardial viability in patients with heart failure. J Nucl Med 2007;48(7):1135–46.

75. Kim RJ, Wu E, Rafael A, et al. The use of contrast-enhanced magnetic resonance imaging to identify reversible myocardial dysfunction. N Engl J Med 2000;343(20):1445–53.

76. Baer FM, Theissen P, Schneider CA, et al. Dobutamine magnetic resonance imaging predicts contractile recovery of chronically dysfunctional myocardium after successful revascularization. J Am Coll Cardiol 1998;31(5):1040–8.

77. Kaandorp TA, Lamb HJ, van der Wall EE, et al. Cardiovascular MR to access myocardial viability in chronic ischaemic LV dysfunction. Heart 2005; 91(10):1359–65.

78. Rehwald WG, Fieno DS, Chen EL, et al. Myocardial magnetic resonance imaging contrast agent concentrations after reversible and irreversible ischemic injury. Circulation 2002;105(2):224–9.

79. Bulow H, Klein C, Kuehn I, et al. Cardiac magnetic resonance imaging: long term reproducibility of the late enhancement signal in patients with chronic coronary artery disease. Heart 2005;91(9):1158–63.

80. Ibrahim T, Nekolla SG, Hornke M, et al. Quantitative measurement of infarct size by contrast-enhanced magnetic resonance imaging early after acute myocardial infarction: comparison with single-photon emission tomography using Tc99m-sestamibi. J Am Coll Cardiol 2005;45(4):544–52.

81. Kwong RY, Chan AK, Brown KA, et al. Impact of unrecognized myocardial scar detected by cardiac magnetic resonance imaging on event-free survival in patients presenting with signs or symptoms of coronary artery disease. Circulation 2006;113(23): 2733–43.

82. Kwong RY, Sattar H, Wu H, et al. Incidence and prognostic implication of unrecognized myocardial scar characterized by cardiac magnetic resonance in diabetic patients without clinical evidence of myocardial infarction. Circulation 2008;118(10): 1011–20.

83. Wellnhofer E, Olariu A, Klein C, et al. Magnetic resonance low-dose dobutamine test is superior to SCAR quantification for the prediction of functional recovery. Circulation 2004;109(18):2172–4.

84. Selvanayagam JB, Kardos A, Francis JM, et al. Value of delayed-enhancement cardiovascular magnetic resonance imaging in predicting myocardial viability after surgical revascularization. Circulation 2004;110(12):1535–41.

85. Lauerma K, Niemi P, Hanninen H, et al. Multimodality MR imaging assessment of myocardial viability: combination of first-pass and late contrast enhancement to wall motion dynamics and comparison with FDG PET-initial experience. Radiology 2000;217(3): 729–36.

86. Bello D, Shah DJ, Farah GM, et al. Gadolinium cardiovascular magnetic resonance predicts reversible myocardial dysfunction and remodeling in patients with heart failure undergoing beta-blocker therapy. Circulation 2003;108(16):1945–53.

87. Bleeker GB, Kaandorp TA, Lamb HJ, et al. Effect of posterolateral scar tissue on clinical and echocardiographic improvement after cardiac resynchronization therapy. Circulation 2006;113(7): 969–76.

88. Coelho-Filho OR, Seabra LF, Mongeon FP, et al. Stress myocardial perfusion imaging by CMR provides strong prognostic value to cardiac events regardless of patient's sex. JACC Cardiovasc Imaging 2011;4(8):850–61.

89. Wilke N, Jerosch-Herold M, Wang Y, et al. Myocardial perfusion reserve: assessment with multisection, quantitative, first-pass MR imaging. Radiology 1997;204(2):373–84.

90. Doyle M, Fuisz A, Kortright E, et al. The impact of myocardial flow reserve on the detection of coronary artery disease by perfusion imaging methods: an NHLBI WISE study. J Cardiovasc Magn Reson 2003;5(3):475–85.

91. Kelm M, Strauer BE. Coronary flow reserve measurements in hypertension. Med Clin North Am 2004; 88(1):99–113.

92. Laine H, Raitakari OT, Niinikoski H, et al. Early impairment of coronary flow reserve in young men with borderline hypertension. J Am Coll Cardiol 1998;32(1):147–53.

93. Weismuller S, Czernin J, Sun KT, et al. Coronary vasodilatory capacity is impaired in patients with dilated cardiomyopathy. Am J Card Imaging 1996;10(3): 154–62.

94. Ingkanisorn WP, Kwong RY, Bohme NS, et al. Prognosis of negative adenosine stress magnetic resonance in patients presenting to an emergency department with chest pain. J Am Coll Cardiol 2006;47(7):1427–32.

95. Kwong RY, Schussheim AE, Rekhraj S, et al. Detecting acute coronary syndrome in the emergency department with cardiac magnetic resonance imaging. Circulation 2003;107(4):531–7.

96. Steel K, Broderick R, Gandla V, et al. Complementary prognostic values of stress myocardial perfusion and late gadolinium enhancement imaging by cardiac magnetic resonance in patients with known or suspected coronary artery disease. Circulation 2009;120(14):1390–400.

97. Jahnke C, Nagel E, Gebker R, et al. Prognostic value of cardiac magnetic resonance stress tests: adenosine stress perfusion and dobutamine stress wall motion imaging. Circulation 2007;115(13):1769–76.

98. Pilz G, Jeske A, Klos M, et al. Prognostic value of normal adenosine-stress cardiac magnetic resonance imaging. Am J Cardiol 2008;101(10): 1408–12.

Automated Quantitative Stress Perfusion in a Clinical Routine

Kristopher D. Knott, MA, MBBS, MRCP[a],
Juliano Lara Fernandes, MD, PhD, MBA[b],
James C. Moon, MB, BCh, MRCP, MD[a,*]

KEYWORDS

- Myocardial perfusion • Stress • Ischemia • MR imaging • Cardiovascular magnetic resonance
- Quantification • Automation

KEY POINTS

- Cardiovascular magnetic resonance (CMR) perfusion can assess ischemia with high accuracy and has been assessed against different modalities in well-designed randomized clinical trials.
- Noninvasive quantification of ischemia has a potential clinical impact in the management of patients with coronary artery disease beyond qualitative evaluation.
- Quantitative CMR perfusion techniques have significantly developed over the years and have shown robust accuracy compared with PET studies or invasive measurements of coronary flow.
- Automated quantitative CMR perfusion allows rapid and accurate creation of pixel-based myocardial blood flow (MBF) maps with in-line processing and improvement in clinical workflow.
- The use of automated CMR MBF maps in clinical routine may allow more accurate diagnosis of coronary artery disease as well as evaluation of the different phenotypic expression of atherosclerosis in both epicardial arteries and microvascular vessels.

INTRODUCTION

Coronary heart disease is the most common cause of morbidity and mortality globally.[1] It is caused by the atherosclerotic narrowing of the coronary arteries and is amenable to treatment with medical therapy and revascularization.[2–4] However, the suitability of a lesion for intervention depends on its functional significance. Coronary stenoses of hemodynamic significance are amenable to percutaneous intervention but intervening on those that are not flow limiting may confer a worse prognosis.[5–7] Furthermore,

the amount of ischemia is important. Subgroup analysis of the COURAGE (Clinical Outcomes Utilizing Revascularization and Aggressive Drug Evaluation) trial has shown that patients with greater than 10% left ventricle (LV) ischemia benefit from revascularization rather than medical therapy alone.[8] The gold standard assessment for suspected coronary artery disease (CAD) is coronary angiography, but this is invasive and therefore associated with risks,[9] and exposes patients to ionizing radiation.[10] Therefore, high-quality assessment of ischemia and

Disclosures: The authors have no conflicts of interest.
[a] Barts Heart Centre, The Cardiovascular Magnetic Resonance Imaging Unit and The Inherited Cardiovascular Diseases Unit, St Bartholomew's Hospital, West Smithfield, 2nd Floor, King George V Block, London EC1A 7BE, UK; [b] Jose Michel Kalaf Research Insitute, Radiologia Clinica de Campinas, Av Jose de Souza Campos 840, Campinas, São Paulo 13092-100, Brazil
* Corresponding author.
E-mail address: james.moon@bartshealth.nhs.uk

Magn Reson Imaging Clin N Am 27 (2019) 507–520
https://doi.org/10.1016/j.mric.2019.04.003
1064-9689/19/© 2019 Elsevier Inc. All rights reserved.

the functional significance of CAD is required to appropriately manage patients.[11–13]

There are various noninvasive techniques to assess ischemia, including stress echocardiography, single-photon emission computed tomography (SPECT), PET, computed tomography with fractional flow reserve (FFR), and cardiovascular magnetic resonance (CMR).[14–20] There are advantages to each and they have high sensitivities and specificities for the detection of coronary heart disease.[14–20] CMR does not use ionizing radiation and is the gold standard for cardiac structure, function, and tissue characterization,[21,22] giving extra useful information to clinicians.

In clinical practice, perfusion CMR is a qualitative technique. Typically, 3 LV short-axis images (base, mid, and apex) are acquired per heartbeat during the first pass of a gadolinium (Gd)-based contrast agent under conditions of vasodilator stress and rest.[23] Experienced observers compare the images and look for areas of relative hypoperfusion at stress, which correspond with functionally significant coronary stenosis. Clinical decisions are then made based on this qualitative assessment. However, truly balanced ischemia caused by disease in all 3 of the coronary artery arteries could cause a global flow reduction that could be missed. Coronary microvascular dysfunction, a cause of chest pain and a common feature in cardiomyopathy, is not well characterized, and visual quantification may have reduced accuracy and reproducibility.[24] Therefore, it is desirable to fully quantify myocardial perfusion and bring this into clinical practice.

Advanced imaging techniques can now quantify myocardial perfusion, the myocardial blood flow (MBF; mL/g/min) at stress and at rest. The myocardial perfusion reserve (MPR; referred to as the coronary flow reserve, CFR, in PET studies) is the ratio of the stress MBF to rest MBF. Relative flow reserve can also be measured by dividing the stress MBF of different myocardial segments. Most of the evidence for quantitative perfusion to date is from the PET literature but quantifying perfusion is also possible with CMR and recent advances have brought this to practice.

This article discusses the benefits of the noninvasive quantification of perfusion, discusses the methods of quantifying perfusion with CMR, and suggests how through automating the process it is possible to introduce quantitative CMR into clinical practice.

THE IMPORTANCE OF QUANTITATIVE PERFUSION IN CLINICAL PRACTICE

CMR quantitative perfusion has historically been time consuming and difficult, which has kept it out of the realms of clinical practice and meant that most of the evidence for quantitative perfusion is in PET studies. Early evidence that MBF could be measured noninvasively came from the initial studies from Gould and colleagues[25] showing the value of quantification to detect significant coronary stenosis. From those initial studies, quantification evolved to show its capability to characterize different levels of CAD severity in a more accurate way than qualitative analysis, especially identifying single-vessel versus 3-vessel disease and microcirculatory involvement. Patients with 3-vessel CAD had more extensive perfusion abnormalities on fully quantitative assessment than patients with single-vessel disease.[26] Similarly, in a small CMR study of 41 patients with suspected CAD, fully quantitative perfusion was able to reliably discriminate between single-vessel and triple-vessel disease, which was not possible with qualitative perfusion.[27] In one PET study, which enrolled 104 patients at moderate risk of CAD, absolute quantification had a significantly higher positive predictive value, negative predictive value, and accuracy for the detection of obstructive disease compared with qualitative perfusion.[28] Furthermore, the interobserver variability of perfusion assessment was lower for the quantitative method. All these findings have important clinical implications where the extent of ischemia influences treatment choices.

Quantitative perfusion also gives additional information compared with qualitative analysis. Absolute stress perfusion and CFR are prognostic. In one study, 256 patients, including 150 with known CAD, underwent ammonia PET evaluation and were followed up for 5.5 years.[29] Those with impaired CFR (<2) had higher rates of death and major adverse cardiovascular events than those with normal CFR (>2). CFR was additive to risk determined by qualitative clinical read. Those with perfusion defects and abnormal CFR had worse clinical outcomes than those with normal CFR.

In patients with impaired LV function, myocardial perfusion is also important. Neglia and colleagues[30] enrolled 67 patients with LV impairment with dipyridamole stress PET and followed them up for 45 months. Patients with severely depressed stress (≤1.36 mL/g/min) and rest perfusion (≤0.65 mL/g/min) had a relative risk of death or the progression of heart failure of 3.5 and 3.3 respectively compared with those with normal perfusion. On multivariate regression analysis, only stress MBF, resting heart rate, and end-diastolic dimensions were independently prognostic: 5-year event-free survival was 35.8% in patients with stress MBF less than or equal to 1.36 mL/g/min compared with 79% in those with MBF greater than 1.36 mL/g/min.

Perfusion may also be impaired in nonischemic cardiomyopathies. Patients with hypertrophic cardiomyopathy (HCM) often present with chest pain and have ischemic features on electrocardiogram thought to be related to microvascular dysfunction.[31] Ischemic damage (both acute/subacute and chronic) is seen at autopsy[32] and ischemia detected by SPECT is associated with ventricular tachycardia.[33] Patient with HCM have impaired stress perfusion compared with healthy controls (even in nonhypertrophied segments) and this is associated with increasing wall thickness and fibrosis.[34] In a prospective cohort study of 51 patients and 12 controls with atypical chest pain, the degree of perfusion impairment was an independent predictor of death and adverse cardiovascular events.[35] Other cardiomyopathies with hypertrophy, such as Fabry disease and amyloidosis, also have impaired perfusion. In Fabry, this has been used to evaluate treatment efficiency.[36] In amyloidosis, microvascular dysfunction has been shown using PET even in the absence of epicardial CAD and with lower stress and rest absolute perfusion values compared with patients with hypertensive LV hypertrophy.[37] Using CMR, semiquantitative perfusion has been shown to differentiate amyloidosis from normal patients and to identify patients with normal and lower LV function.[38]

In summary, fast, efficient quantitative perfusion for clinical practice and research would have advantages for disease identification and characterization, adding prognostic information and increasing reliability and adding the ability to characterize microvascular disease in CAD and cardiomyopathies, potentially aiding therapeutic drug development and treatment monitoring.

QUALITATIVE AND SEMIQUANTITATIVE PERFUSION CARDIOVASCULAR MAGNETIC RESONANCE

The baseline technique, qualitative stress perfusion CMR, is sensitive and specific for CAD detection[16] and a normal CMR scan confers a good prognosis.[39,40] Using the American Heart Association 17 (or 16) segment model, ischemia extent can be evaluated[24] and used to target revascularisation[8] with either 10% or 1.5 ischemic segments defining patients with a worse prognosis.[41] To improve on this, semiquantitative assessment has been used. This method uses time–signal intensity curves in each myocardial segment to estimate the myocardial perfusion (**Fig. 1**). There are various different methods that may be used for estimating perfusion, including contrast enhancement ratio (CER), myocardial to LV upslope index ratio, and upslope integral ratio.[42] The CER is calculated from $(SI_{peak} - SI_{baseline})/SI_{baseline}$ where SI_{peak} is the maximum signal intensity (SI) in the region of interest and $SI_{baseline}$ is the mean baseline SI. The myocardial to LV upslope method is

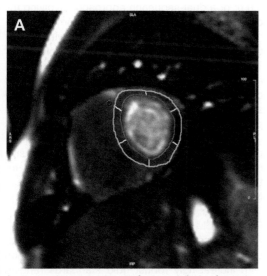
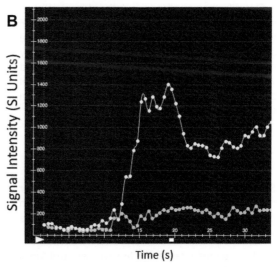

Fig. 1. Semiquantitative perfusion analysis of a patient with a perfusion defect in the inferolateral wall. (*A*) Endocardial (*red*) and epicardial (*green*) contours are drawn for each slice and for each measurement, and the superior right ventricle insertion point is identified. (*B*) Signal intensity is plotted against time for an area of ischemic myocardium (*blue*) and remote myocardium (*yellow*). Subsequent analysis can be performed to calculate perfusion in a semiquantitative fashion.

calculated by dividing the initial upslope of the myocardial time-SI curve by the initial upslope of the LV blood pool myocardial time-SI curve.[43] The upslope integral ratio is the area under the curve (AUC) for the myocardial time-SI curve once the baseline has been adjusted for.[44] The diagnostic accuracy of semiquantitative perfusion has been compared, using PET, with absolute MBF using animal models and microspheres[42] and invasive coronary angiography.[43,45] Compared with absolute MBF as measured using animal models and microspheres, at low flows there is a linear relationship between semiquantitative perfusion and MBF. However, as the absolute flow increases (hyperemic flow), the semiquantitative methods all significantly underestimate flow. The CER and the LV to myocardial upslope method begin to underestimate absolute MBF from 1 mL/g/min. Of the 3, the most linearly associated method is the upslope integral ratio, but even with this method the linearity decreased with flows greater than 3 mL/g/min.

Schwitter and colleagues[43] found that semiquantitative perfusion had a sensitivity, specificity, and AUC of 91%, 94%, and 93% respectively for the detection of CAD with PET as the gold standard but lower compared with quantitative angiography (diameter stenosis >50%): 87%, 85%, and 91% respectively. Not all studies are so positive; for example, Mordini and colleagues[45] compared each of the semiquantitative methods with quantitative coronary angiography, finding CER (57%, 91%, and 78%), the LV to myocardial upslope method (87%, 68%, and 82%), and the upslope integral ratio (83%, 68%, and 75%).

Overall the nonlinear relationship between semiquantitative perfusion and absolute MBF with the underestimation of hyperemic flow make semiquantitative assessment of perfusion only modestly incremental for accuracy compared with qualitative approaches for routine clinical practice, a benefit that is at best marginal given the associated time penalty of the analysis.

QUANTITATIVE CARDIOVASCULAR MAGNETIC RESONANCE PERFUSION

Standardized full quantification is desirable for more accurate measurements of CMR perfusion but has been hard. The steps involved can be described as follows:

1. Precise measurement of the arterial input function (AIF)
2. Precise measurement of myocardial enhancement
3. Sufficient temporal-spatial resolution to detect disease

4. The ability to convert the above signals into contrast concentrations [Gd]
5. A model of blood myocardium contrast behavior
6. The computing power to solve the model to derive MBF
7. The ability to do the above with sufficient accuracy, low time penalty, and in a generalizable way to be useful for clinical care

To perform these steps requires further capabilities. To convert MR signal to Gd concentration requires deep magnetic resonance (MR) imaging sequence knowledge (eg, gradient performance, understanding of prepulse limitations, coil performance, contrast nonlinearity, and signal clipping), the ability to image fast (every heartbeat, pixels across the myocardium, number of slices), the ability to motion correct images (at the varying contrast concentrations present), and the ability to segment the blood pool and therefore the myocardium. For clinical utility, this needs to be automated, but in a way that permits quality control overview by the reporting physician (ie, the display of quality control outputs) and display in a standardized format for clinicians. During first pass, Gd is very concentrated in the blood pool, resulting in T1, T2, and T2* effects not present when diluted during passage into the myocardium. A single measurement (readout) technique cannot be optimized for both. Two approaches are used: a dual-bolus approach, involving stress and rest perfusion done twice, initially with a low dose (eg, 10× lower) of Gd for blood AIF, repeated at normal dose for myocardium; or a dual-sequence approach, involving full coverage optimized for myocardium, 1 slice repeated optimized to measure blood with its high Gd concentrations (this can be low resolution).[46] There are a variety of different models of blood myocardial contrast exchange and a variety of different ways to solve these.[47] Increasing model sophistication requires increasing computational power but supplies more potential accuracy. This domain is not yet standardized and a variety of approaches are available[48] (a more comprehensive review on the models and approaches used for the quantification methods can be found in Katia Menacho and colleagues' article, "T2* Mapping Techniques: Iron Overload Assessment and Other Potential Clinical Applications," in this issue).

To assess the performance of such models requires both animal and human experimentation with increasingly robust gold standards ranging from microsphere experiments (animal models), comparator noninvasive testing (PET), and invasive testing based on coronary angiography, which needs to either quantitate luminal narrowing

Table 1
Cardiovascular magnetic resonance perfusion quantification studies

Study	Field Strength (T)	AIF	Calculation Model	Automation	Software Used	Validation
Costa et al,[51] 2007	1.5	Single bolus	Fermi deconvolution	No	In-house development	FFR
Lockie et al,[52] 2011	3.0	Single bolus	Fermi deconvolution	No	In-house development	FFR
Hsu et al,[57] 2012	1.5	Single bolus, dual sequence	Model-constrained deconvolution	Semiautomated; pixel-wise quantification	In-house development	Microspheres (dogs); Visual invasive coronary angiography (human studies)
Huber et al,[53] 2012	1.5	Single bolus	Model-independent deconvolution	No	In-house development	QCA + FFR
Morton et al,[58] 2012	1.5	Dual bolus	Fermi deconvolution	No	ViewForum Software	PET
Miller et al,[61] 2014	1.5	Single bolus	Fermi, truncated singular valued, Tikhonov regularization	No	In-house development	PET
Mordini et al,[45] 2014	1.5	Dual bolus	Fermi deconvolution	No	In-house development	QCA
Motwani et al,[54] 2014	3.0	Single bolus	Fermi deconvolution	No	In-house development	QCA
Papanastasiou et al,[55] 2016	3.0	Single bolus	Fermi and 1-barrier, 2-region distributed parameter	No	In-house development	FFR
Chung et al,[56] 2016	3.0	Single bolus	Flexible tissue homogeneity and adiabatic tissue homogeneity	No	In-house development	Visual invasive coronary angiography
Kellman et al,[64] 2017	1.5	Single bolus, dual sequence	Fermi + blood tissue exchange	Yes	Gadgetron framework	Phantom, PET
Qayyum et al,[60] 2017	1.5	Single bolus	Tikhonov regularization	No	In-house development	PET
Hsu et al,[69] 2018	1.5	Single bolus, dual sequence	Model-constrained deconvolution	—	In-house development	QCA and CTA

Abbreviation: QCA, quantitative coronary angiography

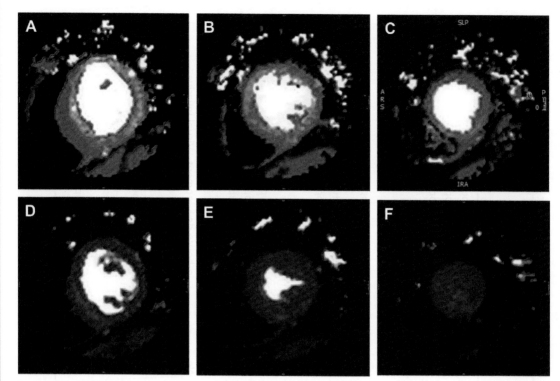

Fig. 2. MBF maps during stress with 0.56 mg/kg of dipyridamole (*A–C*) and at rest (*D–F*). The calculated MBF at stress was 2.23 mL/min/g versus the rest MBF of 0.61 mL/min/g. The MPR was normal at 3.7. First-pass perfusion images (not shown) were also considered normal, without any visual perfusion deficits. Rest and stress slices are in a slightly different location because of patient movement between acquisitions.

(three-dimensional quantitative coronary angiography, or via intracoronary wires with intravascular ultrasonography or optical coherence tomography) or measure intracoronary hemodynamics (FFR or instantaneous wave-free ratio). A summary of quantitative CMR studies using different approaches is listed in **Table 1**. The first studies in 1993 and followed up in 1998 compared MR imaging measurements with microspheres in a dog model.[49,50] These studies used a dual-bolus technique and compared with microsphere data with good correlation within a range of flow up to

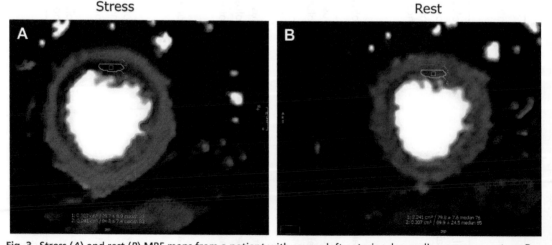

Fig. 3. Stress (*A*) and rest (*B*) MBF maps from a patient with severe left anterior descending coronary artery. During stress, the endocardial MBF in the anteroseptal wall decreased from 0.70 to 0.30 mL/min/g, a significant reduction compared with the epicardial layer, where the MBF almost did not change. The relative perfusion reserve (RPR) during rest was 0.88 but decreased significantly to 0.36 during stress, quantitatively showing the predominance of ischemia affecting the subendocardial layers.

5.0 mL/min/g both at rest and under pharmacologic stress.[42] The first human studies compared quantitative perfusion with functional assessment of stenosis using invasive FFR as the gold standard and showed good sensitivity of 92.9% but low specificity of 56.7% using an MPR cutoff of 2.04.[51] Using a high-resolution sequence at 3.0 T, there was an improvement in the accuracy of quantitative MPR versus FFR using a cutoff of 1.58 with a sensitivity of 0.80 and an improved specificity of 0.89.[52] An example of a normal quantitative stress CMR perfusion examination is shown in **Fig. 2**. Other investigators have also shown that quantitative perfusion may outperform qualitative and semiquantitative approaches with different techniques, either comparing the results with quantitative coronary angiography or invasive FFR as the gold standard.[45,53–57] Compared with PET studies, CMR showed similar accuracy for the detection of significant coronary lesions but the absolute myocardial flow values were only weakly correlated, with mean CMR MBF values slightly different than the ones obtained with PET both for stenotic and nonstenotic territories with the methods used.[58–61] Given the higher spatial resolution provided by CMR, analysis of differences in perfusion between the endocardial and epicardial layers can now be assessed more accurately and quantified, as shown in **Fig. 3** in a patient with a severe left anterior descending artery proximal lesion. This assessment of transmural perfusion gradients quantitatively may become

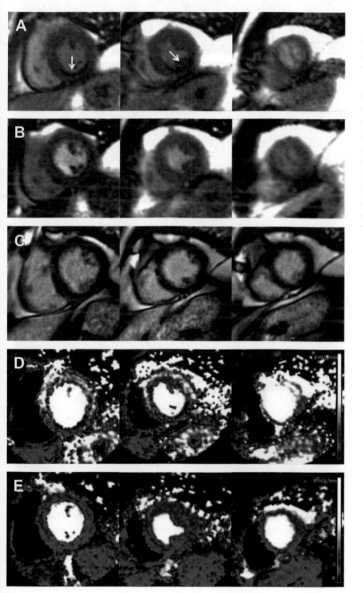

Fig. 4. Stress (A) and rest (B) perfusion in a patient with a severe stenosis of the right coronary artery. There is an adenosine-induced perfusion defect in the basal to mid inferior wall (*white arrows*). Late Gd enhancement images (C) show no associated infarction. Perfusion mapping basal, mid, and apical short-axis views are shown at stress (D) and rest (E). Perfusion is quantified automatically and in-line at the scanner at a voxel level. There is an area of hypoperfusion in the basal and mid inferior wall (0.7 mL/g/min compared with 2.7 mL/g/min in the remote myocardium). The rest flow in the inferior wall is 1.0 mL/g/min.

one of the unique applications made possible by CMR because it depends on high-resolution maps for correct analysis.[62]

FULLY AUTOMATED QUANTITATIVE CARDIOVASCULAR MAGNETIC RESONANCE PERFUSION

Recent developments in all aspects of CMR with advances in computational power have permitted full automation of quantitative perfusion either offline or, most recently, on the fly, generating perfusion maps on the scanner with each pixel color coded in milliliters per gram per minute. Kellman and Sorensen[63] first developed a dual-sequence approach integrated within the Gadgetron framework that allows all reconstruction and processing of images to be done in line and fully automated with results available within

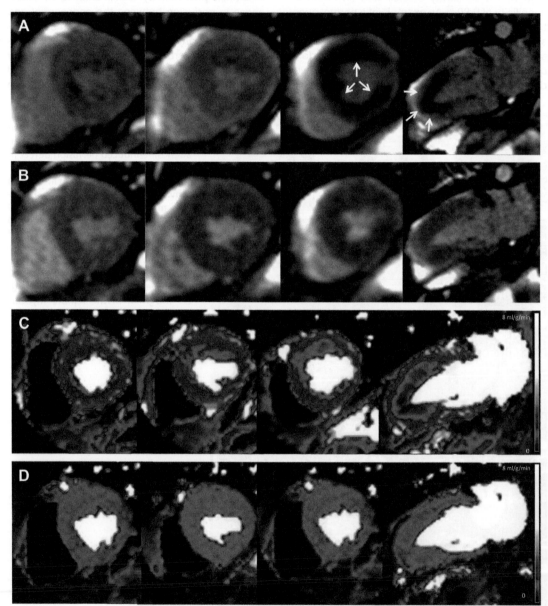

Fig. 5. Stress (*A*) and rest (*B*) perfusion in a patient with apical hypertrophic cardiomyopathy. There is an adenosine-induced perfusion defect in the hypertrophied apex at stress (*white arrows*). Perfusion mapping in the same patient in basal, mid, and apical short-axis and horizontal long-axis views at stress (*C*) and rest (*D*). Perfusion is quantified automatically and inline at the scanner at a voxel level. There is an area of hypoperfusion in the apex at stress (0.5 mL/g/min compared with 2.2 mL/g/min in the remote basal myocardium). The flow in the apex decreases at stress (a perfusion reserve <1) with flows of 1 mL/g/min measured at rest.

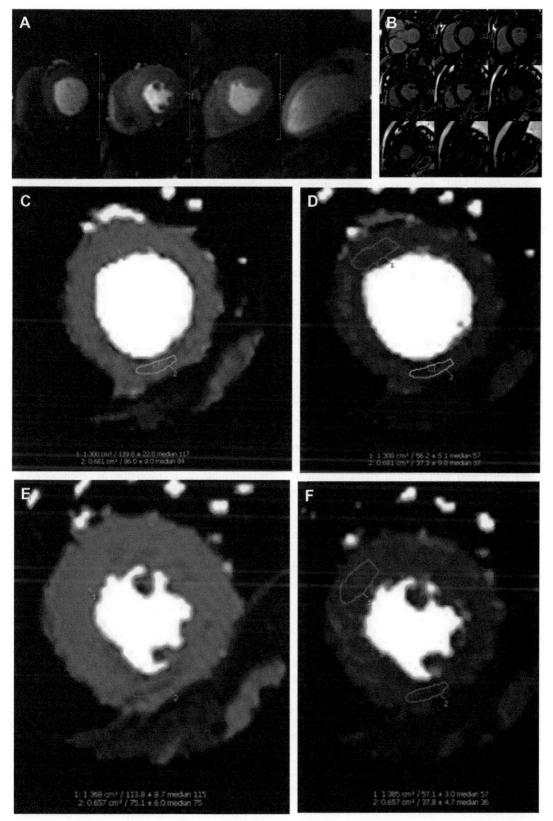

Fig. 6. A woman with known 3-vessel CAD was evaluated with CMR to determine the best treatment strategy. Qualitative first-pass perfusion images (*A*) and late Gd enhancement (*B*) did not show any significant changes.

up to 2 minutes after acquisition using a blood tissue exchange model solved by partial differential equations. The output includes the source SI first-pass images with and without motion correction plus a Gd-concentration image and an MBF map.[64] Additional quality control outputs provide the time between successive R waves on the electrocardiogram (RR interval) through the acquisition, the blood pool segmentation, and the AIF curve. **Fig. 4** shows motion-corrected first-pass images, late Gd enhancement, and the calculated MBF maps in a patient investigated for obstructive CAD with a reversible inferior-wall defect. An advantage of this approach is that the Gadgetron framework is open source and potentially deployable by all scanner manufacturers, making a standardized approach to image reconstruction/analysis possible across health care systems.

This automated method has been validated against PET with good agreement between the two approaches for global/regional perfusion, rest/stress states, and absolute/relative values.[65] The reproducibility of this approach has also been shown to be within the needs for clinical application with within-subject coefficients of variation between 8% and 12%, lower than the reported coefficients described for PET studies of between 9.6% and 21%.[66,67]

Similar automation processes have also been proposed by other investigators showing similar results compared with manual steps for calculating AIF signal and MBF values.[68] From this framework, Hsu and colleagues[69] showed that the full automated approach provided similar accuracy to the manual quantification and allowed high diagnostic performance in detecting significant CAD at both a patient and vessel level against quantitative coronary angiography and CTA.

CLINICAL APPLICATIONS OF CARDIOVASCULAR MAGNETIC RESONANCE QUANTITATIVE PERFUSION

With the wider adoption and ease of use of the newer automated techniques to perform routine CMR perfusion quantification, the clinical applications of this method should increase significantly. Initial data suggested that the diagnostic accuracy of quantitative perfusion would outperform both semiquantitative and qualitative methods of analysis (AUC, 92% vs 82% for semiquantitative methods vs 78% for qualitative; $P<.001$ for both).[45] However, this notion has been challenged more recently using data from the CE-MARC (Cardiovascular magnetic resonance and single-photon emission computed tomography for diagnosis of coronary heart disease) trial, in which investigators did not identify a difference between visual analysis and the quantitative approach.[70] Although this finding may indicate that a qualitative approach is sufficient for clinical use, it has to be taken into account that the visual diagnosis was performed by experienced users and only manual CMR quantification was used, with definite evidence for or against the superior accuracy of quantifying perfusion still not established, especially with the development of newer automated techniques.[71] One example of how quantification can improve the assessment of perfusion defects compared with visual analysis is shown in a study in which investigators showed that MBF is much lower in true perfusion defects versus in areas with dark rim artifacts, allowing easier distinction between these frequent confounding entities.[72] The example shown in **Fig. 3** also illustrates this point because the subendocardial layers had significantly lower MBF values during stress, facilitating the diagnosis of a true perfusion defect. Another example of the use of quantitative CMR perfusion is shown in **Fig. 5** in a patient with apical hypertrophic cardiomyopathy, in which subendocardial hypoperfused areas can sometimes be misinterpreted given the location of these defects.

Three-vessel CAD is a known situation in which quantitative perfusion has shown an increased diagnostic threshold compared with qualitative analysis when PET is compared with SPECT.[26] Although no focused studies with similar comparisons have been made with CMR, individual cases have already been described.[64] One example of such situation is shown in **Fig. 6**, in which a woman with known 3-vessel CAD was evaluated with CMR to determine the best treatment strategy given her poor overall clinical status and need to determine where an invasive approach would derive the best results.

Besides the assessment of diagnostic accuracy, quantitative CMR perfusion has been shown to add prognostic value compared with visual

---

When quantitative analysis was performed using the MBF maps (stress in basal and mid slices in C, E; rest in D, F), global stress MBF was significantly reduced at 1.12 mL/min/g. The relative flow reserve showed a more pronounced reduction in flow in the inferior wall (MBF of 0.75–0.86 mL/min/g) compared with the anterior wall values (MBF of 1.1–1.2 mL/min/g) and a percutaneous intervention was indicated to selectively treat the inferior-wall ischemia in order to minimize the invasive procedure.

assessment alone, with the measurement of ischemic burden either as a continuous variable or using a threshold of MPR less than 1.5 affecting an area greater than 10% of the myocardium and significantly increasing both the AUC for cardiovascular events at 2 years and improving the net reclassification index.[73] Besides that, microvascular disease assessment is another clinical use in which quantitative CMR seems to have a clear diagnostic advantage. In a group of patients without obstructive CAD but positive risk factors for atherosclerosis, reduced MPR and MBF were identified in these subjects versus healthy volunteers using quantitative CMR.[74] No differences were observed regarding native T1 or extracellular volume fraction (ECV) values and perfusion values remained significantly different even after adjusting for ventricular mass, age, and gender. The ability to monitor changes in microvascular disease with quantitative perfusion in the absence of obstructive disease and beyond traditional clinical and other imaging markers is a unique feature of CMR that may prove even more useful in future studies.

SUMMARY

CMR quantitative perfusion has evolved rapidly in recent years from a tool used only in large research centers to an applicable feature that can be used in a routine clinical environment. Accuracy and reliability of CMR perfusion quantification have been validated against many different standards, with evidence pointing to true gains compared with qualitative techniques and laborious semiquantitative approaches. Automation of processes involved in acquisition and analysis are crucial to the more widespread dissemination of these techniques, opening many opportunities for new discoveries in the pathophysiology of coronary circulation with potential novel treatment goals.

ACKNOWLEDGMENTS

The authors thank Dr Peter Kellman (Medical Signal and Image Processing Program; National Heart, Lung, and Blood Institute; NIH) for his valuable comments and suggestions to improve the article and overall support in implementing some of the sequences used in the figures. This work was directly funded by the National Institute for Health Research Biomedical Research Centre at Barts Heart Centre and University College London.

REFERENCES

1. Finegold JA, Asaria P, Francis DP. Mortality from ischaemic heart disease by country, region, and age: statistics from World Health Organisation and United Nations. Int J Cardiol 2013;168(2):934–45.

2. Beller GA, Zaret BL. Contributions of nuclear cardiology to diagnosis and prognosis of patients with coronary artery disease. Circulation 2000;101(12): 1465–78.

3. Shaw LJ, Hachamovitch R, Heller GV, et al. Noninvasive strategies for the estimation of cardiac risk in stable chest pain patients. Am J Cardiol 2000; 86(1):1–7.

4. Iskander S, Iskandrian AE. Risk assessment using single-photon emission computed tomographic technetium-99m sestamibi imaging. J Am Coll Cardiol 1998;32(1):57–62.

5. Tonino PAL, De Bruyne B, Pijls NHJ, et al. Fractional flow reserve versus angiography for guiding percutaneous coronary intervention. N Engl J Med 2009; 360(3):213–24.

6. Pijls NHJ, Fearon WF, Tonino PAL, et al. Fractional flow reserve versus angiography for guiding percutaneous coronary intervention in patients with multivessel coronary artery disease. J Am Coll Cardiol 2010;56(3):177–84.

7. De Bruyne B, Pijls NHJ, Kalesan B, et al. Fractional flow reserve–guided PCI versus medical therapy in stable coronary disease. N Engl J Med 2012; 367(11):991–1001.

8. Shaw LJ, Berman DS, Maron DJ, et al. Optimal medical therapy with or without percutaneous coronary intervention to reduce ischemic burden. Circulation 2008;117(10):1283–91.

9. Arora N, Matheny ME, Sepke C, et al. A propensity analysis of the risk of vascular complications after cardiac catheterization procedures with the use of vascular closure devices. Am Heart J 2007;153(4): 606–11.

10. Einstein AJ. Radiation risk from coronary artery disease imaging: how do different diagnostic tests compare? Heart 2008;94(12):1519–21.

11. Fihn SD, Gardin JM, Abrams J, et al. 2012 ACCF/AHA/ACP/AATS/PCNA/SCAI/STS guideline for the diagnosis and management of patients with stable ischemic heart disease: executive summary. Circulation 2012;126(25):3097–137.

12. Kelion AD, Nicol ED. The rationale for the primacy of coronary CT angiography in the National Institute for Health and Care Excellence (NICE) guideline (CG95) for the investigation of chest pain of recent onset. J Cardiovasc Comput Tomogr 2018;12(6): 516–22.

13. 2013 ESC guidelines on the management of stable coronary artery disease. Eur Heart J 2013;34(38): 2949–3003.

14. Colleran R, Douglas PS, Hadamitzky M, et al. An FFR CT diagnostic strategy versus usual care in patients with suspected coronary artery disease planned for invasive coronary angiography at

German sites: one-year results of a subgroup analysis of the PLATFORM (Prospective Longitudinal Trial of FFR CT : outcome and resource impacts) study. Open Heart 2017;4(1):e000526.

15. Fintel DJ, Links JM, Brinker JA, et al. Improved diagnostic performance of exercise thallium-201 single photon emission computed tomography over planar imaging in the diagnosis of coronary artery disease: a receiver operating characteristic analysis. J Am Coll Cardiol 1989;13(3):600–12.

16. Greenwood JP, Maredia N, Younger JF, et al. Cardiovascular magnetic resonance and single-photon emission computed tomography for diagnosis of coronary heart disease (CE-MARC): a prospective trial. Lancet 2012;379(9814):453–60.

17. Iskandrian AS, Heo J, Kong B, et al. Effect of exercise level on the ability of thallium-201 tomographic imaging in detecting coronary artery disease: Analysis of 461 patients. J Am Coll Cardiol 1989;14(6):1477–86.

18. Maddahi J, van Train K, Prigent F, et al. Quantitative single photon emission computed thallium-201 tomography for detection and localization of coronary artery disease: optimization and prospective validation of a new technique. J Am Coll Cardiol 1989;14(7):1689–99.

19. Nakazato R, Berman DS, Dey D, et al. Automated quantitative Rb-82 3D PET/CT myocardial perfusion imaging: Normal limits and correlation with invasive coronary angiography. J Nucl Cardiol 2011;19(2):265–76.

20. Schwitter J, Wacker CM, van Rossum AC, et al. MR-IMPACT: comparison of perfusion-cardiac magnetic resonance with single-photon emission computed tomography for the detection of coronary artery disease in a multicentre, multivendor, randomized trial. Eur Heart J 2008;29(4):480–9.

21. Bodi V, Sanchis J, Nunez J, et al. Prognostic value of a comprehensive cardiac magnetic resonance assessment soon after a first ST-segment elevation myocardial infarction. JACC Cardiovasc Imaging 2009;2(7):835–42.

22. Wagner A, Bruder O, Lombardi M, et al. European cardiovascular magnetic resonance (EuroCMR) registry - multi national results from 57 centers in 15 countries. J Cardiovasc Magn Reson 2013;15(S1).

23. Kramer CM, Barkhausen J, Flamm SD, et al. Standardized cardiovascular magnetic resonance (CMR) protocols 2013 update. J Cardiovasc Magn Reson 2013;15(1):91.

24. Shaw LJ, Berman DS, Picard MH, et al. Comparative definitions for moderate-severe ischemia in stress nuclear, echocardiography, and magnetic resonance imaging. JACC Cardiovasc Imaging 2014;7(6):593–604.

25. Gould KL, Goldstein RA, Mullani NA, et al. Noninvasive assessment of coronary stenoses by myocardial perfusion imaging during pharmacologic coronary vasodilation. VIII. Clinical feasibility of positron cardiac imaging without a cyclotron using generator-produced rubidium-82. J Am Coll Cardiol 1986;7(4):775–89.

26. Parkash R. Potential utility of rubidium 82 PET quantification in patients with 3-vessel coronary artery disease*1. J Nucl Cardiol 2004;11(4):440–9.

27. Patel AR, Antkowiak PF, Nandalur KR, et al. Assessment of advanced coronary artery disease. J Am Coll Cardiol 2010;56(7):561–9.

28. Kajander SA, Joutsiniemi E, Saraste M, et al. Clinical value of absolute quantification of myocardial perfusion with 15 O-water in coronary artery disease. Circ Cardiovasc Imaging 2011;4(6):678–84.

29. Herzog BA, Husmann L, Valenta I, et al. Long-term prognostic value of 13n-ammonia myocardial perfusion positron emission tomography. J Am Coll Cardiol 2009;54(2):150–6.

30. Neglia D, Michelassi C, Trivieri MG, et al. Prognostic role of myocardial blood flow impairment in idiopathic left ventricular dysfunction. Circulation 2002;105(2):186–93.

31. Maron BJ, Wolfson JK, Epstein SE, et al. Intramural ("small vessel") coronary artery disease in hypertrophic cardiomyopathy. J Am Coll Cardiol 1986;8(3):545–57.

32. Basso C. Hypertrophic cardiomyopathy and sudden death in the young: pathologic evidence of myocardial ischemia. Hum Pathol 2000;31(8):988–98.

33. Dilsizian V, Bonow RO, Epstein SE, et al. Myocardial ischemia detected by thallium scintigraphy is frequently related to cardiac arrest and syncope in young patients with hypertrophic cardiomyopathy. J Am Coll Cardiol 1993;22(3):796–804.

34. Petersen SE, Jerosch-Herold M, Hudsmith LE, et al. Evidence for microvascular dysfunction in hypertrophic cardiomyopathy. Circulation 2007;115(18):2418–25.

35. Cecchi F, Olivotto I, Gistri R, et al. Coronary microvascular dysfunction and prognosis in hypertrophic cardiomyopathy. N Engl J Med 2003;349(11):1027–35.

36. Elliott PM. Coronary microvascular dysfunction in male patients with Anderson-Fabry disease and the effect of treatment with galactosidase A. Heart 2005;92(3):357–60.

37. Dorbala S, Vangala D, Bruyere J Jr, et al. Coronary microvascular dysfunction is related to abnormalities in myocardial structure and function in cardiac amyloidosis. JACC Heart Fail 2014;2(4):358–67.

38. Li R, Yang ZG, Wen LY, et al. Regional myocardial microvascular dysfunction in cardiac amyloid light-chain amyloidosis: assessment with 3T cardiovascular magnetic resonance. J Cardiovasc Magn Reson 2016;18:16.

39. Ingkanisorn WP, Kwong RY, Bohme NS, et al. Prognosis of negative adenosine stress magnetic

resonance in patients presenting to an emergency department with chest pain. J Am Coll Cardiol 2006;47(7):1427–32.

40. Jahnke C, Nagel E, Gebker R, et al. Prognostic value of cardiac magnetic resonance stress tests. Circulation 2007;115(13):1769–76.

41. Vincenti G, Masci PG, Monney P, et al. Stress perfusion CMR in patients with known and suspected CAD: prognostic value and optimal ischemic threshold for revascularization. JACC Cardiovasc Imaging 2017;10(5):526–37.

42. Christian TF, Rettmann DW, Aletras AH, et al. Absolute myocardial perfusion in canines measured by using dual-bolus first-pass MR imaging. Radiology 2004;232(3):677–84.

43. Schwitter J, Nanz D, Kneifel S, et al. Assessment of myocardial perfusion in coronary artery disease by magnetic resonance. Circulation 2001;103(18): 2230–5.

44. Klocke FJ, Simonetti OP, Judd RM, et al. Limits of detection of regional differences in vasodilated flow in viable myocardium by first-pass magnetic resonance perfusion imaging. Circulation 2001; 104(20):2412–6.

45. Mordini FE, Haddad T, Hsu LY, et al. Diagnostic accuracy of stress perfusion CMR in comparison with quantitative coronary angiography: fully quantitative, semiquantitative, and qualitative assessment. JACC Cardiovasc Imaging 2014;7(1):14–22.

46. Feher A, Sinusas AJ. Quantitative assessment of coronary microvascular function: dynamic single-photon emission computed tomography, positron emission tomography, ultrasound, computed tomography, and magnetic resonance imaging. Circ Cardiovasc Imaging 2017;10(8) [pii:e006427].

47. Biglands JD, Magee DR, Sourbron SP, et al. Comparison of the diagnostic performance of four quantitative myocardial perfusion estimation methods used in cardiac MR imaging: CE-MARC substudy. Radiology 2015;275(2):393–402.

48. van Dijk R, van Assen M, Vliegenthart R, et al. Diagnostic performance of semi-quantitative and quantitative stress CMR perfusion analysis: a meta-analysis. J Cardiovasc Magn Reson 2017;19(1):92.

49. Wilke N, Simm C, Zhang J, et al. Contrast-enhanced first pass myocardial perfusion imaging: correlation between myocardial blood flow in dogs at rest and during hyperemia. Magn Reson Med 1993;29(4): 485–97.

50. Jerosch-Herold M, Wilke N, Stillman AE. Magnetic resonance quantification of the myocardial perfusion reserve with a Fermi function model for constrained deconvolution. Med Phys 1998;25(1):73–84.

51. Costa MA, Shoemaker S, Futamatsu H, et al. Quantitative magnetic resonance perfusion imaging detects anatomic and physiologic coronary artery disease as measured by coronary angiography

and fractional flow reserve. J Am Coll Cardiol 2007;50(6):514–22.

52. Lockie T, Ishida M, Perera D, et al. High-resolution magnetic resonance myocardial perfusion imaging at 3.0-Tesla to detect hemodynamically significant coronary stenoses as determined by fractional flow reserve. J Am Coll Cardiol 2011;57(1):70–5.

53. Huber A, Sourbron S, Klauss V, et al. Magnetic resonance perfusion of the myocardium: semiquantitative and quantitative evaluation in comparison with coronary angiography and fractional flow reserve. Invest Radiol 2012;47(6):332–8.

54. Motwani M, Kidambi A, Sourbron S, et al. Quantitative three-dimensional cardiovascular magnetic resonance myocardial perfusion imaging in systole and diastole. J Cardiovasc Magn Reson 2014;16:19.

55. Papanastasiou G, Williams MC, Dweck MR, et al. Quantitative assessment of myocardial blood flow in coronary artery disease by cardiovascular magnetic resonance: comparison of Fermi and distributed parameter modeling against invasive methods. J Cardiovasc Magn Reson 2016;18(1):57.

56. Chung S, Shah B, Storey P, et al. Quantitative perfusion analysis of first-pass contrast enhancement kinetics: application to MRI of myocardial perfusion in coronary artery disease. PLoS One 2016;11(9): e0162067.

57. Hsu LY, Groves DW, Aletras AH, et al. A quantitative pixel-wise measurement of myocardial blood flow by contrast-enhanced first-pass CMR perfusion imaging: microsphere validation in dogs and feasibility study in humans. JACC Cardiovasc Imaging 2012; 5(2):154–66.

58. Morton G, Chiribiri A, Ishida M, et al. Quantification of absolute myocardial perfusion in patients with coronary artery disease: comparison between cardiovascular magnetic resonance and positron emission tomography. J Am Coll Cardiol 2012;60(16): 1546–55.

59. Papanastasiou G, Williams MC, Dweck MR, et al. Multimodality quantitative assessments of myocardial perfusion using dynamic contrast enhanced magnetic resonance and (15)O-labelled water positron emission tomography imaging. IEEE Trans Radiat Plasma Med Sci 2018;2(3):259–71.

60. Qayyum AA, Qayyum F, Larsson HB, et al. Comparison of rest and adenosine stress quantitative and semi-quantitative myocardial perfusion using magnetic resonance in patients with ischemic heart disease. Clin Imaging 2017;41:149–56.

61. Miller CA, Naish JH, Ainslie MP, et al. Voxel-wise quantification of myocardial blood flow with cardiovascular magnetic resonance: effect of variations in methodology and validation with positron emission tomography. J Cardiovasc Magn Reson 2014; 16:11.

62. Chiribiri A, Hautvast GL, Lockie T, et al. Assessment of coronary artery stenosis severity and location: quantitative analysis of transmural perfusion gradients by high-resolution MRI versus FFR. JACC Cardiovasc Imaging 2013;6(5):600–9.

63. Hansen MS, Sorensen TS. Gadgetron: an open source framework for medical image reconstruction. Magn Reson Med 2013;69(6):1768–76.

64. Kellman P, Hansen MS, Nielles-Vallespin S, et al. Myocardial perfusion cardiovascular magnetic resonance: optimized dual sequence and reconstruction for quantification. J Cardiovasc Magn Reson 2017; 19(1):43.

65. Engblom H, Xue H, Akil S, et al. Fully quantitative cardiovascular magnetic resonance myocardial perfusion ready for clinical use: a comparison between cardiovascular magnetic resonance imaging and positron emission tomography. J Cardiovasc Magn Reson 2017;19(1):78.

66. Brown LAE, Onciul SC, Broadbent DA, et al. Fully automated, inline quantification of myocardial blood flow with cardiovascular magnetic resonance: repeatability of measurements in healthy subjects. J Cardiovasc Magn Reson 2018;20(1):48.

67. Kitkungvan D, Johnson NP, Roby AE, et al. Routine clinical quantitative rest stress myocardial perfusion for managing coronary artery disease: clinical relevance of test-retest variability. JACC Cardiovasc Imaging 2017;10(5):565–77.

68. Jacobs M, Benovoy M, Chang LC, et al. Evaluation of an automated method for arterial input function detection for first-pass myocardial perfusion cardiovascular magnetic resonance. J Cardiovasc Magn Reson 2016;18:17.

69. Hsu LY, Jacobs M, Benovoy M, et al. Diagnostic performance of fully automated pixel-wise quantitative myocardial perfusion imaging by cardiovascular magnetic resonance. JACC Cardiovasc Imaging 2018;11(5):697–707.

70. Biglands JD, Ibraheem M, Magee DR, et al. Quantitative myocardial perfusion imaging versus visual analysis in diagnosing myocardial ischemia: a CE-MARC substudy. JACC Cardiovasc Imaging 2018;11(5):711–8.

71. Axel L. Is qualitative cardiac perfusion MRI "Good Enough"? JACC Cardiovasc Imaging 2018;11(5): 719–21.

72. Ta AD, Hsu LY, Conn HM, et al. Fully quantitative pixel-wise analysis of cardiovascular magnetic resonance perfusion improves discrimination of dark rim artifact from perfusion defects associated with epicardial coronary stenosis. J Cardiovasc Magn Reson 2018;20(1):16.

73. Sammut EC, Villa ADM, Di Giovine G, et al. Prognostic value of quantitative stress perfusion cardiac magnetic resonance. JACC Cardiovasc Imaging 2018;11(5):686–94.

74. Zorach B, Shaw PW, Bourque J, et al. Quantitative cardiovascular magnetic resonance perfusion imaging identifies reduced flow reserve in microvascular coronary artery disease. J Cardiovasc Magn Reson 2018;20(1):14.

Comprehensive Assessment of Cardiac Involvement in Muscular Dystrophies by Cardiac MR Imaging

Carlos Eduardo Rochitte, MD, PhD[a,b,*], Gabriela Liberato, MD[a], Marly Conceição Silva, MD, PhD[c]

KEYWORDS

- Muscular dystrophies • Duchenne • Becker • Cardiac MR imaging

KEY POINTS

- Muscular dystrophies are myogenic muscle disorders characterized by degradation and loss of function, with variable distribution and severity.
- Cardiac involvement is manifested predominantly as hypertrophic, dilated, and arrhythmic cardiomyopathy, with high morbidity and mortality.
- Cardiovascular MR imaging may be of considerable value for early detection of cardiac disease before the onset of cardiac symptoms and electrocardiography and echocardiogram abnormalities.

INTRODUCTION

Muscular dystrophies are myogenic muscle disorders characterized by degradation and loss of function, with variable distribution and severity. They are caused by mutations in genes encoding various proteins responsible for muscle contraction and consequent muscle weakness and progressive loss of function.[1] According to the pattern of inheritance and localization of muscle weakness, they can be classified as specific muscular dystrophies.[2,3] The most prevalent dystrophies commonly associated with cardiac complications include Duchenne, Becker, and female patients carrying mutations in the dystrophin gene; and limb-girdle, Emery-Dreifuss, and myotonic muscular dystrophies.[1] These specific muscular dystrophies and their cardiac involvement phenotypes assessed by cardiovascular MR (CMR) imaging are described in **Table 1**.

Cardiac involvement is manifested predominantly as hypertrophic, dilated, and arrhythmic cardiomyopathy, with high morbidity and mortality. Arrhythmias are very frequent and may manifest with the event of the sudden cardiac death.[1] Patients with a molecularly confirmed diagnosis of Duchenne muscular dystrophy have a median survival of 24 years. The cardiac involvement detected by diagnostic imaging usually precedes the clinical symptoms, considering the limited mobility of these

Disclosures: The authors have nothing to disclose.
[a] Heart Institute (InCor), Clinical Hospital HCFMUSP, University of Sao Paulo Medical School, Brazil, Avenida Dr. Enéas de Carvalho Aguiar, 44, Cerqueira César, São Paulo, SP 05403-000, Brazil; [b] Heart Hospital (HCOR), Hospital do Coração, São Paulo, São Paulo, Brazil; [c] Axial Diagnostic Center, Belo Horizonte, Rua Níquel, 181 Apto 301, Serra - Belo Horizonte, Minas Gerais 30220-280, Brazil
* Corresponding author. Heart Institute, InCor, University of Sao Paulo Medical School, Brazil, Cardiovascular Magnetic Resonance and Computed Tomography Department, Avenida Dr. Enéas de Carvalho Aguiar, 44, Cerqueira César, São Paulo, SP 05403-000, Brazil.
E-mail address: rochitte@incor.usp.br

Magn Reson Imaging Clin N Am 27 (2019) 521–531
https://doi.org/10.1016/j.mric.2019.04.009
1064-9689/19/© 2019 Elsevier Inc. All rights reserved.

Table 1
MR imaging characteristics of the types of muscular dystrophy

Dystrophy	Clinical Features	CMR Imaging Features
DMD BMD	Age of onset: 3–7 y Age of onset: teenage years	Subepicardial fibrosis of the inferolateral wall or transmural LGE
Female DMD or BMD mutation carriers	Cardiac screening has been recommended after the teenage years	Myocardial fibrosis similar to DMD patients, including transmural LGE
EDMD	Bimodal distribution: first or second decade, sometimes adult onset	CMR imaging data are limited Normal myocardium is replaced by fibrous and adipose tissue, usually starting in the atria Myocardial fibrosis does not necessarily precede systolic dysfunction Midwall LGE may occur in the basal or mid ventricular septum segments
LGMD	Variable onset (early childhood to adulthood)	AD subtype: midwall LGE of the basal interventricular septum well before the onset of LV dilatation and systolic dysfunction LGMD2I: midwall or subepicardial fibrosis of the septum and inferior wall (extensive lateral wall LGE has also been described)
MD	MD1 Early childhood to adulthood onset, rarely during infancy (congenital form) MD2 adult onset, usually fourth decade	MD patients may present cardiomyopathy (usually more benign in MD2 than in MD1), dilatation, systolic dysfunction, hypertrophy, and (occasionally) noncompaction LGE data are limited, although septum and basal inferolateral midwall fibrosis has been reported

Abbreviations: AD, autosomal dominant inheritance; DMD, Duchenne muscular dystrophy; EDMD, Emery-Dreifuss muscular dystrophy; LGE, late gadolinium enhancement; LGMD, limb-girdle muscular dystrophy; LV, left ventricular; MD, myotonic dystrophy.

patients.[1,4] With the respiratory care improvement, cardiac disorders have become the leading cause of mortality in many of these patients.[5,6] The early detection of cardiac involvement also enables early cardioprotective treatment with consequent reduction of the cardiac remodeling and attenuation of heart failure symptoms, which is presented in several recently published studies, mainly in dystrophinopathies.[7–12]

Electrocardiogram (ECG) and echocardiogram are routinely used in the evaluation of these patients; however, in many of these diseases, their ability to detect early and subclinical involvement of the heart muscle is limited. CMR imaging has contributed to the early diagnosis of cardiac involvement in various muscular dystrophies, allowing early treatment and possibly reduction of mortality.[10–13]

MUSCULAR DYSTROPHIES RELATED TO DYSTROPHINOPATHIES

Duchenne and Becker muscular dystrophies are genetically determined diseases caused by a mutation in the dystrophin gene located on the X chromosome Xp21 locus. Dystrophin connects the muscle fiber cytoskeleton with the extracellular matrix and is responsible for the stability of muscle fibers during the muscular contraction. With reduced amount (Becker) or absence (Duchenne) of dystrophin occur successive sarcolemma microruptures during muscle contraction, with the consequent necrosis and replacement of the fibers by adipose and fibrous tissue. In DMD, after a short motor development period that is apparently normal, there is progressive and irreversible muscle degeneration with consequent muscle weakness.[14]

Duchenne muscular dystrophy (DMD) is the most common of all muscular dystrophies (1 out of 3000–5000) and BMD is 10 times less frequent.[15]

In the natural history of these dystrophies, there is involvement of skeletal muscle groups, such as the lower members and respiratory muscles, and also the myocardium. Symptoms of heart failure may be nonspecific, such as fatigue, weight loss, vomiting, and sleep disorders.[4] These patients often develop arrhythmias and may have complete atrioventricular (AV) block associated with severe systolic dysfunction in the final stage of the disease.[16,17] The main cause of death is respiratory and/or heart failure. However, with the optimization of respiratory care, the main cause of death has been reported to be of cardiac origin.

An approach for early diagnosis of cardiac involvement of these dystrophies is essential to maximize the length and quality of life. Even clinical data such as early diagnosis of blood pressure changes can trigger useful appropriate therapy potentially leading to increased life expectancy.[18] More specifically, echocardiography is routinely used in the diagnosis of cardiomyopathy. Approximately 28% of patients with DMD exhibit cardiac abnormalities detectable by echocardiogram at the age of 14 years and 57% by the age of 18 years.[17] In DMD patients, an echocardiogram may be limited by a poor acoustic window due to kyphoscoliosis associated with disease progression and the chest adiposity in most patients

from the chronic use of corticosteroids. In contrast, CMR imaging is reproducible and allows full access to the evaluation of global and regional ventricular function (a gold standard method) and myocardial tissue characterization.

Previous studies showed that cardiac involvement is insidious and precedes the onset of symptoms of heart failure, occurring usually after adolescence.[4] In 2007, Silva and colleagues[11] reported, for the first time, the presence of myocardial fibrosis (MF) detected by CMR imaging in subjects with DMD and BMD who had no clinical signs of cardiac involvement or cardiac alterations detectable by conventional echocardiogram, chest radiograph, and ECG. Seven of 10 subjects (70%) had MF. Nonischemic late gadolinium enhancement (LGE) with midwall and subepicardial involvement of the left ventricular (LV) lateral segments was the most frequent pattern of fibrosis (89%): midwall in 57.8% and subepicardial in 31.1% (**Fig. 1**).

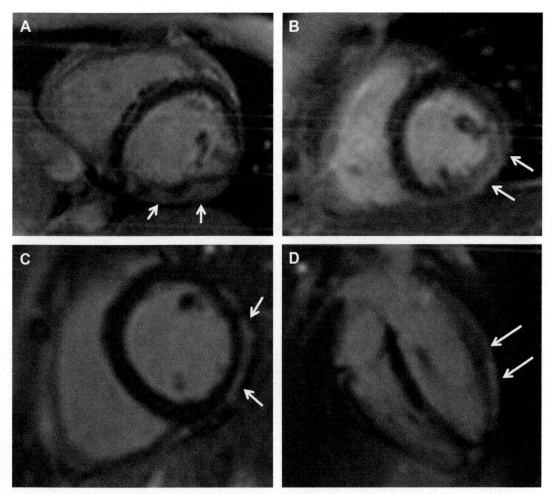

Fig. 1. Myocardial fibrosis in patients with muscular dystrophy. CMR imaging short-axis and long-axis views showing LGE (*arrows*) in the left ventricle. (*A, B*) DMD. (*C, D*) BMD.

In subjects with systolic dysfunction, the agreement between the segmental MF extent and the degree of segmental dysfunction was fair (kappa 0.31, P<.001), emphasizing the importance of fibrosis in the development of cardiomyopathy. Interestingly, MF was detected in very young subjects: in 2 of 4 subjects younger than 10 years old and with a normal echocardiogram. Moreover, of 7 subjects with MF, only 2 had abnormal echocardiography.

LGE is considered the gold standard noninvasive method to detect MF, reaffirming the importance of CMR imaging to detect cardiac involvement and guide early treatment of a variety of cardiomyopathies,[19,20] and has also been advocated as such in muscular dystrophies.[9–12,21] In the specific case of BMD, **Fig. 2** presents an autopsy case with macroscopic and histopathological validation of LGE by CMR imaging accurately indicating the areas with MF by Masson trichrome stain. To the authors' knowledge, this is the first figure demonstration of such a cross-correlation

between LGE by CMR imaging and MF by pathologic assessment in BMD (see **Fig. 2**).

A randomized clinical trial was conducted by Silva and colleagues[10] in 2 centers, and included 76 male subjects with DMD or BMD (mean age at baseline ~13 years) undergoing 2 CMR imaging studies with a 2-year interval for ventricular function and MF assessment. In a non–intent-to-treat trial, 42 subjects with MF and normal LV ejection fraction (LVEF) were randomized (1:1) to receive or not receive angiotensin converting enzyme (ACE) inhibitor therapy. Chest radiography, ECG, and echocardiogram were also carried out in this period.

MF was present in 72% of the subjects and LV systolic dysfunction in only 24% of them. The pattern of MF was mostly midwall and subepicardial, predominantly affecting lateral and inferior LV segments (**Fig. 3**).

MF at baseline was an independent predictor of lower LVEF at follow-up (P = .03). Among subjects with MF and preserved ejection fraction, those randomized to receive ACE inhibitors

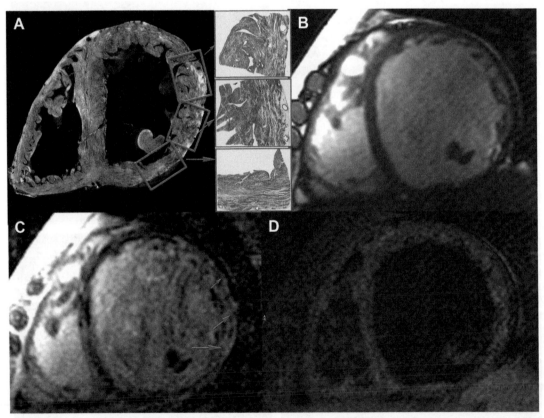

Fig. 2. Patient with BMD who died and underwent autopsy, showing MF by pathologic assessment in the same slice and segments showing LGE by CMR imaging. (A) Macroscopic pathologic assessment of a left ventricle short-axis with corresponding histopathological slides using Masson trichrome stain (*red boxes*). (B) Cine steady-state free precession (SSFP) image at the same level in diastole showing LV dilatation and thin walls. (C) LGE (*red arrows*) corresponding to same areas with myocardial fibrosis seen on pathologic assessment. (D) T2-weighted triple–inversion recovery fast spin echo (IR FSE) image showing no signs of myocardial edema.

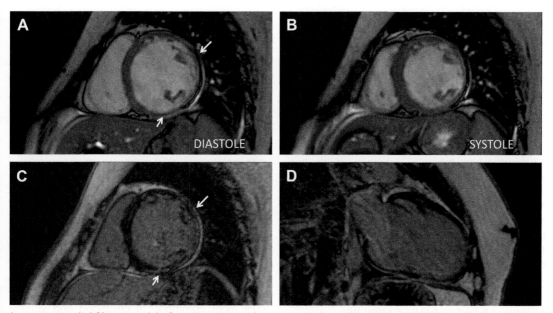

Fig. 3. Myocardial fibrosis and dysfunction in muscular dystrophy by CMR imaging. (*A, B*) Cine sequences in short-axis view. (*C, D*) LGE in short-axis and long-axis views. A patient with DMD showing inferior and lateral myocardial LGE (*arrows* on *C*) along with akinesia of these segments (*arrows* on *A*, note the absence of thickening in the same segments on *B*) and severe global LV dysfunction (comparing A and B).

demonstrated slower MF progression compared with the untreated group (*P* = .001), even though all groups have had MF progression.

There was a significant positive correlation between age and the amount of MF identified by CMR imaging, both at baseline and at follow-up (correlation coefficients, *r* = 0.52 at baseline and *r* = 0.50 at follow-up; *P*<.001 for both). Moreover, all the studied age groups presented MF and progression up to the age of 15 to 16 years, and slower progression after that.

Subjects with MF noted on CMR imaging had a higher probability of cardiovascular events (*P* = .04).

In multivariate analysis, ACE inhibitor therapy was an independent indicator of decreased MF progression (*P* = .04). This study demonstrated that the use of ACE inhibitors in subjects with DMD and BMD diagnosed with MF by CMR imaging caused a reduction of the progression of MF in a period of 2 years. These findings reinforce the need for early diagnosis and treatment of cardiac involvement in subjects with DMD and BMD before the onset of symptoms. ECG, echocardiogram, and chest radiograph showed low sensitivity and negative predictive value for early detection of cardiac involvement in DMD and BMD, reinforcing the usefulness of CMR imaging in this clinical setting.[10]

A key aspect in cardiac involvement in BMD or DMD patients is the genetic profile. Jefferies and colleagues[8] showed a strong association between mutations in exons 12 and 14 to 17 with LV

dysfunction. Additionally, the investigators showed that mutation in exons 51 to 54 and 68 to 71 had a possible cardioprotective effect. Other studies pointed out that some dystrophin isoforms are absent in the myocardium and are transcribed in exons greater than 45 and 56.[22,23] A randomized trial by Silva and colleagues[24,25] was the first to demonstrate that subjects with mutations in exons less than 45 had greater amounts of MF and lower LVEF in both basal and follow-up CMR imaging studies. There was a significant correlation between the site of mutation in the dystrophin gene and MF. Mutations in exons greater than or equal to 45 appear to protect against cardiac involvement. However, the impact of these findings on clinical management remains to be determined.

Ashford and colleagues[26] studied subjects with DMD and demonstrated subclinical cardiac dysfunction using the myocardial tagging technique of CMR imaging with alteration of segmental contractility in the lateral and inferior walls.

A clinical trial was conducted by Raman and colleagues[27] that enrolled boys aged 7 years or older with DMD. It was demonstrated that, at an early stage of myocardial disease (myocardial damage by LGE CMR imaging and preserved ejection fraction), the addition of eplerenone to background ACE inhibitors or angiotensin receptor blocker (ARB) therapy attenuates the progressive decline in LV systolic function (LV circumferential strain; *P* = .020).

A working group of the National Heart, Lung, and Blood Institute (NHLBI) published an update (NHLBI 2015) on the cardiac involvement in DMD.[16] CMR imaging was considered as a noninvasive modality of choice except in young patients who do not cooperate with the maneuvers necessary to accomplish the examination. Echocardiogram should be performed until the age of 6 to 7 years. After this, at least 1 CMR imaging should be performed every 2 years, and annually after 10 years when the risk increases of cardiac involvement (MF, dilated left ventricle and ventricular dysfunction). Traditionally, ACE inhibitors and ARBs have been used as first-line treatment in cardiac patients with DMD or Becker muscular dystrophy. The NHLBI 2014 recommends the use of ACE inhibitors or ARBs in patients 10 years or older with DMD.[16]

CARDIAC INVOLVEMENT IN FEMALE MUSCULAR DYSTROPHY CARRIERS

Female DMD or BMD carriers are mostly free of skeletal muscle symptoms but they are also prone to cardiomyopathy. Florian and colleagues[21] showed that 47% of the carriers of these mutations showed at least 1 positive finding in CMR imaging. LGE was present in 44% of these subjects. The LGE pattern was predominantly subepicardial.[21] In 2018, Birnkrant and colleagues[28] published a recommendation to perform a cardiac evaluation in early adulthood that includes an ECG and CMR imaging and to consider a follow-up every 3 to 5 years.

LIMB-GIRDLE MUSCULAR DYSTROPHIES

The girdle muscular dystrophy type (limb-girdle muscular dystrophies [LGMDs]) comprises a heterogeneous group of genetically determined diseases that present with variable skeletal muscle and cardiac involvement. It is characterized by weakness of the proximal waist members (scapular and pelvic girdle, and trunk). This is an example of nonallelic genetic heterogeneity (ie, resulting in different genes), such as phenotype, and identifies various forms of LGMD.[29] There are different abnormalities of the dystrophin-dystroglycan-sarcoglycan complex that can lead to instability and damage of the muscle fiber, including myocyte.[30,31]

Autosomal dominant (AD) and recessive inheritance patterns have been identified. The more common autosomal recessive subtypes usually have an earlier age of onset and show more rapid disease progression compared with AD variants. The subtypes most commonly associated with cardiac involvement and manifested as conduction defects and/or myocardial disease are LGMD1A, LGMD1B, LGMD2C-F, and LGMD2I and LGMD2B.[29] In 2011, Rosales and colleagues[13] published a CMR imaging study in 16 subjects with the LGMD2I and LGMD2B forms, and found that 47% showed the presence of subclinical MF: in 57% of subjects with LGMDB2I and in 33% of subjects with LGMD2B, usually accompanied by diastolic dysfunction. The LGE pattern was mainly epicardial, similar to other progressive muscular dystrophies. One of the subjects with LGMD2I with advanced cardiomyopathy also presented with extensive MF. These findings reinforce the use CMR imaging for early detection of cardiac involvement and the presence of MF.[13]

EMERY-DREIFUSS MUSCULAR DYSTROPHY

Emery-Dreifuss muscular dystrophy (EDMD) occurs most commonly in childhood and adolescence, and is characterized by signs of chronic myopathy. Most cases of EDMD are inherited as an X-linked recessive trait; however, a rarer AD form has also been described.[32]

The X-linked and AD forms of the disease are clinically similar and are caused by defects of the nuclear membrane proteins emerin and lamins A or C, respectively. Deficiency of these proteins causes muscle weakness and atrophy, joint contracture, and cardiomyopathy, especially associated with AV conduction defects.[32,33]

Cardiac involvement in patients with EDMD is common and usually begins in the third decade with progressive muscle weakness. Owing to the conduction defects, there is a high risk of sudden death, necessitating mandatory careful follow-up of these patients.[34] In EDMD, the normal myocardium is progressively replaced by fibro-fatty tissue, a process that usually begins in the atrium, leading to arrhythmias, and often involves the AV node, requiring implantation of a pacemaker. It eventually affects the ventricles, causing progressive dilatation and systolic dysfunction.[35]

Mutations in the genes that encode lamins A and C have been reported as an important cause of dilated cardiomyopathy.[36] Holmström and colleagues[37] showed 17 subjects with mutations in the gene lamins A and C, and 15 subjects presented with LGE. In all subjects, midwall LGE occurred in the basal or mid ventricular septum segments. Contractility abnormalities were noted in greater than 50% of the segments. All subjects with MF showed an AV conduction defect. Many of them had mild systolic dysfunction and univentricular or biventricular dilatation. The investigators suggest that MF may indicate pacemaker implantation to prevent sudden deaths and early pharmacologic treatment of cardiomyopathy.[37]

MYOTONIC DYSTROPHY

Myotonic dystrophy (MD) produces progressive muscle weakness and abnormal cardiac conduction. Two types are identified: MD1 and MD2. MD1, also known as Steinert dystrophy is the most common form of adult muscular dystrophy with an estimated incidence of 1 in 8500. MD1 is associated with abnormal expansion of the DMPK gene encoding protein kinase.[38]

AV and intraventricular conduction defects are common in both types (MD1 and MD2). The cardiomyopathy is usually more benign in MD2 compared with MD1. Structural heart disease is also frequently observed, with LV hypertrophy or dilation in approximately 20% and systolic dysfunction in 14% of the subjects.[39]

Patients with MD1 usually die from heart or respiratory complications. It has been reported that marked abnormalities on ECG and atrial arrhythmias are independent risk factors for sudden death in patients with MD1; when they are associated, the risk is greatly increased.[34,40]

Hermans and colleagues[41] studied 80 subjects with MD1, 45 male and 35 female, and demonstrated that 44% of subjects had structural or functional cardiac abnormalities detected by CMR imaging. Systolic dysfunction was the most common finding (20 subjects), more common in men than in women, and associated with advanced age. MF detected by LGE technique was observed in 13% of subjects. Septum and basal inferolateral were the segments most affected, and the predominant pattern was midwall.[41] Patients with MF have high risk of ventricular tachycardia and sudden death.[42] Hermans and colleagues[41] described that MF diagnosed by CMR imaging may be a predictor of mortality in MD1 patients.

The most common muscular dystrophy CMR imaging phenotypes, modified from previous publications[13,41,43,44], are shown on **Fig. 4**.

T1 AND T2 MAPPING AND MUSCULAR DYSTROPHY

Parametric mapping is a noninvasive CMR imaging tool for quantifying tissue alterations in myocardial disease. T1 mapping can be used to estimate the myocardial extracellular volume (ECV), a validated surrogate marker of diffuse and interstitial fibrosis in the absence of confounders (eg, infiltration). It is based on the change in T1 values following the injection of conventional extracellular T1-shortening agents (eg, gadolinium-based contrasts). T2-weighted CMR imaging is commonly used to assess myocardial inflammation. However, image quality, reproducibility, and subjective assessment of T2-weighted images have been limiting factors in its clinical adoption. To overcome these challenges, regional myocardial T2 mapping has emerged to directly quantify local myocardial inflammation and edema.[45]

Muscular dystrophy patients are more prone to myocarditis compared with the rest of population because abnormal dystrophin acts as a vehicle for different viruses.[46,47] Heart failure treatment is typically started or intensified when myocardial dysfunction and/or LGE develop. However, even patients with normal LVEF and no LGE have elevated ECV and T1 values.[48] This observation suggests that T1 mapping, and perhaps native T1 more than ECV,[49] may identify the onset of fibrotic remodeling earlier than LGE and ejection fraction, providing an opportunity for a more timely intervention.

Other advanced tissue characterization techniques are available for CMR, but they are either under development or not yet systematically tested in muscular dystrophy patients. Among those are techniques for black-blood myocardial delayed enhancement, with and without fat sat, fat-water separation imaging, blood oxygenated level dependent imaging, spin labeling, and even other nuclei imaging such as sodium-23 imaging. Their potential usefulness should be investigated in the future.

MYOCARDIAL FEATURE TRACKING IMAGING

CMR feature tracking (CMR-FT) imaging can calculate myocardial strains precisely and has been able to detect differences between subjects with DMD and controls not detected by speckle tracking echocardiography–derived strains.

CMR-FT imaging was sensitive enough to differentiate subjects with and without LGE and may be able to identify LGE-positive segments in DMD without the use of gadolinium contrast.[50]

The sensitive approach of CMR-FT imaging may be useful in patients with global preserved LVEF, and may be able to delineate the presence and course of myocardial disease and, therefore, be a useful tool for evaluating new therapies planned to avoid or delay the onset and progression of heart failure.[26]

However, these new and advanced techniques for measuring myocardial contractility are still in their infancy regarding muscular dystrophy. Not only technical development but also and, more

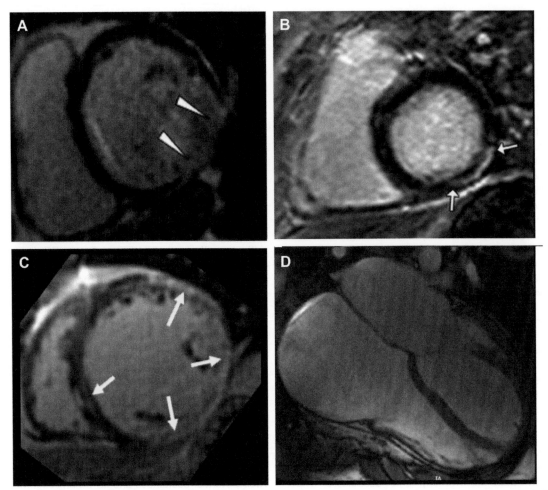

Fig. 4. Muscular dystrophies CMR imaging phenotypes. (*A*) LGE image showing extensive enhancement in the left ventricle inferolateral segment (*arrowheads*) indicating myocardial fibrosis in a female Duchenne carrier. (*B*) A patient with myotonic muscular dystrophy type 1 showing mid-wall inferolateral LGE (*white arrows*). (*C*) A patient with LGMD type 2I and advanced dilated cardiomyopathy with extensive myocardial injury or fibrosis (*yellow arrows*). (*D*) Cine-MR image (SSFP) in a 4-chamber view with severe dilatation of both atria in a patient with EDMD. (*Modified from* [*A*] Rosales XQ, Moser SJ, Tran T, et al. Cardiovascular magnetic resonance of cardiomyopathy in limb girdle muscular dystrophy 2B and 2I. J Cardiovasc Magn Reson 2011;13:39; [*B*] Hermans MC, Faber CG, Bekkers SC, et al. Structural and functional cardiac changes in myotonic dystrophy type 1: a cardiovascular magnetic resonance study. J Cardiovasc Magn Reson 2012;14:48; [*C*] Rodriguez-Torres D, Jimenez-Jaimez J, Macias-Ruiz R, et al. Cardiac manifestations of neuromuscular disease. Rev Esp Cardiol (Engl Ed) 2018;71:580-582; [*D*] Verhaert D, Richards K, Rafael-Fortney JA, et al. Cardiac involvement in patients with muscular dystrophies: magnetic resonance imaging phenotype and genotypic considerations. Circ Cardiovasc Imaging 2011;4:67-76.)

importantly, randomized clinical trials on this specific issue of investigation are mandatory to determine the clinical value of CMR-FT imaging for muscular dystrophy patients.

RECOMMENDED CARDIOVASCULAR MR IMAGING PROTOCOL ACQUISITION

When planning a CMR imaging examination on muscular dystrophy patients, one must keep in mind the clinical conditions of the patient regarding breath holding and standing still

capabilities. Of paramount importance are the thoracic deformities that do not allow patients to lie down for a long period of time in the scanner. In a perfect scenario, the authors recommend at least the following basic protocol:

1. Localizers
2. Cine steady-state free precession (SSFP) short-axis and long-axis planes
3. Edema T2 or T2 mapping
4. T1 mapping (precontrast or native T1 map, 3 short-axis slices)

- Gadolinium contrast–based injection
5. LGE short-axis and long-axis
6. T1 mapping (15 minutes postcontrast, 3 short-axis slices).

Real-time cine techniques or sequences with free breathing may be used as well.

When the complete protocol cannot be performed, the authors suggest

1. Localizers
2. T1 mapping (precontrast, 1 slice); gadolinium contrast–based injection
3. LGE short-axis and long-axis (single-shot as an option, with SSFP readout)
4. Cine SSFP short-axis and long-axis planes (real-time cine can be used).

This entire short protocol can also be acquired with or without breath hold if necessary. In severe cases, the CMR imaging study can be stopped after step 3 (LGE), assuming LV function can be addressed by echocardiography.

SUMMARY

This article focused on the CMR imaging phenotype of muscular dystrophy and showed the central role of CMR imaging in early detection of cardiac involvement. Cardiac injury detected by CMR imaging is a strong prognostic marker. Of note, the presence of LGE in Duchenne and BMD is a mandatory trigger to initiate ACE inhibitor treatment, regardless of LVEF. Patients with MF not promptly treated have a significantly worse prognosis. Nonetheless, the high clinical variability hampers a correlation of cardiac phenotype and genotype, particularly in the more rare types of muscular dystrophy in which the data on CMR imaging are scarce. There is still limited understanding of disease mechanism and heart injury progression. These critical knowledge gaps should trigger strong efforts among scientists in this field to collaborate in well-designed studies to appropriately fill these gaps. It is hoped that new approaches and treatments will emerge from this quest and potentially improve the quality and quantity of life of patients with muscular dystrophy.

ACKNOWLEDGMENTS

This work was partially supported by Zerbini Foundation.

REFERENCES

1. Bushby K, Muntoni F, Bourke JP. 107th ENMC international workshop: the management of cardiac involvement in muscular dystrophy and myotonic dystrophy. 7th-9th June 2002, Naarden, the Netherlands. Neuromuscul Disord 2003;13:166–72.

2. Cox GF, Kunkel LM. Dystrophies and heart disease. Curr Opin Cardiol 1997;12:329–43.

3. English KM, Gibbs JL. Cardiac monitoring and treatment for children and adolescents with neuromuscular disorders. Dev Med Child Neurol 2006;48:231–5.

4. American Academy of Pediatrics Section on Cardiology and Cardiac Surgery. Cardiovascular health supervision for individuals affected by Duchenne or Becker muscular dystrophy. Pediatrics 2005;116:1569–73.

5. Bach JR. Update and perspective on noninvasive respiratory muscle aids. Part 2: the expiratory aids. Chest 1994;105:1538–44.

6. Ishikawa Y, Miura T, Ishikawa Y, et al. Duchenne muscular dystrophy: survival by cardio-respiratory interventions. Neuromuscul Disord 2011;21:47–51.

7. Duboc D, Meune C, Lerebours G, et al. Effect of perindopril on the onset and progression of left ventricular dysfunction in Duchenne muscular dystrophy. J Am Coll Cardiol 2005;45:855–7.

8. Jefferies JL, Eidem BW, Belmont JW, et al. Genetic predictors and remodeling of dilated cardiomyopathy in muscular dystrophy. Circulation 2005;112:2799–804.

9. Mavrogeni S, Markousis-Mavrogenis G, Papavasiliou A, et al. Cardiac involvement in Duchenne and Becker muscular dystrophy. World J Cardiol 2015;7:410–4.

10. Silva MC, Magalhaes TA, Meira ZM, et al. Myocardial fibrosis progression in Duchenne and Becker muscular dystrophy: a randomized clinical trial. JAMA Cardiol 2017;2:190–9.

11. Silva MC, Meira ZM, Gurgel Giannetti J, et al. Myocardial delayed enhancement by magnetic resonance imaging in patients with muscular dystrophy. J Am Coll Cardiol 2007;49:1874–9.

12. Tandon A, Villa CR, Hor KN, et al. Myocardial fibrosis burden predicts left ventricular ejection fraction and is associated with age and steroid treatment duration in duchenne muscular dystrophy. J Am Heart Assoc 2015;4.

13. Rosales XQ, Moser SJ, Tran T, et al. Cardiovascular magnetic resonance of cardiomyopathy in limb girdle muscular dystrophy 2B and 2I. J Cardiovasc Magn Reson 2011;13:39.

14. Cohn RD, Campbell KP. Molecular basis of muscular dystrophies. Muscle Nerve 2000;23:1456–71.

15. Zundel WS, Tyler FH. The muscular dystrophies. N Engl J Med 1965;273:537–43. CONTD.

16. McNally EM, Kaltman JR, Benson DW, et al. Contemporary cardiac issues in Duchenne muscular dystrophy. Working Group of the National Heart, Lung, and Blood Institute in collaboration with Parent Project Muscular Dystrophy. Circulation 2015;131:1590–8.

17. Nigro G, Comi LI, Politano L, et al. The incidence and evolution of cardiomyopathy in Duchenne muscular dystrophy. Int J Cardiol 1990;26:271–7.

18. Marui F, Bianco HT, Bombig MTN, et al. Behavior of blood pressure variables in children and adolescents with Duchenne muscular dystrophy. Arq Bras Cardiol 2018;110:551–7.

19. Rochitte CE, Tassi EM, Shiozaki AA. The emerging role of MRI in the diagnosis and management of cardiomyopathies. Curr Cardiol Rep 2006;8: 44–52.

20. Senra T, Ianni BM, Costa ACP, et al. Long-term prognostic value of myocardial fibrosis in patients with Chagas cardiomyopathy. J Am Coll Cardiol 2018; 72:2577–87.

21. Florian A, Rosch S, Bietenbeck M, et al. Cardiac involvement in female Duchenne and Becker muscular dystrophy carriers in comparison to their first-degree male relatives: a comparative cardiovascular magnetic resonance study. Eur Heart J Cardiovasc Imaging 2016;17:326–33.

22. Mehler MF. Brain dystrophin, neurogenetics and mental retardation. Brain Res Brain Res Rev 2000; 32:277–307.

23. Taylor PJ, Betts GA, Maroulis S, et al. Dystrophin gene mutation location and the risk of cognitive impairment in Duchenne muscular dystrophy. PLoS One 2010;5:e8803.

24. Silva MC, Rassi CH, Meira ZM, et al. Association between specific dystrophin gene mutations and myocardial fibrosis by cardiovascular magnetic resonance imaging in patients with Duchenne and Becker muscular dystrophy. J Cardiovasc Magn Reson 2014;16(Suppl 1):419–20.

25. Silva MC. Diagnóstico da cardiomiopatia na distrofia muscular progressiva por ressonância magnética cardiovascular - correlação com tratamento, prognóstico e preditores genéticos. Faculdade de Medicina da Universidade de São Paulo [Tese]. São Paulo (Brazil): University of São Paulo; 2013.

26. Ashford MW Jr, Liu W, Lin SJ, et al. Occult cardiac contractile dysfunction in dystrophin-deficient children revealed by cardiac magnetic resonance strain imaging. Circulation 2005;112:2462–7.

27. Raman SV, Hor KN, Mazur W, et al. Eplerenone for early cardiomyopathy in Duchenne muscular dystrophy: a randomised, double-blind, placebo-controlled trial. Lancet Neurol 2015;14:153–61.

28. Birnkrant DJ, Bushby K, Bann CM, et al. Diagnosis and management of Duchenne muscular dystrophy, part 2: respiratory, cardiac, bone health, and orthopaedic management. Lancet Neurol 2018;17: 347–61.

29. Norwood F, de Visser M, Eymard B, et al. EFNS guideline on diagnosis and management of limb girdle muscular dystrophies. Eur J Neurol 2007;14: 1305–12.

30. Bushby KM. Making sense of the limb-girdle muscular dystrophies. Brain 1999;122(Pt 8): 1403–20.

31. Guglieri M, Straub V, Bushby K, et al. Limb-girdle muscular dystrophies. Curr Opin Neurol 2008;21: 576–84.

32. Emery AE. Emery-Dreifuss muscular dystrophy - a 40 year retrospective. Neuromuscul Disord 2000; 10:228–32.

33. Emery AE. The muscular dystrophies. Lancet 2002; 359:687–95.

34. Buckley AE, Dean J, Mahy IR. Cardiac involvement in Emery Dreifuss muscular dystrophy: a case series. Heart 1999;82:105–8.

35. Karkkainen S, Peuhkurinen K. Genetics of dilated cardiomyopathy. Ann Med 2007;39:91–107.

36. Arbustini E, Pilotto A, Repetto A, et al. Autosomal dominant dilated cardiomyopathy with atrioventricular block: a lamin A/C defect-related disease. J Am Coll Cardiol 2002;39:981–90.

37. Holmstrom M, Kivisto S, Helio T, et al. Late gadolinium enhanced cardiovascular magnetic resonance of lamin A/C gene mutation related dilated cardiomyopathy. J Cardiovasc Magn Reson 2011;13:30.

38. Ranum LP, Cooper TA. RNA-mediated neuromuscular disorders. Annu Rev Neurosci 2006;29: 259–77.

39. Bhakta D, Lowe MR, Groh WJ. Prevalence of structural cardiac abnormalities in patients with myotonic dystrophy type I. Am Heart J 2004;147:224–7.

40. Bhakta D, Groh MR, Shen C, et al. Increased mortality with left ventricular systolic dysfunction and heart failure in adults with myotonic dystrophy type 1. Am Heart J 2010;160:1137–41, 1141.e1.

41. Hermans MC, Faber CG, Bekkers SC, et al. Structural and functional cardiac changes in myotonic dystrophy type 1: a cardiovascular magnetic resonance study. J Cardiovasc Magn Reson 2012;14:48.

42. Assomull RG, Prasad SK, Lyne J, et al. Cardiovascular magnetic resonance, fibrosis, and prognosis in dilated cardiomyopathy. J Am Coll Cardiol 2006; 48:1977–85.

43. Rodriguez-Torres D, Jimenez-Jaimez J, Macias-Ruiz R, et al. Cardiac manifestations of neuromuscular disease. Rev Esp Cardiol (Engl Ed) 2018;71: 580–2.

44. Verhaert D, Richards K, Rafael-Fortney JA, et al. Cardiac involvement in patients with muscular dystrophies: magnetic resonance imaging phenotype and genotypic considerations. Circ Cardiovasc Imaging 2011;4:67–76.

45. Messroghli DR, Moon JC, Ferreira VM, et al. Correction to: Clinical recommendations for cardiovascular magnetic resonance mapping of T1, T2, T2* and extracellular volume: a consensus statement by the Society for Cardiovascular Magnetic Resonance (SCMR) endorsed by the European Association for

Cardiovascular Imaging (EACVI). J Cardiovasc Magn Reson 2018;20:9.

46. Mavrogeni S, Papavasiliou A, Spargias K, et al. Myocardial inflammation in Duchenne Muscular Dystrophy as a precipitating factor for heart failure: a prospective study. BMC Neurol 2010;10:33.

47. Badorff C, Knowlton KU. Dystrophin disruption in enterovirus-induced myocarditis and dilated cardiomyopathy: from bench to bedside. Med Microbiol Immunol 2004;193:121–6.

48. Soslow JH, Damon SM, Crum K, et al. Increased myocardial native T1 and extracellular volume in patients with Duchenne muscular dystrophy. J Cardiovasc Magn Reson 2016;18:5.

49. Olivieri LJ, Kellman P, McCarter RJ, et al. Native T1 values identify myocardial changes and stratify disease severity in patients with Duchenne muscular dystrophy. J Cardiovasc Magn Reson 2016;18:72.

50. Siegel B, Olivieri L, Gordish-Dressman H, et al. Myocardial strain using cardiac MR feature tracking and speckle tracking echocardiography in duchenne muscular dystrophy patients. Pediatr Cardiol 2018;39:478–83.

Assessment of Cardiotoxicity of Cancer Chemotherapy
The Value of Cardiac MR Imaging

Thiago Ferreira de Souza, MD, MSc[a],
Thiago Quinaglia, MD, PhD[a], Tomas G. Neilan, MD, MPH[b],
Otávio R. Coelho-Filho, MD, PhD, MPH[a,c],*

KEYWORDS

- Cardiovascular magnetic resonance • Myocardial remodeling • Cardiotoxicity • Chemotherapy

KEY POINTS

- Several strengths of cardiac magnetic resonance (CMR) imaging, including its ability to accurately assess cardiac morphology, function, and scar, as well as myocardial tissue remodeling, have been supporting its use to investigate myocardial injury in cancer survivals.
- Because CMR incorporates several different types of imaging strategies, it provides a very comprehensive evaluation of the cardiovascular system, which is very helpful in patients with cancer.
- Novel CMR techniques, incorporating T1 and T2 mapping, have the potential not only to improve the current knowledge of cardiotoxicity, but also has the promising capability to detect early markers of left ventricular remodeling, which may facilitate development of prevention and therapeutic interventions.

INTRODUCTION

There have been marked improvements in outcomes among patients diagnosed with cancer. These improvements are related, in part, to the improved understanding of cancer biology leading to the development of more effective therapies. However, as the number of cancer survivors increases, there has been a renewed focus on the potential cardiotoxic effects of cancer therapies. In addition, the types of therapies available for cancer treatment have expanded from traditional radiation and chemotherapy to targeted and

Disclosures: The authors have nothing to disclose.
Sources of Funding: Dr Coelho-Filho is supported by National Council for Scientific and Technological Development (CNPq) Productivity in Research award grant (303366/2015-0) and travel award grant (453960/2016-2). Dr Coelho-Filho is also supported by a Young Investigators grant from The São Paulo Research Foundation (2015/15402-2). Dr Neilan has the following support: The Kohlberg Foundation, National Institutes of Health/ National Heart, Lung, and Blood Institute (1R01HL130539-01A1; 1R01HL137562 - 01A1) and National Institutes of Health/ Harvard Center for AIDS Research (P30 AI060354).
[a] Faculdade de Ciências Médicas - Universidade Estadual de Campinas, Rua Tessália Vieira de Camargo, 126, Campinas, São Paulo 13083-887, Brasil; [b] Cardio-Oncology Program and Cardiac MR PET CT Program, Massachusetts General Hospital, Harvard Medical School, 55 Fruit Street, Boston, MA 02114, USA; [c] Division of Cardiology, Department of Medicine, State University of Campinas (UNICAMP), Rua Tessália Vieira de Camargo, 126, Campinas, São Paulo 13083-887, Brasil
* Corresponding author. Division of Cardiology, Department of Medicine, State University of Campinas (UNICAMP), Rua Tessália Viera de Camargo, 126 Campinas, São Paulo 13083-887, Brasil.
E-mail addresses: orcfilho@unicamp.br; tavicocoelho@gmail.com
; @Otavio_Coelho_F (O.R.C.-F.)

mri.theclinics.com

immune therapies. There are more than 15 million cancer survivors in the United States, and this number is projected to increase.[1] Both preexisting risk factors for cardiovascular (CV) disease and possible cardiotoxic effects of cancer therapy contribute to enlarge the likelihood of CV disease development and exacerbation to these individuals.[2,3] Moreover, the number of older patients with multiple risk factors for CV disease who receive a diagnosis of a malignancy has considerably increased during the past 3 decades.[4] The combination of the increased complexities of these cancer therapies, the increased number of cancer survivors, and the recognition of the increased risk of CV disease among cancer survivors has led to the development of a specialty called cardio-oncology or onco-cardiology.[5]

CV complications may occur after many types of cancer therapies, including traditional chemotherapy, radiotherapy, and targeted and immune therapy regimens.[6–8] The manifestations of CV disease among patients with cancer are broad and although cardiac injury is more frequently observed in the myocardium as left ventricular (LV) systolic dysfunction, it also may appear at other heart structures such as valves, coronary arteries, pericardium, great arteries, and electrical system.[9]

Despite advances, the effective detection and quantification of cancer therapy–related cardiotoxicity is challenged by several factors. First, in many cases, cardiac dysfunction occurs only after many years of chemotherapy and in the absence of clinical symptoms, confounding its association with cancer therapy.[10] In addition, although the definition of cardiotoxicity has proven its clinical utility (a decrease in LV ejection fraction [LVEF] of $\geq$5% to <55% in the presence of symptoms of heart failure (HF) or an asymptomatic decrease in LVEF by $\geq$10% to <55%),[11] this definition relies exclusively on longitudinal monitoring of LV systolic function and ejection fraction, commonly performed by standard transthoracic echocardiogram, which has several limitations, such as poor reproducibility, lack to provide tissue characterization and to identify LV remodeling beyond systolic dysfunction. Finally, reductions in LVEF frequently take place within the normal range, indicating that subtle myocardial injury may occur before LV dysfunction.[12,13]

Consistent data have established that cardiac magnetic resonance (CMR) is one of the most accurate imaging modalities for the assessment of cardiac toxicity and adverse LV remodeling. Its ability to assess cardiac morphology and function is highly accurate and reproducible.[14] CMR also integrates different types of imaging sequences (eg, cine imaging for morphology, T2-weighted imaging for myocardial edema, perfusion for ischemia assessment, late gadolinium enhancement [LGE] for scar, and tagging for myocardial strain imaging), providing a very comprehensive evaluation of the LV remodeling associated with cancer therapy. More recently, different groups[15–17] have applied more novel sequences to characterize the effects of cancer therapy, such as the use of T1 and T2 mapping techniques; providing not only data regarding the early abnormalities in myocardial tissue composition, but also improving the current mechanistic understanding of cancer-related cardiotoxicity.

MECHANISMS OF THE MOST COMMON CHEMOTHERAPY-INDUCED CARDIOTOXICITY
Anthracyclines

Anthracyclines are commonly implicated as a cause of CV toxicity among patients with cancer. The risk of HF with anthracyclines is related to cumulative dose, with the risk increasing with higher cumulative doses. The cardiotoxicity of anthracyclines is far higher than the rates of clinical HF. Specifically, rates of subclinical cardiotoxicity are higher, occurring even with lower cumulative doses, particularly when more than 350 mg/m^2.[18,19] In a retrospective analysis, Swain and colleagues[20] identified an increased risk of cardiotoxicity even with doses previously considered safe ($\leq$300 mg/m^2). Once HF is established, Mortality from HF secondary to anthracycline therapy ranges from 30% to 70%.[21] There may be a long latency period between anthracycline and clinical HF, especially among young patients; however, among adults, toxicity generally appears early, with 90% of cases occurring within the first year.[10] The cardiotoxicity of anthracyclines is likely a multifactorial process, related to oxidative stress, mitochondriopathy, changes in iron and calcium homeostasis, and in respiratory chain components.[22,23] Zhang and colleagues[24] proposed a unifying mechanism of cardiotoxicity, implicating topoisomerase-IIβ as an essential driver in this mechanism, because in its presence, doxorubicin activates the DNA response and apoptosis pathways and affects oxidative phosphorylation and mitochondrial biogenesis in cardiomyocytes.

Trastuzumab

Trastuzumab is a monoclonal antibody and inhibits the human epidermal growth factor by the receptor tyrosine-protein kinase erbB-2 pathway. ErbB-2 is also present in cardiomyocytes and downstream pathways that regulate apoptosis, mitosis, cell hypertrophy and elongation, cellular adhesion, angiogenesis, and sensitivity to adrenergic signaling,[25] being potentially deleterious to myocardial tissue. Trastuzumab has been associated with an increased incidence of cardiac dysfunction of 3% to 7%.[11] The risk rises with concomitant use of paclitaxel (13%) and even more when concomitantly administered with anthracyclines and/or cyclophosphamide (27%). Trastuzumab-induced cardiotoxicity is not dose-dependent (as when determined by anthracyclines) but is often reversible, although it is difficult to predict which patients are at risk of developing toxicity.[26]

Mitoxantrone

Mitoxantrone, an anthracenedione agent, is a DNA-topoisomerase II inhibitor with antineoplastic activity and potent anti-inflammatory and immuno-modulating properties. It acts intercalating into DNA, reducing DNA repair and interfering with RNA synthesis.[27] Mitoxantrone is associated with cumulative dose-related cardiotoxicity, and myocytes exposed to it experience similar alterations at electron microscopy to those seen with anthracycline.[28] Mitoxantrone-induced cardiotoxicity manifests as systolic and diastolic dysfunction.[29] It is recognized that approximately 2% of patients with cancer treated with drug will develop cardiotoxicity. Although this condition is asymptomatic in most cases, it may transition to congestive HF–related symptoms and may transition to congestive cardiac failure, increasing the risk of death.[30]

Cyclophosphamide

Cyclophosphamide is a nitrogen mustard-alkylating agent with potent antineoplastic, immunosuppressive, and immunomodulatory properties. Although the precise mechanism of cyclophosphamide-induced cardiac toxicity has not been entirely established, the metabolites can cause oxidative stress and endothelial damage. Cyclophosphamide cardiac toxicity is associated with cumulative doses and typically manifests as a fulminant myocarditis.

Tyrosine Kinase Inhibitors

Sunitinib targets the vascular endothelial growth factor molecular pathway through tyrosine kinase inhibition. A recent review indicated that sunitinib was the preferred initial therapeutic option for metastatic renal cell carcinoma.[31] However, sunitinib affects the AMP-activated protein kinase and platelet-derived growth factor receptor, which are critical for cardiomyocyte function and

survival,[32,33] leading to hypertension, LV dysfunction, and HF.[34–36]

INITIAL MANAGEMENT

Cardiac complication after cancer therapy may manifest in different ways, including cardiac systolic dysfunction, cardiac ischemia, arrhythmias, pericarditis, and electrical repolarization abnormalities. A close interaction and cooperation between oncology and cardiology is required to improve care of many patients with cancer at risk of developing cancer-related cardiac complications. Patients considered for antineoplastic therapy should undergo initial CV evaluation to diagnose preexisting cardiac diseases, including physical examination, electrocardiogram, and analysis of ventricular function, identifying those with conditions that can be readily treated or might require more surveillance. Serial imaging assessment of cardiac function is suggested, even in asymptomatic patients, as discontinuation of cardiotoxic chemotherapy might allow reversible improvement in cardiac function when LV systolic dysfunction is identified in this group.[37]

CARDIAC MAGNETIC RESONANCE IMAGING
Morphologic and Functional Parameters

CMR is the method of choice for assessing changes in cardiac morphology and function caused by cancer treatment and cardiotoxicity.[38–40] Its high contrast-to-noise ratio, superior accuracy, and excellent reproducibility allow detection of slight changes that may benefit from preventive therapies. Both LV and right ventricle (RV) volumes and mass can be precisely obtained using standard cine CMR images, independently of any assumption of ventricle shape and the degree of remodeling.[41] Commonly used steady-state free-precession (SSFP) pulse sequences, which deliver high signal-to-noise and tissue-to-blood contrast (**Fig. 1**), provide precise data on both global and regional wall motion, capturing even subtle functional changes.[42] Drafts and coworkers[15] demonstrated that CMR cine images were able to detect early and significant abnormalities in cardiac structure and function secondary to cardiotoxicity therapy, even after moderate to low doses of anthracycline chemotherapy. Performing a series of CMR examinations, before and up to 6 months after anthracycline therapy, the investigators showed that reduction in LVEF occurred as early as 1 month after chemotherapy initiation, identifying individuals at high risk to maintain significant later decline in LV function. Interestingly, they also demonstrated that the decrease in LV

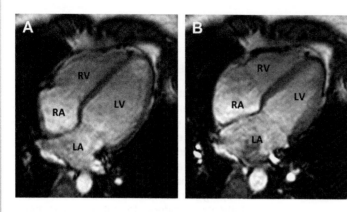

Fig. 1. Four-chamber SSFP showing the high resolution and excellent soft tissue contrast of cardiac MR imaging in end diastole (A) and end systole (B). LA, left atrium; RA, right atrium.

function was associated with LV enlargement, highlighting the potential negative effect of anthracycline-based chemotherapy on systolic function. Using LGE imaging, new areas with infarcts or scar were not seen, suggesting that anthracycline-induced cardiotoxicity appeared not to be caused by myocardial ischemia or myocardial infarction. A study comparing different imaging approaches for screening adult survivors of childhood cancer treated with anthracycline chemotherapy and/or radiation therapy,[43] has shown that 2-dimensional (2D) echocardiogram, using the biplane method, may not achieve a clinically reasonable accuracy for detecting LVEF less than 50% measured by CMR, demonstrating in this scenario limited sensitivity (25%) with high rates of false-positives (75%). Although 3D echocardiogram may improve sensitivity (53%), this approach also fails to accomplish results comparable to CMR imaging.[43] LV mass can also change

during cancer therapy and especially after anthracycline-based chemotherapy.[15] Nearby 50% of childhood cancer survivors have been shown to have LV mass ≥2 standard deviations below the mean normative values.[43] Neilan and colleagues,[44] examining 91 individuals with decreased LVEF after anthracycline-based chemotherapy at a median follow-up 88 months, found that indexed LV mass measured by CMR had a negative correlation with the cumulative given dose of anthracycline (**Fig. 2**A). In the same study, LV mass was shown to be a strong predictor of major CV events, and patients with indexed LV mass less than 57 g/m² had significantly higher rates of CV deaths, appropriate implantable cardioverter-defibrillator therapies, and admissions for decompensated HF compared with those with indexed LV mass ≥57 g/m² (**Fig. 2**B). A recent study, using novel CMR markers of myocardial tissue remodeling, indicates that LV atrophy could be

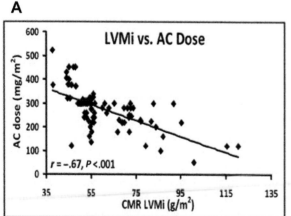 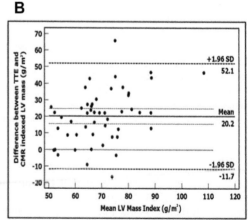

Fig. 2. (A) Association of LV mass derived by CMR with anthracycline dose. (B) Kaplan-Meier curves showing event-free probability according to LV mass index by CMR (≥57 or <57 g/m²). AC, anthracycline; LVMi, left ventricule mass index; TTE, transthoracic echocardiogram. (From Neilan TG, Coelho-Filho OR, Pena-Herrera D, et al. Left ventricular mass in patients with a cardiomyopathy after treatment with anthracyclines. Am J Cardiol. 2012;110(11):1679–86; with permission).

accounted not only for the expansion of the extra-cellular space, but also by a reduction in cardio-myocyte size.[17] In addition, Jordan and colleagues[45] suggested not only that the decrease in LV mass occurs early after anthracycline initiation, but also may take place regardless of factors that increase myocardial wall tension and stress. They also showed that a reduction in LV mass was associated with worsening HF symptoms.

Although few observations have specifically focused on the effects of cancer therapy on RV, recent reports have demonstrated significant decline in RV systolic function after anthracycline alone or in combination with trastuzumab.[46–48] RV failure has been associated with significant morbidity and mortality in patients with HF with both reduced and preserved ejection fraction.[49] Because the RV is a thin and complex structure compared with the LV, noninvasive imaging may be challenging. CMR has been shown to be very accurate[50] and reproducible[51] to assess RV volumes and function,[52,53] having several advantages over 2D echocardiography, including outstanding spatial resolution, volumetric quantification, and definition of complex structures and anatomy.

Tissue Characterization

Myocardial edema
CMR has the advantage to offer information on myocardial tissue remodeling complementary to traditional morphologic and functional measurements. Compelling evidence indicates that myocardial edema, inflammation, abnormal strain, and expansion of interstitial fibrosis occur before cardiac dysfunction develops. Indeed, experimental[54] and clinical observation[15,17,55] have shown that a multiple-parametric CMR protocol, incorporating recently developed T1 and T2 mapping techniques, may detect very early signs of myocardial tissue remodeling, improving the current understanding of chemotherapy-induced cardiotoxicity, facilitating future development and implementation of potential preventive treatments. Detection of myocardial edema and inflation, which are mostly based on increased ratio of T2-weighted signal intensity of myocardium normalized to skeletal muscle, has been successfully applied to ischemic[56] and nonischemic cardiomyopathy.[57–59] In a well-designed animal study, comprising baseline and post-doxorubicin multiple-parametric CMR examination, Farhad and colleagues[54] demonstrated that both myocardial edema and expansion of interstitial fibrosis occurred prematurely, having also a significant association with animal mortality rates. Using widely available black-blood T2-weighted sequences,

Ferreira de Souza and colleagues[17] observed a significant rise in myocardial T2-weighted signal intensity ratio to skeletal muscle early after a moderate cumulative dose of doxorubicin (total dose of 240 mg/m^2) (**Figs. 3** and **4**). Also, data suggest that myocardial edema, assessed by myocardial T2-weighted signal intensity normalized to skeletal muscle has been shown to be significantly associated with decreased RV systolic function, 12 months after anthracycline and/or trastuzumab treatment.[47] Various groups are currently investigating the role of novel T2 mapping sequences to serially detect myocardial edema after cancer therapy, but up to now, T2-weighted imaging has not been broadly studied to establish the usefulness of edema quantification to monitor patients after cancer therapy.

Myocardial fibrosis
Although LGE imaging has been shown to precisely recognize both myocardial scar and replacement fibrosis,[60,61] this technique may only accomplish partial assessment of the myocardial fibrosis burden.[62] Because LGE imaging relies on relative signal intensity differences after gadolinium-based contrast administration, it can fail to identify interstitial myocardial fibrosis. In numerous reports, including retrospective and prospective studies, LGE was not uniformly detected after anthracycline-based chemotherapy.[15,63,64] Actually, a negative LGE imaging study, frequently seen in anthracycline-induced cardiomyopathy (**Fig. 5**), may not represent true

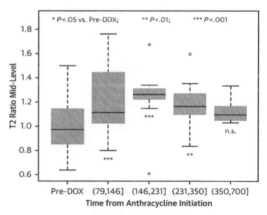

Fig. 3. The T2-weighted signal intensity ratio (myocardium/skeletal muscle) significantly increased early after anthracycline therapy, maintaining significantly higher until the third follow-up quartile compared with baseline (all *P*<.05). DOX, doxorubicin. (*From* Ferreira de Souza T, Quinaglia A C Silva T, Osorio Costa F, et al. Anthracycline therapy is associated with cardiomyocyte atrophy and preclinical manifestations of heart disease. JACC Cardiovasc Imaging. 2018;11(8):1045–1055; with permission).

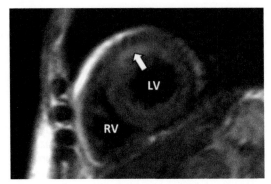

Fig. 4. Short-axis T2-weighted imaging exhibiting myocardial edema in anterior wall (*white arrow*) in patient with breast cancer treated with anthracycline-based chemotherapy.

absence of fibrosis, highlighting the limitation of LGE imaging in this setting. Although Fallah-Rad and colleagues[65] showed evidence of subepicardial LGE in all patients who developed

trastuzumab-induced cardiac dysfunction, several subsequent studies reveled conflicting results,[66] with a report from Lawley and colleagues[67] showing LGE in only 8% of the 25 women treated with trastuzumab. In addition, Neilan and colleagues[44] also observed that LGE is an infrequent finding in patients treated with anthracycline-cardiomyopathy, occurring in only 6% of cases.

Myocardial T1 mapping

Recently developed CMR techniques, based on T1 measurements done before and after administration of usual dose of gadolinium-based contrast agents, allow accurate quantification of the extracellular volume fraction (ECV), a marker of myocardial interstitial fibrosis. Even before the advent of T1 mapping approaches, Wassmuth and colleagues,[63] using T1-weighted sequences, were able to demonstrate abnormal myocardial accumulation of gadolinium within the myocardium of cancer survivors. Although this approach

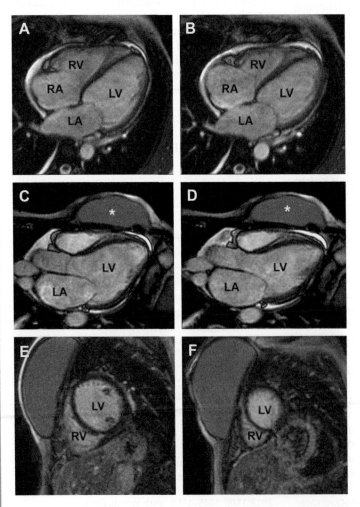

Fig. 5. 46-year-old women with breast cancer with anthracycline-induced cardiomyopathy. Four-chamber and 3-chamber views SSFP in diastole (*A, C*) and systole (*B, D*) showing severe LV dysfunction and an absence of scar on LGE images (*E, F*). Asterisk, breast prosthesis; LA, left atrium; RA, right atrium.

has several important limitations, this study confirmed that T1 measurements after gadolinium administration might detect subclinical cardiotoxic effects of chemotherapy. Most proposed T1 mapping techniques measure the longitudinal relaxation[68] before and after gadolinium administration, which induces more prominent changes in the areas of the myocardium with increased interstitial fibrosis. Using precontrast and postcontrast T1 measurements, signal intensity versus time curves for the myocardium and the blood pool were used to determine partition coefficient for gadolinium. ECV can then be obtained correcting blood pool measurements for patient's hematocrit. Both animal[69–71] and clinical[72–76] studies, using slightly different approaches and pulse sequences to measure T1 in myocardium and blood pool, have shown excellent agreement between the ECV derived from CMR with fibrosis quantification measured by histology. Numerous studies have examined the usefulness of CMR T1 mapping to investigate myocardial tissue remodeling after cancer therapy. In a pediatric cohort of cancer survivors treated with anthracycline, Tham and colleagues[77] showed a positive association of ECV measured by CMR with the chemotherapy dose. Interestingly, although the entire cohort has preserved LVEF, the CMR measurements of interstitial fibrosis were also associated with impaired physical capacity measured by cardiopulmonary exercise testing. These unique findings indicate that ECV is directly related to the total anthracycline dose, being also an early marker of cardiotoxicity, which also predicts physical impairment.[63] Data from another cohort study[16] revealed that patients previously exposed to anthracyclines had significantly higher ECV compared with age-matched controls, which also correlated with LV volume and diastolic function. In an interesting study, Jordan and colleagues[78] investigated a relatively large cohort of patients with cancer, including patients not yet treated (n = 37) and treated with anthracycline (n = 27) or nonanthracycline (n = 17) chemotherapy. Native T1 was significantly higher in patients with cancer pretreatment (1058 ± 7 ms) and posttreatment (1040 ± 7 ms) compared with cancer-free individuals (965 ± 3 ms; $P<.0001$). The investigators also demonstrated that ECV was elevated in anthracycline-treated patients with cancer (30.4% ± 0.7%) compared with pretreatment cancer (27.8% ± 0.7%; $P<.01$) or controls (26.9% ± 0.2%; $P<.0001$). In the same study, using multivariable models, they could confirm that both native T1 and ECV remained elevated in cancer survivors after adjusting to previous risk

factors for CV disease. Finally, changes in ECV occurred in parallel to reduction in LV systolic function.

Our group has shown that quantification of the intracellular lifetime of water (τ_{ic}) in the myocardium provides an innovative approach to detect changes in cardiomyocyte size, thereby expanding the capability for myocardial tissue profiling by CMR.[79] Both intracellular lifetime of water (τ_{ic}) and ECV can be simultaneously measured by CMR T1 mapping over a range of contrast concentrations. Ferreira de Souza and colleagues,[17] using this novel CMR approach, revealed that anthracycline therapy was associated with cardiomyocyte atrophy and early signs of heart disease. In this study, 27 patients with breast cancer were studied before and serially after anthracycline (240 mg/m²), including CMR imaging and biomarkers. At 351 to 700 days after anthracycline, LVEF declined by 12% to 58% ± 6% ($P<.001$), and LV mass index by 19 g/m² to 36 ± 6 g/m² ($P<.001$) and ECV increased by 0.037 to 0.36 ± 0.04 ($P<.004$), whereas intracellular lifetime of water (τ_{ic}) decreased by 62 ms to 119 ± 54 ms ($P<.004$) (Fig. 6). One of the main findings of this study is that anthracycline-induced remodeling is associated with a decline in cardiomyocyte size, suggesting that not only interstitial fibrosis and/or myocardial interstitial edema[19] can increase ECV. These findings support further investigations of the role for this novel CMR-based tissue characterization in patients treated with anthracycline-based chemotherapy.

Left Ventricular Strain

Strain and strain rate are sensitive and reproducible measurements of systolic changes, with proved prognostic significance. CMR strain methods perform better then echocardiography for applications focused on segmental function,[80] with the advantage to also demonstrate tissue abnormalities, such as myocardial fibrosis or edema. Jolly and colleagues[81] used an automated method in 72 patients undergoing chemotherapy to measure 3-month serial changes in LV mean mid-wall circumferential strain through the analysis of cine white blood images. The results indicated that circumferential strain worsened from −18.8 ± 2.89 at baseline to −17.6 ± 3.08 at 3-month visit, had strong correlation with subclinical declines in LVEF, and do not require extra image acquisition. CMR strain techniques are not widely clinically available, and future studies are needed to assess the prognostic value of CMR strain in cardio-oncology patients. More recently

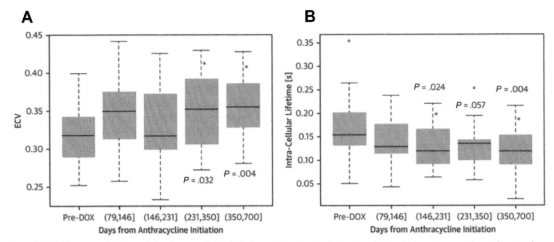

Fig. 6. ECV increased (*A*) and the intracellular lifetime of water (τ_{ic}) declined (*B*) after anthracycline. The *P* values in (*A*) and (*B*) are for the fixed effect of follow-up time (in quartiles) versus baseline in linear mixed-effects models for ECV and τ_{ic}, respectively. (*From* Ferreira de Souza T, Quinaglia A C Silva T, Osorio Costa F, et al. Anthracycline therapy is associated with cardiomyocyte atrophy and preclinical manifestations of heart disease. JACC Cardiovasc Imaging. 2018;11(8):1045–1055; with permission).

developed CMR strain methods using feature tracking assessing global longitudinal, radial, and circumferential strain have been proposed and its feasibility has also been proved in small studies. Additional well-conducted long-term follow-up trials are necessary to further investigate the role of CMR strain imaging in cancer survivals. Because this method can detect early signs of myocardial dysfunction, occurring before LV dysfunction, it may be suitable to identify those at higher risk to develop cardiotoxicity, allowing earlier intervention that can potentially improve clinical outcomes.

Vascular Remodeling

Cancer therapy may also impact vasculature and contribute to CV events. Anthracycline can be deleterious to the CV system, with direct cardiotoxic effect by suppression of endothelin-1 production, leading to apoptosis.[82] Although the nature of vascular remodeling remains not entirely understood, some reports have shown that the pulse wave velocity in the aortic arch determined by CMR, which is a measure of aortic stiffness, increased 4 months after anthracycline therapy.[83] In the same study, patients with elevated pulse wave velocity had 3 times more chance to experience a CV event.

Recommendation in Cardiovascular Imaging

Cardiotoxicity screening and detection include cardiac imaging and biomarkers, and the choice of modality should consider reproducibility, likelihood to provide additional clinical information, availability throughout the treatment pathway, and a high-quality radiation-free imaging.[39] A comparison between the most commonly used imaging modalities is shown in **Fig. 7**. The ideal imaging modality should identify those at high risk for future CV events, guide the initiation of protective therapies, and be economically viable. To assist referring physicians make the most appropriate imaging decision and enhance quality of care, in a joint report, the American College of Radiology and the American College of Cardiology wrote an evidence-based document determining the appropriate use of CV imaging in patients with HF,[84] in which echocardiography, radionuclide ventriculography, and CMR are appropriate in evaluation of patients with malignancy on current or planned cardiotoxic therapy and no prior imaging evaluation.

A statement from the American Heart Association[85] suggested that echocardiography is likely to be the mainstay of monitoring given its widespread availability; however, CMR offers several advantages over it. Evaluation of ventricular mass and function are highly reproducible, even in challenging cases for other modalities, when low image quality and assumptions of cardiac geometry are important limitations. The use of CMR tissue characterization capability can identify edema, inflammation, scarring, perfusion abnormalities, and even diffuse fibrosis, quantification of extracellular volume fraction, and cardiomyocyte size, as previously discussed. It also evaluates pericardium and great vessels and characterizes cardiac masses.

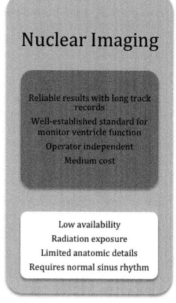

Fig. 7. Comparison between imaging modalities with advantages in upper gray boxes and disadvantages in bottom white boxes.

SUMMARY

Several strengths of CMR imaging, including its ability to accurately assess cardiac morphology, function, and scar, as well as myocardial tissue remodeling, have been supporting its use to investigate myocardial injury in cancer survivals. Because CMR incorporates several different types of imaging strategies, it provides a comprehensive evaluation of the CV system, which is very helpful in patients with cancer. Novel CMR techniques, incorporating T1 and T2 mapping, have the potential to not only improve the current knowledge of cardiotoxicity, but also the promising capability to detect early markers of LV remodeling that may facilitate developing of prevention and therapeutic interventions. Future clinical studies, investigating both widely availed and novel CMR methods in a broad cancer population are required to further explore its clinical role.

REFERENCES

1. U.S. Department of Health and Human Services. 2018. Available at: https://www.cancer.gov/about-Cancer/understanding/statistics. Accessed November 4, 2018.

2. Hooning MJ, Botma A, Aleman BM, et al. Long-term risk of cardiovascular disease in 10-year survivors of breast cancer. J Natl Cancer Inst 2007;99(5): 365–75.

3. Swerdlow AJ, Higgins CD, Smith P, et al. Myocardial infarction mortality risk after treatment for Hodgkin disease: a collaborative British cohort study. J Natl Cancer Inst 2007;99(3):206–14.

4. Hayat MJ, Howlader N, Reichman ME, et al. Cancer statistics, trends, and multiple primary cancer analyses from the Surveillance, Epidemiology, and End Results (SEER) Program. Oncologist 2007;12(1): 20–37.

5. Hong RA, Iimura T, Sumida KN, et al. Cardio-oncology/onco-cardiology. Clin Cardiol 2010; 33(12):733–7.

6. Steinherz LJ, Graham T, Hurwitz R, et al. Guidelines for cardiac monitoring of children during and after anthracycline therapy: report of the Cardiology Committee of the Children's Cancer Study Group. Pediatrics 1992;89(5 Pt 1):942–9.

7. Mahmood SS, Fradley MG, Cohen JV, et al. Myocarditis in patients treated with immune checkpoint inhibitors. J Am Coll Cardiol 2018;71(16): 1755–64.

8. Chen MH, Kerkela R, Force T. Mechanisms of cardiac dysfunction associated with tyrosine kinase inhibitor cancer therapeutics. Circulation 2008;118(1): 84–95.

9. Watts RG, George M, Johnson WH Jr. Pretreatment and routine echocardiogram monitoring during chemotherapy for anthracycline-induced cardiotoxicity rarely identifies significant cardiac dysfunction or alters treatment decisions: a 5-year review at a single pediatric oncology center. Cancer 2012; 118(7):1919–24.

10. Steinherz LJ, Steinherz PG, Tan CT, et al. Cardiac toxicity 4 to 20 years after completing anthracycline therapy. JAMA 1991;266(12):1672–7.

11. Seidman A, Hudis C, Pierri MK, et al. Cardiac dysfunction in the trastuzumab clinical trials experience. J Clin Oncol 2002;20(5):1215–21.

12. Ewer MS, Lenihan DJ. Left ventricular ejection fraction and cardiotoxicity: is our ear really to the ground? J Clin Oncol 2008;26(8):1201–3.

13. Eidem BW. Identification of anthracycline cardiotoxicity: left ventricular ejection fraction is not enough. J Am Soc Echocardiogr 2008;21(12):1290–2.

14. Mor-Avi V, Jenkins C, Kuhl HP, et al. Real-time 3-dimensional echocardiographic quantification of left ventricular volumes: multicenter study for validation with magnetic resonance imaging and investigation of sources of error. JACC Cardiovasc Imaging 2008;1(4):413–23.

15. Drafts BC, Twomley KM, D'Agostino R Jr, et al. Low to moderate dose anthracycline-based chemotherapy is associated with early noninvasive imaging evidence of subclinical cardiovascular disease. JACC Cardiovasc Imaging 2013;6(8):877–85.

16. Neilan TG, Coelho-Filho OR, Shah RV, et al. Myocardial extracellular volume by cardiac magnetic resonance imaging in patients treated with anthracycline-based chemotherapy. Am J Cardiol 2013;111(5):717–22.

17. Ferreira de Souza T, Quinaglia ACST, Osorio Costa F, et al. Anthracycline therapy is associated with cardiomyocyte atrophy and preclinical manifestations of heart disease. JACC Cardiovasc Imaging 2018;11(8):1045–55.

18. Alexander J, Dainiak N, Berger HJ, et al. Serial assessment of doxorubicin cardiotoxicity with quantitative radionuclide angiocardiography. N Engl J Med 1979;300(6):278–83.

19. Buzdar AU, Marcus C, Smith TL, et al. Early and delayed clinical cardiotoxicity of doxorubicin. Cancer 1985;55(12):2761–5.

20. Swain SM, Whaley FS, Ewer MS. Congestive heart failure in patients treated with doxorubicin: a retrospective analysis of three trials. Cancer 2003; 97(11):2869–79.

21. Aiken MJ, Suhag V, Garcia CA, et al. Doxorubicin-induced cardiac toxicity and cardiac rest gated blood pool imaging. Clin Nucl Med 2009;34(11): 762–7.

22. Minotti G, Menna P, Salvatorelli E, et al. Anthracyclines: molecular advances and pharmacologic developments in antitumor activity and cardiotoxicity. Pharmacol Rev 2004;56(2):185–229.

23. Menna P, Paz OG, Chello M, et al. Anthracycline cardiotoxicity. Expert Opin Drug Saf 2012;11(Suppl 1): S21–36.

24. Zhang S, Liu X, Bawa-Khalfe T, et al. Identification of the molecular basis of doxorubicin-induced cardiotoxicity. Nat Med 2012;18(11):1639–42.

25. De Keulenaer GW, Doggen K, Lemmens K. The vulnerability of the heart as a pluricellular paracrine organ: lessons from unexpected triggers of heart failure in targeted ErbB2 anticancer therapy. Circ Res 2010;106(1):35–46.

26. Rushton M, Johnson C, Dent S. Trastuzumab-induced cardiotoxicity: testing a clinical risk score in a real-world cardio-oncology population. Curr Oncol 2017;24(3):176–80.

27. Murray TJ. The cardiac effects of mitoxantrone: do the benefits in multiple sclerosis outweigh the risks? Expert Opin Drug Saf 2006;5(2):265–74.

28. Benjamin RS, Chawla SP, Ewer MS, et al. Evaluation of mitoxantrone cardiac toxicity by nuclear angiography and endomyocardial biopsy: an update. Invest New Drugs 1985;3(2):117–21.

29. Shaikh AY, Suryadevara S, Tripathi A, et al. Mitoxantrone-induced cardiotoxicity in acute myeloid leukemia—a velocity vector imaging analysis. Echocardiography 2016;33(8):1166–77.

30. Ghalie RG, Edan G, Laurent M, et al. Cardiac adverse effects associated with mitoxantrone (Novantrone) therapy in patients with MS. Neurology 2002;59(6):909–13.

31. Jonasch E, Signorovitch JE, Lin PL, et al. Treatment patterns in metastatic renal cell carcinoma: a retrospective review of medical records from US community oncology practices. Curr Med Res Opin 2014; 30(10):2041–50.

32. Rainer PP, Doleschal B, Kirk JA, et al. Sunitinib causes dose-dependent negative functional effects on myocardium and cardiomyocytes. BJU Int 2012;110(10):1455–62.

33. Force T, Krause DS, Van Etten RA. Molecular mechanisms of cardiotoxicity of tyrosine kinase inhibition. Nat Rev Cancer 2007;7(5):332–44.

34. Schmidinger M, Zielinski CC, Vogl UM, et al. Cardiac toxicity of sunitinib and sorafenib in patients with metastatic renal cell carcinoma. J Clin Oncol 2008; 26(32):5204–12.

35. Chu TF, Rupnick MA, Kerkela R, et al. Cardiotoxicity associated with tyrosine kinase inhibitor sunitinib. Lancet 2007;370(9604):2011–9.

36. Qi WX, He AN, Shen Z, et al. Incidence and risk of hypertension with a novel multi-targeted kinase inhibitor axitinib in cancer patients: a systematic review and meta-analysis. Br J Clin Pharmacol 2013; 76(3):348–57.

37. Guarneri V, Lenihan DJ, Valero V, et al. Long-term cardiac tolerability of trastuzumab in metastatic breast cancer: the M.D. Anderson Cancer Center experience. J Clin Oncol 2006;24(25): 4107–15.

38. Goenka AH, Flamm SD. Cardiac magnetic resonance imaging for the investigation of cardiovascular disorders. Part 1: current applications. Tex Heart Inst J 2014;41(1):7–20.

39. Zamorano JL, Lancellotti P, Rodriguez Munoz D, et al. 2016 ESC Position Paper on cancer treatments and cardiovascular toxicity developed under the auspices of the ESC Committee for Practice Guidelines: The Task Force for cancer treatments and cardiovascular toxicity of the European Society of Cardiology (ESC). Eur Heart J 2016;37(36): 2768–801.

40. Armenian SH, Lacchetti C, Lenihan D. Prevention and monitoring of cardiac dysfunction in survivors of adult cancers: American Society of Clinical Oncology clinical practice guideline summary. J Oncol Pract 2017;13(4):270–5.

41. Walsh TF, Hundley WG. Assessment of ventricular function with cardiovascular magnetic resonance. Cardiol Clin 2007;25(1):15–33, v.

42. Sarwar A, Shapiro MD, Abbara S, et al. Cardiac magnetic resonance imaging for the evaluation of ventricular function. Semin Roentgenol 2008;43(3): 183–92.

43. Armstrong GT, Plana JC, Zhang N, et al. Screening adult survivors of childhood cancer for cardiomyopathy: comparison of echocardiography and cardiac magnetic resonance imaging. J Clin Oncol 2012; 30(23):2876–84.

44. Neilan TG, Coelho-Filho OR, Pena-Herrera D, et al. Left ventricular mass in patients with a cardiomyopathy after treatment with anthracyclines. Am J Cardiol 2012;110(11):1679–86.

45. Jordan JH, Castellino SM, Melendez GC, et al. Left ventricular mass change after anthracycline chemotherapy. Circ Heart Fail 2018;11(7):e004560.

46. Cottin Y, Touzery C, Coudert B, et al. Diastolic or systolic left and right ventricular impairment at moderate doses of anthracycline? A 1-year follow-up study of women. Eur J Nucl Med 1996;23(5): 511–6.

47. Grover S, Leong DP, Chakrabarty A, et al. Left and right ventricular effects of anthracycline and trastuzumab chemotherapy: a prospective study using novel cardiac imaging and biochemical markers. Int J Cardiol 2013;168(6):5465–7.

48. Calleja A, Poulin F, Khorolsky C, et al. Right ventricular dysfunction in patients experiencing cardiotoxicity during breast cancer therapy. J Oncol 2015; 2015:609194.

49. Ghio S, Guazzi M, Scardovi AB, et al. Different correlates but similar prognostic implications for right ventricular dysfunction in heart failure patients with reduced or preserved ejection fraction. Eur J Heart Fail 2017;19(7):873–9.

50. Grothues F, Moon JC, Bellenger NG, et al. Interstudy reproducibility of right ventricular volumes, function, and mass with cardiovascular magnetic resonance. Am Heart J 2004;147(2):218–23.

51. Mooij CF, de Wit CJ, Graham DA, et al. Reproducibility of MRI measurements of right ventricular size and function in patients with normal and dilated ventricles. J Magn Reson Imaging 2008;28(1):67–73.

52. Foppa M, Arora G, Gona P, et al. Right ventricular volumes and systolic function by cardiac magnetic resonance and the impact of sex, age, and obesity in a longitudinally followed cohort free of pulmonary and cardiovascular disease: the Framingham heart study. Circ Cardiovasc Imaging 2016;9(3):e003810.

53. Crean AM, Maredia N, Ballard G, et al. 3D Echo systematically underestimates right ventricular volumes compared to cardiovascular magnetic resonance in adult congenital heart disease patients with moderate or severe RV dilatation. J Cardiovasc Magn Reson 2011;13:78.

54. Farhad H, Staziaki PV, Addison D, et al. Characterization of the changes in cardiac structure and function in mice treated with anthracyclines using serial cardiac magnetic resonance imaging. Circ Cardiovasc Imaging 2016;9(12) [pii:e003584].

55. Melendez GC, Jordan JH, D'Agostino RB Jr, et al. Progressive 3-month increase in LV myocardial ECV after anthracycline-based chemotherapy. JACC Cardiovasc Imaging 2017;10(6):708–9.

56. Abdel-Aty H, Zagrosek A, Schulz-Menger J, et al. Delayed enhancement and T2-weighted cardiovascular magnetic resonance imaging differentiate acute from chronic myocardial infarction. Circulation 2004;109(20):2411–6.

57. Torreao JA, Ianni BM, Mady C, et al. Myocardial tissue characterization in Chagas' heart disease by cardiovascular magnetic resonance. J Cardiovasc Magn Reson 2015;17:97.

58. Zagrosek A, Abdel-Aty H, Boye P, et al. Cardiac magnetic resonance monitors reversible and irreversible myocardial injury in myocarditis. JACC Cardiovasc Imaging 2009;2(2):131–8.

59. Carbone I, Childs H, Aljizeeri A, et al. Importance of reference muscle selection in quantitative signal intensity analysis of T2-weighted images of myocardial edema using a T2 ratio method. BioMed Research International 2015;2015:232649.

60. Kim RJ, Fieno DS, Parrish TB, et al. Relationship of MRI delayed contrast enhancement to irreversible injury, infarct age, and contractile function. Circulation 1999;100(19):1992–2002.

61. Assomull RG, Prasad SK, Lyne J, et al. Cardiovascular magnetic resonance, fibrosis, and prognosis in dilated cardiomyopathy. J Am Coll Cardiol 2006; 48(10):1977–85.

62. Mewton N, Liu CY, Croisille P, et al. Assessment of myocardial fibrosis with cardiovascular magnetic resonance. J Am Coll Cardiol 2011;57(8): 891–903.

63. Wassmuth R, Lentzsch S, Erdbruegger U, et al. Subclinical cardiotoxic effects of anthracyclines as assessed by magnetic resonance imaging—a pilot study. Am Heart J 2001;141(6):1007–13.

64. Ylanen K, Poutanen T, Savikurki-Heikkila P, et al. Cardiac magnetic resonance imaging in the evaluation of the late effects of anthracyclines among long-term survivors of childhood cancer. J Am Coll Cardiol 2013;61(14):1539–47.

65. Fallah-Rad N, Walker JR, Wassef A, et al. The utility of cardiac biomarkers, tissue velocity and strain imaging, and cardiac magnetic resonance imaging in predicting early left ventricular dysfunction in patients with human epidermal growth factor receptor II-positive breast cancer treated with adjuvant trastuzumab therapy. J Am Coll Cardiol 2011;57(22):2263–70.

66. Wassmuth R, Schulz-Menger J. Late gadolinium enhancement in left ventricular dysfunction after trastuzumab. J Am Coll Cardiol 2011;58(25):2697–8 [author reply: 9-700].

67. Lawley C, Wainwright C, Segelov E, et al. Pilot study evaluating the role of cardiac magnetic resonance imaging in monitoring adjuvant trastuzumab therapy for breast cancer. Asia Pac J Clin Oncol 2012;8(1):95–100.

68. Biglands JD, Radjenovic A, Ridgway JP. Cardiovascular magnetic resonance physics for clinicians: Part II. J Cardiovasc Magn Reson 2012;14:66.

69. Coelho-Filho OR, Mongeon FP, Mitchell R, et al. Role of transcytolemmal water-exchange in magnetic resonance measurements of diffuse myocardial fibrosis in hypertensive heart disease. Circ Cardiovasc Imaging 2013;6(1):134–41.

70. Coelho-Filho OR, Shah RV, Neilan TG, et al. Cardiac magnetic resonance assessment of interstitial myocardial fibrosis and cardiomyocyte hypertrophy in hypertensive mice treated with spironolactone. J Am Heart Assoc 2014;3(3):e000790.

71. Messroghli DR, Nordmeyer S, Dietrich T, et al. Assessment of diffuse myocardial fibrosis in rats using small-animal Look-Locker inversion recovery T1 mapping. Circ Cardiovasc Imaging 2011;4(6):636–40.

72. Sibley CT, Noureldin RA, Gai N, et al. T1 Mapping in cardiomyopathy at cardiac MR: comparison with endomyocardial biopsy. Radiology 2012;265(3):724–32.

73. Jerosch-Herold M, Sheridan DC, Kushner JD, et al. Cardiac magnetic resonance imaging of myocardial contrast uptake and blood flow in patients affected with idiopathic or familial dilated cardiomyopathy. Am J Physiol Heart Circ Physiol 2008;295(3):H1234–42.

74. Flett AS, Hayward MP, Ashworth MT, et al. Equilibrium contrast cardiovascular magnetic resonance for the measurement of diffuse myocardial fibrosis: preliminary validation in humans. Circulation 2010;122(2):138–44.

75. Iles L, Pfluger H, Phrommintikul A, et al. Evaluation of diffuse myocardial fibrosis in heart failure with cardiac magnetic resonance contrast-enhanced T1 mapping. J Am Coll Cardiol 2008;52(19):1574–80.

76. Vita T, Grani C, Abbasi SA, et al. Comparing CMR mapping methods and myocardial patterns toward heart failure outcomes in nonischemic dilated cardiomyopathy. JACC Cardiovasc Imaging 2018. [Epub ahead of print].

77. Tham EB, Haykowsky MJ, Chow K, et al. Diffuse myocardial fibrosis by T1-mapping in children with subclinical anthracycline cardiotoxicity: relationship to exercise capacity, cumulative dose and remodeling. J Cardiovasc Magn Reson 2013;15:48.

78. Jordan JH, Vasu S, Morgan TM, et al. Anthracycline-associated T1 mapping characteristics are elevated independent of the presence of cardiovascular comorbidities in cancer survivors. Circ Cardiovasc Imaging 2016;9(8) [pii:e004325].

79. Coelho-Filho OR, Shah RV, Mitchell R, et al. Quantification of cardiomyocyte hypertrophy by cardiac magnetic resonance: implications for early cardiac remodeling. Circulation 2013;128(11):1225–33.

80. Amzulescu MS, Langet H, Saloux E, et al. Head-to-head comparison of global and regional two-dimensional speckle tracking strain versus cardiac magnetic resonance tagging in a multicenter validation study. Circ Cardiovasc Imaging 2017;10(11) [pii:e006530].

81. Jolly MP, Jordan JH, Melendez GC, et al. Automated assessments of circumferential strain from cine CMR correlate with LVEF declines in cancer patients early after receipt of cardio-toxic chemotherapy. J Cardiovasc Magn Reson 2017;19(1):59.

82. Keltai K, Cervenak L, Mako V, et al. Doxorubicin selectively suppresses mRNA expression and production of endothelin-1 in endothelial cells. Vascul Pharmacol 2010;53(5–6):209–14.

83. Chaosuwannakit N, D'Agostino R Jr, Hamilton CA, et al. Aortic stiffness increases upon receipt of anthracycline chemotherapy. J Clin Oncol 2010;28(1):166–72.

84. Patel MR, White RD, Abbara S, et al. 2013 ACCF/ACR/ASE/ASNC/SCCT/SCMR appropriate utilization of cardiovascular imaging in heart failure: a joint report of the American College of Radiology Appropriateness Criteria Committee and the American College of Cardiology Foundation Appropriate Use Criteria Task Force. J Am Coll Cardiol 2013;61(21):2207–31.

85. Lipshultz SL, Adams MJ, Colan SD, et al. Long-term cardiovascular toxicity in children, adolescents, and young adults who receive cancer therapy: pathophysiology, course, monitoring, management, prevention, and research directions: a scientific statement from the American Heart Association. Circulation 2013;128(17):1927–95.

The Prognostic Value of Late Gadolinium Enhancement in Nonischemic Heart Disease

Zorana Mrsic, MD[a,b], Negareh Mousavi, MD[c],
Edward Hulten, MD, MPH[b,d],
Marcio Sommer Bittencourt, MD, MPH, PhD[e,f,g],*

KEYWORDS

- Late gadolinium enhancement • Myocardial disease • Diagnosis • Prognosis
- Nonischemic myocardial disease

KEY POINTS

- Cardiac magnetic resonance late gadolinium enhancement (LGE) is a robust imaging sequence that has become routine in the investigation of myocardial diseases.
- LGE is useful for diagnosis of the etiology in many myocardial diseases.
- The presence and extent of LGE have important prognostic implications in patients presenting with heart failure for most etiologies.

TECHNICAL ASPECTS OF LATE GADOLINIUM ENHANCEMENT

Gadolinium is a paramagnetic ion that has T1-shortening effects. When injected intravenously, it transits through the blood, into the myocardial extracellular volume (ECV), then washes out and recirculates to some degree before ultimately leaving the body unmetabolized via urinary excretion. Normal myocytes are tightly compacted with a small ECV, but pathologic myocardium affected by inflammation, infiltration, or infarction may expand the ECV, allowing for gadolinium accumulation upon its first passage through the myocardium (**Fig. 1**). With appropriate timing appreciative of gadolinium kinetics and MR

Disclosure Statement: All authors report no conflict of interest.

Disclaimer: The identification of specific products or scientific instrumentation is considered an integral part of the scientific endeavor and does not constitute endorsement or implied endorsement on the part of the author, Department of Defense, or any component agency. The views expressed in this abstract are those of the author and do not reflect the official policy of the Department of the Army, Department of Defense, or US government.

[a] Department of Cardiology, Walter Reed National Military Medical Center, 8901 Rockville Pike, Bethesda, MD 20814, USA; [b] Uniformed Services University School of Health Sciences, Bethesda, MD, USA; [c] McGill University Health Centre, Royal Victoria Hospital, 1001 Decarie Boulevard, D05.5115, Montreal, Quebec H4A 3J1, Canada; [d] Cardiopulmonary Clinic, Department of Medicine, Evans Army Community Hospital, 1650 Cochrane Circle, Fort Carson, CO 80913, USA; [e] Delboni - DASA, São Paulo, Brazil; [f] Hospital Israelita Albert Einstein & School of Medicine, Faculdade Israelita de Ciência da Saúde Albert Einstein, São Paulo, Brazil; [g] Center for Clinical and Epidemiological Research, University Hospital & Sao Paulo State Cancer Institute, University of Sao Paulo, Av. Lineu Prestes, 2565 – Butanta, São Paulo 05412-003, Brazil

* Corresponding author. Center for Clinical and Epidemiological Research, University Hospital & Sao Paulo State Cancer Institute, University of Sao Paulo, Av. Lineu Prestes, 2565 – Butanta, São Paulo 05412-003, Brazil.
E-mail address: mbittencourt@hu.usp.br

Normal myocardium   Acute infarction   Scar

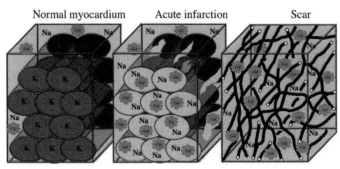

Intact cell membrane   Ruptured cell membrane   Collagen matrix

Fig. 1. The volume of distribution of gadolinium is increase in both acute and chronic infarcts. (*From* Higgins, CB; de Roos, Albert. Cardiovascular MRI and MRA. LWW. 2002; with permission.)

imaging hardware, including cardiac gating, and software, especially sequences that maximize T1-weighted signal to noise, healthy myocardium may be differentiated from cardiomyopathy involving expanded ECV, as with infiltration, inflammation, or infarction, via late gadolinium enhancement or LGE imaging (**Fig. 2**).

In order to perform late gadolinium enhancement (LGE) imaging for myocardial tissue characterization, the most common techniques approved for clinical use today have not deviated significantly from the classic T1-weighted gradient echo inversion recovery sequence read out several minutes after gadolinium infusion as initially described.[1] Although other contrast agents have been tested, standard gadolinium contrast agents are used in the vast majority of clinical cases. Similarly, the timing delay after gadolinium infusion may differ depending upon the MR imaging hardware and sequence, but typically ranges from 10 to 20 minutes after gadolinium infusion. The gadolinium is dosed by weight, which varies according to each specific product and may be infused as a rapid bolus or over several seconds, but should not be infused slowly over many minutes in order to avoid gadolinium washout before the entire contrast dose has been administered. The gadolinium administration intended for LGE purposes can also be used to perform some clinically useful first-pass imaging acquisition during the infusion. Often this might be vasodilator stress and rest perfusion imaging, which complement infarct imaging, especially for patients with symptoms of possible angina or being considered for coronary revascularization. Other options to take advantage of the gadolinium infusion might include coronary or thoracic angiography or selective slice plane imaging of a cardiac mass for first-pass perfusion.[2] The CE-MARC trial[3] evaluated the incremental value of routinely performing coronary magnetic resonance angiography (MRA) with the gadolinium infusion in addition to vasodilator stress perfusion CMR. However, the coronary MRA did not add diagnostic value to perfusion CMR in CE-MARC, and the MRA requires navigator gating to correct for respiratory motion and so is relatively time consuming (5 to 20 minutes) on contemporary scanners. Therefore, most sites do not routinely perform coronary MRA when conducting stress perfusion CMR with LGE viability for clinical indications.

Cardiac MR imaging centers most commonly rely upon 2-dimensional short axis slices through the ventricular myocardium for LGE imaging. Longitudinal slices, such as 4 chambers, 2 chambers, or 3 chambers, are often obtained either in single slices or stacks through each plane. Typically, the inversion time and field of view are optimized for left ventricular (LV) myocardial imaging. Classically, the standard protocol has involved the MR imaging technician starting with a standard inversion time, or TI, such as 200 milliseconds depending upon the particular magnet and field strength, and then adjusting the TI at small increments such as 30 milliseconds to reduce artifacts and optimize signal to noise. A semiautomated approach involves a series of snapshots at incremental TI, called a look locker. The technician simply selects the optimal TI from the look locker sequence and proceeds with the remainder of the LGE imaging. The right ventricle may also be evaluated, but attention must be paid to ensure that the inversion time is correct, as the right ventricle inversion time may be 50 to 100 milliseconds different from the LV inversion time, although newer scanners can overcome this difficulty automatically. For example, phase-sensitive inversion recovery (PSIR) sequences available on new MR imaging hardware and software essentially eliminate the need to adjust TI or use a look locker and provide a faster, more accurate, and simpler approach to LGE imaging.[4] However, PSIR LGE images still require review in order to ensure no images need to be repeated because of artifacts.[5]

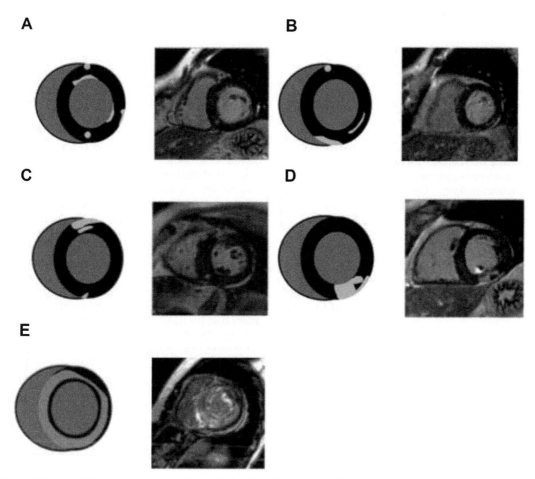

Fig. 2. Differing LGE patterns of cardiomyopathies. (*A*) Idiopathic Cardiomyopathy with a subendocardial and a midwall LGE pattern. (*B*) Sarcoidosis with a patchy LGE pattern and non-specific enhancement at the right ventricular insertion points. (*C*) Hypertrophic Cardiomyopathy with LGE pattern at the right ventricular insertion points. (*D*) Severe Myocarditis with a transmural LGE pattern. (*E*) Amyloidosis with the inability to adequately null the myocardium.

Alternative sequences have been performed and include steady-state free precession, or SSFP, readouts. In addition, newer MR imaging scanners are capable of performing free-breathing 3-dimensional LGE imaging of the whole heart using navigator techniques to eliminate respiratory motion, although the acquisition may require 3 to 10 minutes, depending upon the equipment. More recently, a black blood LGE technique[6] has been reported to be more sensitive at differentiating subendocardial infarcts from that blood pool that has typically been bright on classic LGE imaging, which may obscure small infarcts and unfortunately results in false-negative LGE images.

Gadolinium contrast agents for LGE imaging in general are widely regarded as safe and low risk. Because gadolinium is a toxic heavy metal ion,

clinical contrast agents chelate the gadolinium that is excreted in the urine. Nephrogenic systemic fibrosis (NSF), also known as nephrogenic fibrosing dermopathy, is a painful and debilitating chronic skin disease that has been rarely reported after gadolinium use for MR imaging.[7] However, NSF has been almost exclusively reported in patients with glomerular filtration rates below 30 mL/s/m², particularly patients on dialysis. Therefore, the US Food and Drug Administration (FDA) generally prohibits clinical use of gadolinium for those patients. Also, most cases of NSF were reported in association with gadolinium compounds with a linear molecular structure in contrast to newer agents with a cyclic molecule, which are safer. Gadolinium does cross the placenta and should not be administered to pregnant patients because of the risk of fetal toxicity. Rarely, anaphylaxis may occur. The American College of Radiology has published a summary of contrast agent safety that addresses these important topics.[8]

DIAGNOSTIC IMPLICATIONS OF LATE GADOLINIUM ENHANCEMENT IN NONISCHEMIC CARDIOMYOPATHY

CMR is an extremely valuable tool for the evaluation of patients with cardiomyopathy and has an important impact on diagnosis, prognosis, and therapeutic decision-making.[9] CMR plays a major role in determining the etiology of the underlying cardiomyopathy through its ability to characterize the myocardial tissue by using different techniques. Although this is usually performed with a combination of CMR sequences, tissue characterization generally includes late LGE, as it has been validated against histologic findings in a wide range of clinical scenarios. In particular, the pattern of LGE in the myocardium can help differentiate underlying etiology of nonischemic cardiomyopathies.[9] An example of the impact of CMR data on the diagnosis of dilated cardiomyopathy is presented in **Fig. 3**.[9] A detailed list of diagnostic and prognostic implications of CMR is presented in **Table 1**.

DILATED CARDIOMYOPATHY

Dilated cardiomyopathy likely represents an end-stage manifestation of multiple nonischemic disorders that can damage the myocardium. Approximately one-third of patients with dilated cardiomyopathy (DCM) will have evidence of replacement myocardial fibrosis by LGE in the midwall of the interventricular septum,[10,11] which can be related to chronic healing phase of myocarditis. CMR including LGE is useful in defining the etiology of DCM. It can differentiate ischemic from nonischemic LGE, including nonischemic patterns that may indicate other causes as will be further detailed.[9]

Interestingly, in a large study of patients with nonobstructive dilated cardiomyopathy, 13% displayed LGE in an infarct pattern, despite the absence of obstructive coronary artery disease.[10] This ischemic pattern may be a nonischemic pathology mimicking infarction or the result of transient occlusion caused by a nonobstructive unstable plaque, coronary vasoconstriction, or other transient myocardial ischemia.[12] Nevertheless, most CMR studies have demonstrated that LGE was a highly effective diagnostic tool, with a significant impact as a gatekeeper to coronary angiography by excluding major 3-vessel coronary artery disease (CAD) or left main disease in individuals with DCM.[13,14]

Moreover, the presence of LGE is associated with abnormalities in contractility and serves as a potential substrate for re-entrant ventricular arrhythmia.[9] The presence of LGE identifies a cohort of patients who do not respond as well to optimal medical therapy,[15] a finding independent of other standard clinical parameters such as QRS complex duration and N-terminal pro–B-type natriuretic peptide levels. Based on this evidence, some authors have proposed the use of LGE as a criterion for advanced therapy such as ICD, although current guidelines do not support such strategy.

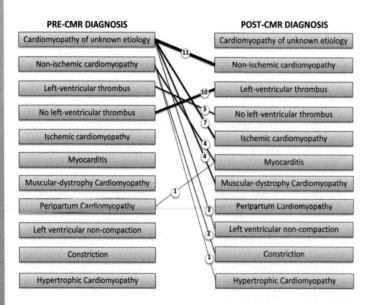

Fig. 3. Changes in diagnosis from pre versus post CMR. (*From* Abbasi SA, Ertel A, Shah RV, et al. Impact of cardiovascular magnetic resonance on management and clinical decision-making in heart failure patients. Journal of cardiovascular magnetic resonance: official journal of the Society for Cardiovascular Magnetic Resonance 2013;15:89; with permission.)

Table 1
Summary of the typical late gadolinium enhancement patterns, distribution, and their value for the diagnosis and prognosis in each clinical condition

Condition	Typical Pattern of LGE	Diagnosis	Prognosis/ Risk Stratification
Valvular disease	Heterogeneous: focal, subendocardial, midwall, or extensive diffuse; aortic stenosis LGE often anteroseptal; VHD with pulmonary hypertension LGE may affect RV septal insertion	+	+
Sarcoidosis	Patchy, multifocal, may be intensely bright because of granuloma formation, usually sparing subendocardium, anteroseptal LGE extending into RV free wall = hook sign	+	+
HCM	Patchy, midmyocardial, spares subendocardium, LGE in regions of wall thickening	+	+
Amyloidosis	Global transmural or subendocardial, difficulty nulling myocardium, atrial walls, and interatrial septum	+	+
Chagas	Heterogeneous, predominantly inferolateral, inferior, and apical LV segments	+	+
Muscular dystrophy	Subepicardial, primarily inferolateral wall	+	+
Systemic Sclerosis	Midwall, patchy or linear, basal and mid-LV segments	+	Uncertain
Lupus	Localized, midwall, primarily interventricular septum	+	Uncertain
Postinfectious	Subepicardial or midwall, inferior, lateral, and basal anteroseptal	+	+
ARVC	RV LGE, subepicardial inferior, and lateral LV wall	-	+
Postchemotherapy	Subepicardial linear LGE, lateral LV wall	+	Uncertain

MYOCARDITIS

Myocarditis commonly presents as an acute inflammatory disease. In this setting, the presence of LGE identifies acute inflammation, although later in the course of the disease LGE may be associated with areas of irreversible necrosis or fibrosis. Although the LGE distribution in myocarditis may be variable, the finding of LGE in the mid-wall and subepicardium of the left ventricle seems specific for viral myocarditis and has been validated against histology.[16] Additionally, some studies suggest the LGE distribution might be related to the type of virus.[17]

Older studies suggested that early postcontrast T1-weighted enhancement of the myocardium could be a marker of inflammation in myocarditis.[18] In addition, T2-weighted imaging demonstrating myocardial edema can be a diagnostic sign. Thus, the Lake Louise consensus group in 2009 provided recommendations on the use of CMR in patients with suspected myocarditis suggesting that positivity of 2 of 3 techniques (early enhancement ratio, LGE, and/or increased T2 signal) may be an ideal diagnostic approach for myocarditis.[18,19] Hence, combination of these techniques may be the best way to accurately identify acute myocarditis, although depending on the clinical presentation, LGE alone may suffice to confirm the diagnosis.

Additionally, some studies have suggested that the evaluation of myocarditis should also include T1 or T2 mapping. In a study of 61 patients with acute myocarditis and 67 patients with chronic myocarditis, diagnostic accuracy of native T1, that is, T1 mapping before contrast, was 99%, compared with 86% for LGE alone and 72% for increased T2-weighted signal for diagnosing acute myocarditis.[20] In chronic myocarditis, LGE alone performed better than T1 mapping (94% vs 84% accuracy), but the combination of the 2 techniques significantly improved overall accuracy. Nevertheless, T1 and T2 mapping are not yet included in myocarditis imaging guidelines.

HYPERTROPHIC CARDIOMYOPATHY

Hypertrophic cardiomyopathy (HCM) is the most common genetic myocardial disease and an important cause of sudden cardiac death in young people and athletes.[21] Although echocardiography remains as the initial test in suspected HCM, CMR provides a more comprehensive evaluation, including a more sensitive assessment of myocardial hypertrophy. However, the most meaningful use of CMR in HCM is the ability to identify and quantify myocardial fibrosis with the use of LGE in this patient population. LGE has been reported in 63% to 67% of patients with HCM.[22,23] In those individuals, LGE represents areas of focal interstitial expansion caused by myocardial replacement fibrosis,[24] and it typically presents with patchy enhancement involving myocardial walls with the greatest hypertrophy and at the right ventricular (RV) septal insertion sites.

AMYLOIDOSIS

Cardiac amyloidosis (CA) is a rare infiltrative disorder in which abnormally folded amyloid proteins are deposited within the myocardium, and CMR can be a valuable tool for its detection. Presence of amyloid proteins in myocardial interstitium is associated with characteristic patterns of LGE, usually related to marked expansion of the ECV.[25]

LGE may appear for CA patients as a widespread circumferential subendocardial enhancement most pronounced at the base and middle of the ventricle, matching the distribution of amyloid protein on histology. Validation against endomyocardial biopsy was performed in 33 patients with diastolic dysfunction, and features concerning for amyloid and diffuse subendocardial LGE had a specificity of nearly 95% for CA diagnosis.[26,27] Although circumferential subendocardial LGE is present in the majority of patients with CA, alternative patterns of LGE such as midwall, subepicardial, and interatrial septum enhancement are also commonly encountered (see **Fig. 2**).[27] It is important to note that the interpretation of LGE images in this population can often be challenging because of the diffuse nature of LGE and the inability to adequately null the myocardial signal because of prolonged and significant gadolinium deposition into the expanded ECV.

CMR can also be used to discriminate light chain (AL) amyloidosis from the transthyretin (ATTR) CA forms. Not only are the morphologic features generally different between AL and ATTR, as ATTR is more associated with severely thickened myocardium, but also a study comparing LGE findings in 46 patients with biopsy-proven AL and 51 with ATTR amyloidosis,= noted that LGE was much more extensive in ATTR, with 90% demonstrating transmural LGE compared with only 37% in AL.[28] These investigators developed an LGE scoring system that differentiated the 2 types with 87% sensitivity and 96% specificity.

SARCOIDOSIS

Sarcoidosis is a multiorgan inflammatory disorder characterized by noncaseating granulomatous infiltration. The diagnosis of cardiac sarcoidosis may be challenging and delayed, particularly in patients without known extracardiac sarcoidosis, which may be underdiagnosed.[29] Because of these complexities several diagnostic guidelines have been proposed, including the one from the Japanese Ministry of Health in 2006, the United States National Institute of Health algorithm from 2014, the World Association for Sarcoidosis and Other Granulomatous Disorders (WASOG) recommendations for initial diagnosis of cardiac sarcoidosis, and the Heart Rhythm Society 2014 clinical algorithm for determining probable cardiac sarcoidosis, defined as greater than 50% likelihood of cardiac sarcoid.[30]

Challenges with all of the existing clinical diagnostic criteria include that history, physical examination, electrocardiogram (ECG), and echocardiography lack sensitivity and specificity; thus most imaging centers use either positron emission tomography/computed tomography (PET/CT) or CMR for evaluation of suspected cardiac sarcoidosis depending upon institutional expertise, with a trend toward CMR, as it involves no ionizing radiation and is not technically reliant upon patient glucose and insulin manipulation for diagnostic images. Both the WASOG and HRS criteria for sarcoidosis include CMR LGE, although the JMH criteria have not yet incorporated LGE. Several investigators have shown that CMR can readily identify individuals with CS by the identification of small areas of myocardial involvement using LGE.[31] Furthermore, CMR and PET/CT offer complementary information such that both tests may be considered in some patients, as CMR best identifies area of fibrosis but is relatively incapable of identifying active inflammation or staging disease activity among sarcoid patients, as with PET-CT (**Fig. 4**).[32]

The LGE pattern in CS is variable, but it most commonly affects the basal to mid anteroseptum with a classic pattern of midwall or epicardial enhancement. Often the LGE is focal and bright because of localized expansion of ECV with noncaseating granulomatous inflammation and fibrosis. Focal basal to midanteroseptal LGE with concomitant RV LGE has been termed the hook sign and is consistent usually with CS. Subendocardial or transmural enhancement in almost any coronary distribution can also be present, which may mimic infarction. One CMR study of 58 patients with biopsy-proven pulmonary sarcoidosis found 19 patients with evidence of

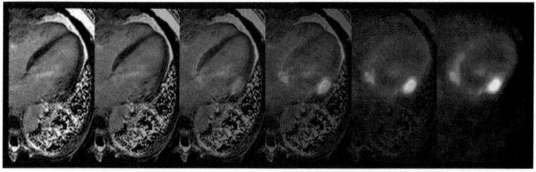

Cardiac MRI LGE ⟶ PDG PET inflammation

Fig. 4. Coregistration of CMR and cardiac PET, with a region of focal LGE on the basal anterolateral wall on CMR and active inflammation in the same area in addition to an area of less intense inflammation in the basal anteroseptum that did not have significant LGE. (*From* Hulten E, Aslam S, Osborne M, Abbasi S, Bittencourt MS, Blankstein R. Cardiac sarcoidosis—state of the art review. Cardiovascular Diagnosis and Therapy 2016;6(1):50–63; with permission.)

LGE, mostly in the basal and lateral myocardium, a higher prevalence than identified by standard Japanese Ministry of Health (JMH) guidelines.[33] Cardiac sarcoidosis is a protean disease, the evaluation of which benefits from careful integration of all clinical history and diagnostic studies with LGE CMR.

ARRHYTHMOGENIC VENTRICULAR CARDIOMYOPATHY

ARVC is an inherited cardiomyopathy that is associated with arrhythmias and sudden death. Because of its ability to accurately assess RV structure and function, MR imaging has become an integral part of the diagnosis of ARVC.[34] The presence of RV LGE has been described in up to 60% of cases.[35]

Diagnostic findings in this disease include RV dilatation and global or regional dysfunction including focal RV systolic dyskinesis or aneurysm.[34] CMR is the gold standard method for the diagnosis of arrhythmogenic ventricular cardiomyopathy. Although in some cases, LGE of the RV free wall has been reported,[35] this can be difficult to distinguish from myocardial fat. LV LGE, on the other hand can delineate different patterns of AVC. In the classic form, midwall LGE is seen in the inferolateral and inferior wall, while the left-dominant phenotype, often misdiagnosed as DCM, may include prominent LV midwall enhancement affecting the septum with preserved RV function.[36] LGE is evaluated and often noted in patients undergoing evaluation for possible diagnosis of AVC, but RV LGE lacks accuracy and reliability. Thus, despite initial enthusiasm for RV LGE, this criterion was removed from the most recent AVD diagnostic guidelines in favor of RV volumes and systolic function.

CHAGAS

Chagas disease (CD) is a chronic disease caused by *Trypanosoma cruzi* infection and is an important cause of heart failure and mortality that predominantly affects Latin American countries. CD has 3 clinical phases: acute, indeterminate, and chronic. In its chronic form, CD can affect the gastrointestinal tract and/or the cardiovascular system. Chronic chagas cardiomyopathy (CCM) is both the most common and the deadliest manifestation of chronic infection. Although the clinical presentation and disease progression are highly variable, from minor rhythm disturbances to advanced heart failure, many of the complications associated with it are atrioventricular blocks and ventricular arrhythmias that can lead to sudden cardiac death (SCD). Myocardial delayed enhancement on cardiac MR imaging has surfaced as a diagnostic and prognostic tool for cardiac involvement in CD, as it has demonstrated higher sensitivity than electrocardiography and echocardiography.[37] However, because the confirmation of CD is based on serologic evaluation, the role of LGE in the diagnosis of CD is mostly in the documentation of cardiac involvement from the systemic disease.

OTHER NONISCHEMIC CARDIOMYOPATHIES

CMR is also able to diagnose a variety of other nonischemic cardiomyopathies, including takotsubo cardiomyopathy demonstrating myocardial edema without LGE,[38] iron-overload cardiomyopathy (using T2* mapping),[39] and Anderson-Fabry disease with characteristic findings of basal lateral LGE.[40] Although LGE can be present in most myocardial diseases, the pattern of distribution might not be diagnostic in many, and its findings may solely be interpreted as an indication of structurally abnormal myocardium.

PROGNOSTIC IMPLICATIONS OF LATE GADOLINIUM ENHANCEMENT IN NONISCHEMIC CARDIOMYOPATHY
Dilated Cardiomyopathy

Presence and extent of LGE in DCM have been linked to increased risk of SCD and ventricular arrhythmias independent of other markers of risk such as reduced LV ejection fraction (LVEF).[41,42] In a prospective longitudinal study in 472 patients with dilated cardiomyopathy over a median follow-up of 5.3 years,[43] patients with mid-wall fibrosis were significantly more likely to die (27% vs 11%) or have a significant arrhythmic event (30% vs 7%) when compared with patients without LGE. After adjustment for LVEF and other conventional prognostic factors, both the presence of fibrosis (HR, 2.43 [95% CI, 1.50–3.92]) and its extent (HR, 1.11 [95% CI, 1.06–1.16]) were independently and incrementally associated with mortality.

In a prospective study of 137 patients being considered for ICD placement, myocardial scarring detected by cardiac MR imaging was an independent predictor of adverse outcomes.[44] In patients with LVEF greater than 30%, significant scarring (>5% left ventricle) identifies a high-risk cohort similar in risk to those with LVEF of no more than 30%. Conversely, in patients with LVEF of less than or equal to 30%, minimal or no scarring identifies a low-risk cohort similar to those with LVEF greater than 30%.

In another prospective study enrolling 399 patients with dilated cardiomyopathy and an LVEF greater than 40%, a midwall LGE pattern was present in 25% of individuals and was associated with a ninefold increase in the risk of SCD or aborted SCD when compared with patients without LGE.[45] In this study, the estimated hazard ratios (HRs) for SCD or aborted SCD for patients with an LGE extent of 0% to 2.5%, 2.5% to 5%, and greater than 5% compared with those without LGE were 10.6 (95% confidence interval [CI], 3.9–29.4), 4.9 (95% CI, 1.3–18.9), and 11.8 (95% CI, 4.3–32.3), respectively.

Hypertrophic Cardiomyopathy

Several studies have examined the relationship between the presence of LGE and outcome in HCM.[22,23] Among 243 patients with HCM over a follow-up period of 3 years, LGE was seen in 67% of patients, with an odds ratio (OR) of 5.5 for all-cause mortality and 8.0 for cardiac mortality.[20] A meta-analysis with 2993 patients over a median follow-up of 3 years demonstrated that the presence of LGE was associated with a 3.4-fold increase in risk for SCD, a 1.8-fold increase in all-cause mortality, a 2.9-fold increase in cardiovascular mortality, and a trend for heart failure death.[46] Given the high prevalence of LGE, its presence alone cannot be used as an indication for ICD. Interestingly, the extent of LGE may have more discriminatory value than its presence. In this meta-analysis, after adjusting for baseline characteristics, the extent of LGE was strongly associated with the risk of SCD with an HR of 1.36 for every 10% increase in LGE extent.[46]

In another study with 1293 patients followed for 3.3 years, a continuous relationship was evident between LGE involvement by percent LV mass and SCD event risk in HCM patients, and an LGE of at least 15% of LV mass was associated with a twofold increase in SCD event risk in those patients otherwise considered to be at lower risk, with an estimated likelihood for SCD events of 6% at 5 years.[47]

Valvular Heart Disease

Valvular heart disease is an important public health problem, and it is a growing concern with the increasing in prevalence in the aging population, particularly for aortic stenosis (AS).[48] Although the current valvular guidelines recommend using CMR for evaluation of patients in whom echocardiography is not diagnostic,[49] there is evidence that CMR can detect early signs of cardiac dysfunction and assist in risk stratification of patients with valvular diseases beyond usual care.

In patients with severe aortic valve disease, the chronic pressure or volume overload results in progressive myocardial injury, myocyte degeneration, and interstitial myocardial fibrosis. This was previously described in histopathological studies in patients with AS and aortic insufficiency (AI) who underwent valve replacement surgery.[50] The process of myocyte degeneration and IM fibrosis was later correlated to decline in LV systolic function and heart failure.[51] In patients with AS and AI, the amount of fibrosis correlates with increase in LV end diastolic volumes, end systolic volumes, and mass, as well as an inverse relationship with LVEF.[52]

Weideman and colleagues[53] were the first to evaluate how myocardial fibrosis on CMR relates to prognosis in patients with severe symptomatic AS. They evaluated 58 patients who were followed for 9 months after aortic valve replacement (AVR) with clinical evaluation and repeat imaging. In their cohort, the extent and severity of fibrosis measured by LGE correlated with baseline New York Heart Association (NYHA) functional class, as well as postoperative prognosis and function. After a 9-month follow up, the degree of LGE remained unchanged in all groups. Although patients with no LGE experienced a significant improvement in NYHA functional class, patients with severe LGE demonstrated no functional improvement. Additionally, mortality during follow-up occurred only in patients with severe LGE, suggesting that the fibrosis is irreversible and a marker of poor prognosis in this population. Dweck and colleagues[54] also assessed the relationship of LGE and prognosis in patients with AS. They evaluated 143 patients with moderate to severe AS, followed them up for a mean of 2 years, and demonstrated that patients with a midwall LGE pattern, compared to matched patients with no LGE, had an eightfold increase in all-cause mortality. The risk of mortality also had a linear correlation with the LGE burden such that every 1% increase in LGE mass increased the risk of mortality by 5%. Although AVR improved survival in all patients, it did not lead to reversal of LGE, and the increased mortality associated with LGE persisted despite the intervention, with an incidence of 53.8 cases per 1000 patient-years in patients with LGE versus 13.7 cases per 1000 patient-years in patients without LGE. The association between presence of LGE and perioperative outcomes was also evaluated in the 63 patients who underwent AVR.[55] Compared with no LGE, the presence of midwall LGE was associated with a significantly increased 30-day composite endpoint of death, myocardial infarction, and cerebrovascular accident (CVA), and this was largely driven by CVA. The patients with midwall pattern LGE also had 3 times higher rates of heart block and a trend toward higher rates of ventricular tachycardia compared to patients with no LGE. Survival in patients with severe AS and evidence of LGE undergoing surgical and transcatheter AVR was examined by Barone-Rochette and colleagues.[56] In their cohort of 154 patients, 44 had preoperative evidence of LGE, which was associated with a significantly increased all-cause mortality and cardiovascular mortality over a median 2.9-year follow-up. In the largest cohort to date, Chin and colleagues[57] evaluated the association of myocardial fibrosis and outcomes in patients with aortic stenosis in 166 patients with AS followed for 2.9 plus or minus 0.8 years. In their cohort, LGE was associated with more severe AS, increased LV mass, impaired LV performance, and impaired functional status. LGE was also associated with a significantly higher mortality versus individuals with no LGE, with 71 deaths per 1000 patient-years versus 8 deaths per 1000 patient years. Additionally, although there was an association between the degree of AS and presence of LGE, about one-third of the patients with LGE had moderate AS, with similar outcomes to those with severe AS, suggesting that LGE

prognostic value is independent of the degree of stenosis.

Similar findings have been reported by Azevedo and colleagues[58] in a study of 54 individuals, 28 with predominant AS and 26 with predominant AI, who were undergoing AVR. They obtained baseline and repeated CMR at 27 months and extended follow-up to 4.3 plus or minus 1.4 years. On follow-up imaging, there was no change in the degree of LGE following AVR. Patients with more extensive LGE had significantly less postoperative improvement in LV systolic function. Additionally, presence of LGE was associated with a 1.26 times higher risk of mortality in a multivariate analysis, suggesting once more an association between LGE.

In mitral regurgitation (MR), LV remodeling and myocardial fibrosis may occur before the development of symptoms. In a study that evaluated LGE in 41 patients with at least moderate asymptomatic primary MR,[59] 31% of patients had evidence of LGE on MR imaging. LGE was present in both infarct and midwall patterns and correlated to increased LV end systolic and end diastolic volumes. Similar findings were seen in a cohort of 35 asymptomatic patients with at least moderate primary MR,[60] 31% of whom were found to have midwall pattern LGE, which correlated with significantly increased left atrial volumes compared to patients without LGE. These findings suggest that LV remodeling can be detected by CMR prior to development of LV dysfunction and clinical symptoms. Han and colleagues[61] evaluated patients with mitral valve prolapse (MVP) with CMR and found that 94% of their cohort had LGE on the mitral valve or the mitral annulus, while 63%, were found to have papillary muscle LGE, which strongly correlated to presence of complex ventricular arrhythmias, although this analysis was limited by a small number of events. In a more recent study of patients with MVP and moderate-to-severe MR,[62] the authors found no correlation between presence of LGE and arrhythmias by symptoms or ambulatory monitoring in patients with positive papillary muscle LGE. With respect to LGE and perioperative prognosis, Chaikriangkrai and colleagues[63] evaluated 48 patients with chronic severe primary and secondary MR undergoing mitral valve repair and followed them for a median of 11 months. They observed LGE in 40% of patients, which was associated with a 4.8-fold increased risk of permanent pacemaker implantation, repeat hospitalization, and ICU readmission.

Sarcoidosis

Over a median follow-up of 84 months, LGE on CMR was the only independent predictor of the composite endpoint of all-cause mortality, symptomatic life-threatening arrhythmia, unplanned hospitalization for heart failure, and cardiac transplantation HR: 5.7 (95% CI: 1.7–18.5) in a study of 312 individuals with proven sarcoidosis. A meta-analysis of prognostic CMR studies patients with known or suspected cardiac sarcoidosis demonstrated that the presence of LGE was associated with a 3.1% versus 0.6% annualized all-cause mortality (relative risk [RR]: 3.4, P=.04), 1.9% versus 0.3% cardiovascular mortality (RR: 10.7, P=.03), as well as ventricular arrhythmia occurring in 41 LGE-positive versus 0 LGE-negative patients (RR: 19.5, P=.003, **Fig. 5**).[64] More of this topic will be discussed in Hélder Jorge Andrade Gomes and colleagues' article, "The Value of T1 Mapping Techniques in the Assessment of Myocardial Interstitial Fibrosis," in this issue of this text.

Amyloidosis

The prognosis of immunoglobulin light-chain (AL) and transthyretin (ATTR) amyloidosis is influenced by presence and severity of cardiac involvement, which is used to help guide therapy. Although

the diagnostic performance of CMR has been well-validated for CA, its prognostic value has not been well-established, with several studies yielding mixed results.

Maceira and colleagues[25] prospectively evaluated CMR in 29 biopsy-confirmed patients with echocardiographic criteria for cardiac amyloidosis (25 AL, 4 TTR), compared with 16 controls. Among the patients with amyloidosis, those with LGE had significantly higher LV mass index, RV mass index, and lower LVEF. The same cohort was followed for a median 1.7 years but showed no significant difference in survival based on presence or absence of LGE.[65] Ruberg and colleagues[66] also found that the presence of LGE did not predict mortality in their cohort of 28 patients with systemic amyloidosis followed for 29 months.

In a retrospective study of 29 patients with AL amyloid,[67] the association of LGE on CMR and survival was evaluated. Despite an association with several markers of dysfunction and presence of congestive heart failure, the higher mortality associated with the presence of LGE was only noted in a univariate analysis (P=.002), and lost significance after adjustment for confounding.

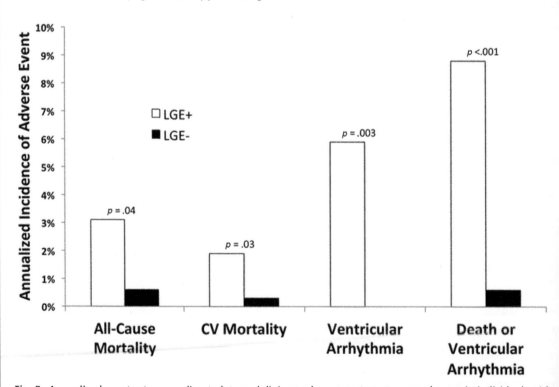

Fig. 5. Annualized event rates according to late gadolinium enhancement presence or absence in individuals with Sardoidosis. (*From* Hulten E, Agarwal V, Cahill M, et al. Presence of late gadolinium enhancement by cardiac magnetic resonance among patients with suspected cardiac sarcoidosis is associated with adverse cardiovascular prognosis clinical perspective: a systematic review and meta-analysis. Circulation: Cardiovascular Imaging 2016;9(9); with permission.)

Those findings were further corroborated by a prospective study with 44 patients with biopsy-proven AL amyloid followed for 62.7 months, which showed that LGE was associated with lower survival but was not found to be an independent predictor of mortality after adjustment.[68]

Subsequent larger studies, however, had different findings. In retrospective review of 76 patients with biopsy-proven AL amyloid followed for a median of 34.4 months, Boynton and colleagues[69] found a predominantly global pattern LGE (42%), which was associated with higher all-cause mortality (HR: 2.93, P<.001) compared with no LGE. Austin and colleagues[70] examined a cohort of 25 patients with biopsy-confirmed amyloidosis and reported a significantly decreased survival in those with LGE, which was the strongest predictor of mortality. Another prospective study included 90 individuals with suspected cardiac amyloid diffuse LGE who had a 2-year survival rate of only 21% compared with 81% in those without LGE. In a multivariate analysis, the presence of LGE was the strongest predictor of all-cause mortality (HR: 7.9, 95% CI: 3.1–20.1).[71] For the secondary endpoint of composite of death, cardiac transplantation, or hospital admission for heart failure, presence of LGE (HR: 6.5, 95% CI: 2.6–16.0) was the strongest predictor in multivariable models. Fontana and colleagues[72] followed 250 patients with AL and ATTR with CMR for 24 plus or minus 13 months. In their cohort, increasing LGE (none, subendocardial, transmural) was associated in AL and ATTR with lower systolic blood pressure, electrocardiogram (ECG) changes, increased NT-pro-BNP, structural and functional changes, increasingly elevated native T1 and extracellular volume (ECV), and more severe echocardiographic diastolic dysfunction. In ATTR, increasing LGE was also associated with decreased functional capacity. At follow-up, the survival curves indicated a 92% chance of survival in patients with no LGE, 81% for patients with subendocardial LGE, and 61% for patients with transmural LGE. Transmural LGE was a significant predictor of mortality (HR, 5.4; 95% CI, 2.1–13.7) and remained significant after adjustment for other relevant disease variables and treatment status.

Conflicting results of early studies of LGE prognosis in cardiac amyloid appear to be related to an inability to detect diffuse enhancement that is a hallmark of this disease process. Newer CMR tissue characterization techniques can overcome these limitations and provide more concrete data on prognostic implication of MR imaging in cardiac amyloid.

Chagas Disease

The pattern of LGE in Chagas cardiomyopathy is heterogeneous, but tends to involve the inferolateral, inferior, and apical LV segments.[73–75] The presence and extent of LGE have demonstrated a positive correlation with disease severity and NYHA class, as well as a negative correlation with LVEF.

Contrast-enhanced MR imaging has been used to stratify arrhythmia risk in patients with CCM, specifically ventricular tachycardia (VT). In a study of 41 patients,[76] the presence of 2 or more contiguous segments of transmural LGE but not the overall extent of LGE was an independent predictor of VT and was associated with a 4.1-fold higher risk of arrhythmia. In a subsequent study of 61 patients with CCM,[75] myocardial fibrosis detected by CMR was the most significant predictor of ventricular arrhythmia, with 12% of myocardial fibrosis derived as a cutoff point delineating significant increase in arrhythmia risk. Two recent studies have further corroborated the independent prognostic value of LGE on CMR for the long-term prognosis of individuals with CD.[77,78]

Muscular Dystrophy

Muscular dystrophy is characterized by progressive weakness and degeneration of skeletal muscles but can affect smooth and cardiac muscle also. Duchenne muscular dystrophy (DMD) is an X-linked recessive disorder, leading to reduced/abnormal dystrophin. Becker muscular dystrophy (BMD) is a milder form, caused by the same mutation, with a nearly normal life expectancy, but with a high incidence of cardiac involvement.[79] Cardiac involvement carries not only an increased morbidity but also an increased risk of mortality in patients with suffering from muscular dystrophy, and MR imaging has demonstrated high sensitivity in determining the extent of cardiac involvement in muscular dystrophy patients.[80–82]

Numerous studies have established the prognostic value of LGE with respect to LV systolic function, heart failure, arrhythmias, and death.[80,83–86] Tandon and colleagues[83] demonstrated a significant correlation of LGE and decline in LV systolic function. In their cohort of 98 DMD patients, the presence of LGE had the strongest correlation with LVEF, and the development of LGE was associated with a 2.2% annual decline in LV systolic function. Similar findings were seen in a study of 27 BMD patients, in which the number of LGE-positive segments correlated well to the LVEF.[85] LGE extent is also related to the occurrence of arrhythmias (odds ratio OR]: 5.34, CI: 1.19-23.919). In a 4-year follow-up, the presence of transmural LGE was associated with increased rates of hospitalization for heart failure and ventricular arrhythmias in patients with DMD/BMD.[84]

Increased mortality in patients with DMD and LGE was first reported by Hor and colleagues[86] in a cohort of 314 DMD patients. They demonstrated a 10% mortality in patients with LGE compared to a single death among patients without LGE. The findings were confirmed in a subsequent study of 32 patients with DMD in whom increasing LGE was an independent predictor of mortality.[80]

These studies highlight the utility of cardiac MR imaging in diagnosing and risk stratifying patients with muscular dystrophy. Further studies are needed to evaluate if earlier detection of subtle abnormalities and earlier treatment can alter the prognosis.

Systemic Sclerosis

Systemic sclerosis (SSc), also known as systemic scleroderma, is an autoimmune connective tissue disorder characterized by vascular dysfunction and multiorgan fibrosis. Cardiac involvement, which can take many forms including myocardial fibrosis, is common and carries a poor prognosis.[87,88]

The use of cardiac MR imaging to detect myocardial fibrosis in SSc was described in numerous studies,[89–92] with a prevalence ranging from 12% to 53%, mostly with midwall patchy or linear pattern, with predominant involvement of the basal and mid segments of the LV.

There is limited information in the literature regarding the effect of LGE on outcomes in SSC, however. In a letter published in JACC,[93] Mousseaux and colleagues reported their findings in a cohort of 58 patients with SSc followed for a mean 19 months. In their report, the presence of LGE was independently associated with MACE (HR: 3.48; 95% CI: 1.01–12.67). Further research is needed to confirm those findings.

Postinfectious

In a study of 202 consecutive biopsy-proven viral myocarditis patients followed for a median 4.7 years,[94] the presence of LGE was the best independent predictor of all-cause mortality and cardiac mortality and carried an 8.4-fold increase in all-cause mortality and a 12.8-fold increase in cardiac mortality, independent of clinical symptoms. In another prospective study of 405 patients followed for more than 4 years,[95] the OR for LGE presence for the combined endpoint of cardiac death, sudden cardiac death, aborted sudden cardiac death, and appropriate implantable cardiac defibrillator (ICD) discharges was 10.9 (P<.001). The extent

of LGE[96] and the location outside of inferolateral wall at diagnosis were also demonstrated to be independent predictors of adverse cardiac outcomes with an HR of 1.42 (P=.027) and 5.88 (P<.01), respectively.[97] On serial CMR, absence of LGE has also been associated with recovery of LVEF, and resolution of LGE has a better prognosis than those patients with persistent LGE. The involvement of the anteroseptal wall rather than other LV segments appears to be associated with the highest risk for the combined endpoint of cardiac death, appropriate ICD discharge, resuscitated cardiac arrest, and hospitalization for heart failure (OR: 2.73; 95% CI: 1.20–5.90).[98] In a large prospective study of 670 patients with suspected myocarditis followed for a median of 4.7 years, Gräni and colleagues[99] demonstrated that LGE extent per 10% increase was associated with a 79% increase in risk of MACE, highlighting that both the presence and extent of LGE have significant implications on patient outcomes in acute myocarditis.

Arrhythmogenic Ventricular Cardiomyopathy

LGE has been found to correlate with several markers of risk in AVC. In 8 patients who had detectible RV LGE, sustained VT could be induced in 6 patients on EP study, while none of the patients without LGE had inducible VT.[35] Additionally, Cheng and colleagues[100] demonstrated that LGE is an independent predictor of syncope in patients with ARVC (OR 8.827, 95% CI 1.945–40.068, P=.005). In a prospective study of 369 patients who met at least 1 diagnostic criterion for ARVC,[101] the presence of LGE was associated with a 19.3-fold increased risk of achieving the composite endpoint of cardiac death, sustained VT, VF, and appropriate ICD discharge over 51 months, while a normal CMR had a negative predictive value of 99% for major clinical events.

Although the Task Force Criteria for AVC do not include the presence of LGE in diagnostic criteria, the presence of LGE, however, when reliably identified, does have significant prognostic implications, and its absence is associated with high event-free survival rates, which can provide reassurance to patients and providers.

Postchemotherapy

Cardio-oncology is an ever-growing field with the primary focus of assessment and management of cardiovascular diseases in patients with cancer, as well as cancer survivors. Several cardiac abnormalities may arise in cancer patients and cancer survivors, and cardiac MR imaging had increasingly been used to assist in diagnosis, risk stratification, and management in this patient population.

Among other clinical scenarios in cardio-oncology, the evaluation of postchemotherapy cardiotoxicity is one of the most frequent clinical presentations in this scenario.

In addition to evaluation of subtle changes in LV dimensions, volumes, and systolic function, myocardial fibrosis as evidenced by LGE has been described in patients with chemotherapy-induced cardiomyopathy. In a study of 10 patients with Trastuzumab-related cardiomyopathy,[102] all patients had evidence of subepicardial linear LGE in the lateral portion of the LV, while none of the patients treated with anthracyclines had evidence of LGE despite persistent myocardial dysfunction.[103] Although early follow-up studies suggested persistent LGE despite normalization of LV function in patients treated with Trastuzumab,[102] a long-term follow-up study[104] found no evidence of LGE in 26 patients 5 months following treatment with Trastuzumab and anthracycline. LGE on CMR has also been instrumental in identifying evidence of myocarditis related to immunotherapy,[105,106] although current data suggest that LGE patterns do not predict outcomes in this population.

Cardiac MR imaging can effectively evaluate cardiac structure and function with minimal inter-observer variability of echocardiography; however, the data on prognostic implications of LGE in the various clinical scenarios of cardio-oncology patients are scarce and warrant further investigation. An in-depth analysis of this question is offered in Thiago Quinaglia A.C. Silva and colleagues' article, "State-of-the-Art Quantitative Assessment of Myocardial Ischemia by Stress Perfusion CMR," in this issue of this text.

SUMMARY

LGE has become part of the routine imaging protocol for CMR on the evaluation of nonischemic cardiomyopathy. Its presence, extent, and pattern of distribution have important clinical implications for the diagnosis and prognosis of several different causes of nonischemic cardiomyopathy. Additionally, LGE information is useful to guide medical and interventional therapies, including implantation of ICDs and ablation of arrhythmias in various clinical scenarios.

REFERENCES

1. Kim RJ, Wu E, Rafael A, et al. The use of contrast-enhanced magnetic resonance imaging to identify reversible myocardial dysfunction. N Engl J Med 2000;343(20):1445–53.
2. Hundley WG, Bluemke DA, Finn JP, et al. ACCF/ACR/AHA/NASCI/SCMR 2010 expert consensus document on cardiovascular magnetic resonance A Report of the American College of Cardiology Foundation Task Force on Expert Consensus Documents. J Am Coll Cardiol 2010;55(23):2614–62.
3. Greenwood JP, Maredia N, Younger JF, et al. Cardiovascular magnetic resonance and single-photon emission computed tomography for diagnosis of coronary heart disease (CE-MARC): a prospective trial. Lancet 2012;379(9814):453–60.
4. Kido T, Kido T, Nakamura M, et al. Three-dimensional phase-sensitive inversion recovery sequencing in the evaluation of left ventricular myocardial scars in ischemic and non-ischemic cardiomyopathy: comparison to three-dimensional inversion recovery sequencing. Eur J Radiol 2014;83(12):2159–66.
5. Kramer CM, Barkhausen J, Flamm SD, et al. Standardized cardiovascular magnetic resonance (CMR) protocols 2013 update. J Cardiovasc Magn Reson 2013;15(1):91.
6. Kim HW, Rehwald WG, Jenista ER, et al. Dark-blood delayed enhancement cardiac magnetic resonance of myocardial infarction. JACC Cardiovasc Imaging 2018;11(12):1758–69.
7. Grobner T. Gadolinium–a specific trigger for the development of nephrogenic fibrosing dermopathy and nephrogenic systemic fibrosis? Nephrol Dial Transplant 2006;21(4):1104–8.
8. Radiology ACo. ACR manual on contrast media, version 9. 2013 2015. Available at: https://www.acr.org/-/media/ACR/Files/Clinical-Resources/Contrast_Media.pdf.
9. Abbasi SA, Ertel A, Shah RV, et al. Impact of cardiovascular magnetic resonance on management and clinical decision-making in heart failure patients. J Cardiovasc Magn Reson 2013;15:89.
10. McCrohon JA, Moon JC, Prasad SK, et al. Differentiation of heart failure related to dilated cardiomyopathy and coronary artery disease using gadolinium-enhanced cardiovascular magnetic resonance. Circulation 2003;108(1):54–9.
11. Mahrholdt H, Wagner A, Judd RM, et al. Delayed enhancement cardiovascular magnetic resonance assessment of non-ischaemic cardiomyopathies. Eur Heart J 2005;26(15):1461–74.
12. Pasupathy S, Air T, Dreyer RP, et al. Systematic review of patients presenting with suspected myocardial infarction and non-obstructive coronary arteries (MINOCA). Circulation 2015;131(10):861–70.
13. Assomull RG, Shakespeare C, Kalra PR, et al. Role of cardiovascular magnetic resonance as a gatekeeper to invasive coronary angiography in patients presenting with heart failure of unknown etiology. Circulation 2011;124(12):1351–60.
14. Pilz G, Bernhardt P, Klos M, et al. Clinical implication of adenosine-stress cardiac magnetic

resonance imaging as potential gatekeeper prior to invasive examination in patients with AHA/ACC class II indication for coronary angiography. Clin Res Cardiol 2006;95(10):531–8.

15. Iles L, Pfluger H, Lefkovits L, et al. Myocardial fibrosis predicts appropriate device therapy in patients with implantable cardioverter-defibrillators for primary prevention of sudden cardiac death. J Am Coll Cardiol 2011;57(7):821–8.

16. Mahrholdt H, Goedecke C, Wagner A, et al. Cardiovascular magnetic resonance assessment of human myocarditis: a comparison to histology and molecular pathology. Circulation 2004;109(10):1250–8.

17. Mahrholdt H, Wagner A, Deluigi CC, et al. Presentation, patterns of myocardial damage, and clinical course of viral myocarditis. Circulation 2006;114(15):1581–90.

18. Friedrich MG, Strohm O, Schulz-Menger J, et al. Contrast media-enhanced magnetic resonance imaging visualizes myocardial changes in the course of viral myocarditis. Circulation 1998;97(18):1802–9.

19. Friedrich MG, Sechtem U, Schulz-Menger J, et al. Cardiovascular magnetic resonance in myocarditis: a JACC white paper. J Am Coll Cardiol 2009;53(17):1475–87.

20. Hinojar R, Foote L, Arroyo Ucar E, et al. Native T1 in discrimination of acute and convalescent stages in patients with clinical diagnosis of myocarditis: a proposed diagnostic algorithm using CMR. JACC Cardiovasc Imaging 2015;8(1):37–46.

21. Semsarian C, Ingles J, Maron MS, et al. New perspectives on the prevalence of hypertrophic cardiomyopathy. J Am Coll Cardiol 2015;65(12):1249–54.

22. Bruder O, Wagner A, Jensen CJ, et al. Myocardial scar visualized by cardiovascular magnetic resonance imaging predicts major adverse events in patients with hypertrophic cardiomyopathy. J Am Coll Cardiol 2010;56(11):875–87.

23. O'Hanlon R, Grasso A, Roughton M, et al. Prognostic significance of myocardial fibrosis in hypertrophic cardiomyopathy. J Am Coll Cardiol 2010;56(11):867–74.

24. Maron MS, Maron BJ, Harrigan C, et al. Hypertrophic cardiomyopathy phenotype revisited after 50 years with cardiovascular magnetic resonance. J Am Coll Cardiol 2009;54(3):220–8.

25. Maceira AM, Joshi J, Prasad SK, et al. Cardiovascular magnetic resonance in cardiac amyloidosis. Circulation 2005;111(2):186–93.

26. Vogelsberg H, Mahrholdt H, Deluigi CC, et al. Cardiovascular magnetic resonance in clinically suspected cardiac amyloidosis: noninvasive imaging compared to endomyocardial biopsy. J Am Coll Cardiol 2008;51(10):1022–30.

27. Selvanayagam JB, Hawkins PN, Paul B, et al. Evaluation and management of the cardiac amyloidosis. J Am Coll Cardiol 2007;50(22):2101–10.

28. Dungu JN, Valencia O, Pinney JH, et al. CMR-based differentiation of AL and ATTR cardiac amyloidosis. JACC Cardiovasc Imaging 2014;7(2):133–42.

29. Okada DR, Bravo PE, Vita T, et al. Isolated cardiac sarcoidosis: a focused review of an under-recognized entity. J Nucl Cardiol 2018;25(4):1136–46.

30. Birnie DH, Sauer WH, Bogun F, et al. HRS expert consensus statement on the diagnosis and management of arrhythmias associated with cardiac sarcoidosis. Heart Rhythm 2014;11(7):1305–24.

31. Smedema JP, Snoep G, van Kroonenburgh MP, et al. Evaluation of the accuracy of gadolinium-enhanced cardiovascular magnetic resonance in the diagnosis of cardiac sarcoidosis. J Am Coll Cardiol 2005;45(10):1683–90.

32. Vita T, Okada DR, Veillet-Chowdhury M, et al. Complementary value of cardiac magnetic resonance imaging and positron emission tomography/computed tomography in the assessment of cardiac sarcoidosis CLINICAL PERSPECTIVE. Circ Cardiovasc Imaging 2018;11(1):e007030.

33. Smedema JP, Snoep G, van Kroonenburgh MP, et al. The additional value of gadolinium-enhanced MRI to standard assessment for cardiac involvement in patients with pulmonary sarcoidosis. Chest 2005;128(3):1629–37.

34. Marcus FI, McKenna WJ, Sherrill D, et al. Diagnosis of arrhythmogenic right ventricular cardiomyopathy/dysplasia: proposed modification of the task force criteria. Circulation 2010;121(13):1533–41.

35. Tandri H, Saranathan M, Rodriguez ER, et al. Noninvasive detection of myocardial fibrosis in arrhythmogenic right ventricular cardiomyopathy using delayed-enhancement magnetic resonance imaging. J Am Coll Cardiol 2005;45(1):98–103.

36. Sen-Chowdhry S, Syrris P, Prasad SK, et al. Left-dominant arrhythmogenic cardiomyopathy: an under-recognized clinical entity. J Am Coll Cardiol 2008;52(25):2175–87.

37. Lee-Felker S, Thomas M, Felker E, et al. Value of cardiac MRI for evaluation of chronic Chagas disease cardiomyopathy. Clin Radiol 2016;71(6):618.e1-7.

38. Eitel I, von Knobelsdorff-Brenkenhoff F, Bernhardt P, et al. Clinical characteristics and cardiovascular magnetic resonance findings in stress (takotsubo) cardiomyopathy. JAMA 2011;306(3):277–86.

39. Kirk P, Roughton M, Porter JB, et al. Cardiac T2* magnetic resonance for prediction of cardiac complications in thalassemia major. Circulation 2009;120(20):1961–8.

40. Moon JC, Sachdev B, Elkington AG, et al. Gadolinium enhanced cardiovascular magnetic resonance in Anderson-Fabry disease. Evidence for a disease specific abnormality of the myocardial interstitium. Eur Heart J 2003;24(23):2151–5.

41. Assomull RG, Prasad SK, Lyne J, et al. Cardiovascular magnetic resonance, fibrosis, and prognosis in dilated cardiomyopathy. J Am Coll Cardiol 2006; 48(10):1977–85.

42. Lehrke S, Lossnitzer D, Schob M, et al. Use of cardiovascular magnetic resonance for risk stratification in chronic heart failure: prognostic value of late gadolinium enhancement in patients with non-ischaemic dilated cardiomyopathy. Heart 2011;97(9):727–32.

43. Gulati A, Jabbour A, Ismail TF, et al. Association of fibrosis with mortality and sudden cardiac death in patients with nonischemic dilated cardiomyopathy. JAMA 2013;309(9):896–908.

44. Klem I, Weinsaft JW, Bahnson TD, et al. Assessment of myocardial scarring improves risk stratification in patients evaluated for cardiac defibrillator implantation. J Am Coll Cardiol 2012; 60(5):408–20.

45. Halliday BP, Gulati A, Ali A, et al. Association between midwall late gadolinium enhancement and sudden cardiac death in patients with dilated cardiomyopathy and mild and moderate left ventricular systolic dysfunction. Circulation 2017;135(22): 2106–15.

46. Weng Z, Yao J, Chan RH, et al. Prognostic value of LGE-CMR in HCM: a meta-analysis. JACC Cardiovasc Imaging 2016;9(12):1392–402.

47. Chan RH, Maron BJ, Olivotto I, et al. Prognostic value of quantitative contrast-enhanced cardiovascular magnetic resonance for the evaluation of sudden death risk in patients with hypertrophic cardiomyopathy. Circulation 2014;130(6):484–95.

48. Benjamin EJ, Virani SS, Callaway CW, et al. Heart disease and stroke statistics—2018 update: a report from the American Heart Association. Circulation 2018;137(12):e67–492.

49. Nishimura RA, Otto CM, Bonow RO, et al. 2014 AHA/ACC guideline for the management of patients with valvular heart disease: a report of the American College of Cardiology/American Heart Association Task Force on Practice Guidelines. J Am Coll Cardiol 2014;63(22): e57–185.

50. Krayenbuehl HP, Hess OM, Monrad ES, et al. Left ventricular myocardial structure in aortic valve disease before, intermediate, and late after aortic valve replacement. Circulation 1989;79(4): 744–55.

51. Hein S, Arnon E, Kostin S, et al. Progression from compensated hypertrophy to failure in the pressure-overloaded human heart: structural deterioration and compensatory mechanisms. Circulation 2003;107(7):984–91.

52. Nigri M, Azevedo CF, Rochitte CE, et al. Contrast-enhanced magnetic resonance imaging identifies focal regions of intramyocardial fibrosis in patients with severe aortic valve disease: correlation with quantitative histopathology. Am Heart J 2009; 157(2):361–8.

53. Weidemann F, Herrmann S, Störk S, et al. Impact of myocardial fibrosis in patients with symptomatic severe aortic stenosis. Circulation 2009;120(7): 577–84.

54. Dweck MR, Joshi S, Murigu T, et al. Midwall fibrosis is an independent predictor of mortality in patients with aortic stenosis. J Am Coll Cardiol 2011;58(12): 1271–9.

55. Quarto C, Dweck MR, Murigu T, et al. Late gadolinium enhancement as a potential marker of increased perioperative risk in aortic valve replacement. Interact Cardiovasc Thorac Surg 2012;15(1): 45–50.

56. Barone-Rochette G, Piérard S, de Ravenstein CDM, et al. Prognostic significance of LGE by CMR in aortic stenosis patients undergoing valve replacement. J Am Coll Cardiol 2014;64(2):144–54.

57. Chin CW, Everett RJ, Kwiecinski J, et al. Myocardial fibrosis and cardiac decompensation in aortic stenosis. JACC Cardiovasc Imaging 2017;10(11): 1320–33.

58. Azevedo CF, Nigri M, Higuchi ML, et al. Prognostic significance of myocardial fibrosis quantification by histopathology and magnetic resonance imaging in patients with severe aortic valve disease. J Am Coll Cardiol 2010;56(4):278–87.

59. Van De Heyning CM, Magne J, Piérard LA, et al. Late gadolinium enhancement CMR in primary mitral regurgitation. Eur J Clin Invest 2014;44(9): 840–7.

60. Edwards NC, Moody WE, Yuan M, et al. Quantification of left ventricular interstitial fibrosis in asymptomatic chronic primary degenerative mitral regurgitation CLINICAL PERSPECTIVE. Circ Cardiovasc Imaging 2014;7(6):946–53.

61. Han Y, Peters DC, Salton CJ, et al. Cardiovascular magnetic resonance characterization of mitral valve prolapse. JACC Cardiovasc Imaging 2008; 1(3):294–303.

62. Bui AH, Roujol S, Foppa M, et al. Diffuse myocardial fibrosis in patients with mitral valve prolapse and ventricular arrhythmia. Heart 2017;103(3): 204–9.

63. Chaikriangkrai K, Lopez-Mattei JC, Lawrie G, et al. Prognostic value of delayed enhancement cardiac magnetic resonance imaging in mitral valve repair. Ann Thorac Surg 2014;98(5):1557–63.

64. Hulten E, Agarwal V, Cahill M, et al. Presence of late gadolinium enhancement by cardiac magnetic

resonance among patients with suspected cardiac sarcoidosis is associated with adverse cardiovascular prognosis clinical perspective: a systematic review and meta-analysis. Circ Cardiovasc Imaging 2016;9(9):e005001.

65. Maceira AM, Prasad SK, Hawkins PN, et al. Cardiovascular magnetic resonance and prognosis in cardiac amyloidosis. J Cardiovasc Magn Reson 2008;10(1):54.

66. Ruberg FL, Appelbaum E, Davidoff R, et al. Diagnostic and prognostic utility of cardiovascular magnetic resonance imaging in light-chain cardiac amyloidosis. Am J Cardiol 2009;103(4):544–9.

67. Mekinian A, Lions C, Leleu X, et al. Prognosis assessment of cardiac involvement in systemic AL amyloidosis by magnetic resonance imaging. Am J Med 2010;123(9):864–8.

68. Migrino RQ, Harmann L, Christenson R, et al. Clinical and imaging predictors of 1-year and long-term mortality in light chain (AL) amyloidosis: a 5-year follow-up study. Heart Vessels 2014;29(6):793–800.

69. Boynton SJ, Geske JB, Dispenzieri A, et al. LGE provides incremental prognostic information over serum biomarkers in AL cardiac amyloidosis. JACC Cardiovasc Imaging 2016;9(6):680–6.

70. Austin BA, Tang WW, Rodriguez ER, et al. Delayed hyper-enhancement magnetic resonance imaging provides incremental diagnostic and prognostic utility in suspected cardiac amyloidosis. JACC Cardiovasc Imaging 2009;2(12):1369–77.

71. White JA, Kim HW, Shah D, et al. CMR imaging with rapid visual T1 assessment predicts mortality in patients suspected of cardiac amyloidosis. JACC Cardiovasc Imaging 2014;7(2):143–56.

72. Fontana M, Pica S, Reant P, et al. Prognostic value of late gadolinium enhancement cardiovascular magnetic resonance in cardiac amyloidosis. Circulation 2015;132(16):1570–9.

73. Rochitte CE, Oliveira PF, Andrade JM, et al. Myocardial delayed enhancement by magnetic resonance imaging in patients with Chagas' disease: a marker of disease severity. J Am Coll Cardiol 2005;46(8):1553–8.

74. Regueiro A, García-Álvarez A, Sitges M, et al. Myocardial involvement in Chagas disease: insights from cardiac magnetic resonance. Int J Cardiol 2013;165(1):107–12.

75. Tassi EM, Continentino MA, Nascimento FMD, et al. Relationship between fibrosis and ventricular arrhythmias in Chagas heart disease without ventricular dysfunction. Arq Bras Cardiol 2014;102(5):456–64.

76. Mello RPD, Szarf G, Schvartzman PR, et al. Delayed enhancement cardiac magnetic resonance imaging can identify the risk for ventricular tachycardia in chronic Chagas' heart disease. Arq Bras Cardiol 2012;98(5):421–30.

77. Volpe GJ, Moreira HT, Trad HS, et al. Left ventricular scar and prognosis in chronic chagas cardiomyopathy. J Am Coll Cardiol 2018;72(21):2567.

78. Senra T, Ianni BM, Costa ACP, et al. Long-term prognostic value of myocardial fibrosis in patients with chagas cardiomyopathy. J Am Coll Cardiol 2018;72(21):2577.

79. Verhaert D, Richards K, Rafael-Fortney JA, et al. Cardiac involvement in patients with muscular dystrophies: magnetic resonance imaging phenotype and genotypic considerations. Circ Cardiovasc Imaging 2011;4(1):67–76.

80. Menon SC, Etheridge SP, Liesemer KN, et al. Predictive value of myocardial delayed enhancement in Duchenne muscular dystrophy. Pediatr Cardiol 2014;35(7):1279–85.

81. Silva MC, Meira ZMA, Giannetti JG, et al. Myocardial delayed enhancement by magnetic resonance imaging in patients with muscular dystrophy. J Am Coll Cardiol 2007;49(18):1874–9.

82. Yilmaz A, Gdynia H-J, Baccouche H, et al. Cardiac involvement in patients with Becker muscular dystrophy: new diagnostic and pathophysiological insights by a CMR approach. J Cardiovasc Magn Reson 2008;10(1):50.

83. Tandon A, Villa CR, Hor KN, et al. Myocardial fibrosis burden predicts left ventricular ejection fraction and is associated with age and steroid treatment duration in duchenne muscular dystrophy. J Am Heart Assoc 2015;4(4):e001338.

84. Florian A, Ludwig A, Engelen M, et al. Left ventricular systolic function and the pattern of late-gadolinium-enhancement independently and additively predict adverse cardiac events in muscular dystrophy patients. J Cardiovasc Magn Reson 2014;16(1):81.

85. Florian A, Ludwig A, Rösch S, et al. Myocardial fibrosis imaging based on T1-mapping and extracellular volume fraction (ECV) measurement in muscular dystrophy patients: diagnostic value compared with conventional late gadolinium enhancement (LGE) imaging. Eur Heart J Cardiovasc Imaging 2014;15(9):1004–12.

86. Hor KN, Taylor MD, Al-Khalidi HR, et al. Prevalence and distribution of late gadolinium enhancement in a large population of patients with Duchenne muscular dystrophy: effect of age and left ventricular systolic function. J Cardiovasc Magn Reson 2013;15(1):107.

87. Clements PJ, Lachenbruch PA, Furst DE, et al. A semiquantitative measure of cardiac involvement that improves prediction of prognosis in systemic sclerosis. Arthritis Rheum 1991;34(11):1371–80.

88. Kahan A, Allanore Y. Primary myocardial involvement in systemic sclerosis. Rheumatology 2006; 45(suppl_4):iv14–7.

89. Barison A, Gargani L, De Marchi D, et al. Early myocardial and skeletal muscle interstitial remodelling in systemic sclerosis: insights from extracellular volume quantification using cardiovascular magnetic resonance. Eur Heart J Cardiovasc Imaging 2014;16(1):74–80.

90. Hachulla A-L, Launay D, Gaxotte V, et al. Cardiac magnetic resonance imaging in systemic sclerosis: a cross-sectional observational study of 52 patients. Ann Rheum Dis 2009;68(12):1878–84.

91. Di Cesare E, Battisti S, Di Sibio A, et al. Early assessment of sub-clinical cardiac involvement in systemic sclerosis (SSc) using delayed enhancement cardiac magnetic resonance (CE-MRI). Eur J Radiol 2013;82(6):e268–73.

92. Ntusi NA, Piechnik SK, Francis JM, et al. Subclinical myocardial inflammation and diffuse fibrosis are common in systemic sclerosis–a clinical study using myocardial T1-mapping and extracellular volume quantification. J Cardiovasc Magn Reson 2014;16(1):21.

93. Mousseaux E, Agoston-Coldea L, Marjanovic Z, et al. Left ventricle replacement fibrosis detected by CMR associated with cardiovascular events in systemic sclerosis patients. J Am Coll Cardiol 2018;71(6):703–5.

94. Grün S, Schumm J, Greulich S, et al. Long-term follow-up of biopsy-proven viral myocarditis: predictors of mortality and incomplete recovery. J Am Coll Cardiol 2012;59(18):1604–15.

95. Schumm J, Greulich S, Wagner A, et al. Cardiovascular magnetic resonance risk stratification in patients with clinically suspected myocarditis. J Cardiovasc Magn Reson 2014;16(1):14.

96. Mewton N, Dernis A, Bresson D, et al. Myocardial biomarkers and delayed enhanced cardiac magnetic resonance relationship in clinically suspected myocarditis and insight on clinical outcome. J Cardiovasc Med 2015;16(10):696.

97. Filippetti L, Mandry D, Venner C, et al. Long-term outcome of patients with low/intermediate risk myocarditis is related to the presence of left ventricular remodeling in addition to the mri pattern of delayed gadolinium enhancement. JACC Cardiovasc Imaging 2018;11(9):1367–9.

98. Aquaro GD, Perfetti M, Camastra G, et al. Cardiac MR with late gadolinium enhancement in acute myocarditis with preserved systolic function: ITAMY study. J Am Coll Cardiol 2017;70(16): 1977–87.

99. Gräni C, Eichhorn C, Bière L, et al. Prognostic value of cardiac magnetic resonance tissue characterization in risk stratifying patients with suspected myocarditis. J Am Coll Cardiol 2017; 70(16):1964–76.

100. Cheng H, Lu M, Hou C, et al. Comparative study of CMR characteristics between arrhythmogenic right ventricular cardiomyopathy patients with/without syncope. Int J Cardiovasc Imaging 2014;30(7): 1365–72.

101. Deac M, Alpendurada F, Fanaie F, et al. Prognostic value of cardiovascular magnetic resonance in patients with suspected arrhythmogenic right ventricular cardiomyopathy. Int J Cardiol 2013;168(4): 3514–21.

102. Fallah-Rad N, Lytwyn M, Fang T, et al. Delayed contrast enhancement cardiac magnetic resonance imaging in trastuzumab induced cardiomyopathy. J Cardiovasc Magn Reson 2008;10(1):5.

103. Ylänen K, Poutanen T, Savikurki-Heikkilä P, et al. Cardiac magnetic resonance imaging in the evaluation of the late effects of anthracyclines among long-term survivors of childhood cancer. J Am Coll Cardiol 2013;61(14):1539–47.

104. Kimball A, Patil S, Koczwara B, et al. Late characterisation of cardiac effects following anthracycline and trastuzumab treatment in breast cancer patients. Int J Cardiol 2018;261:159–61.

105. Johnson DB, Balko JM, Compton ML, et al. Fulminant myocarditis with combination immune checkpoint blockade. N Engl J Med 2016;375(18): 1749–55.

106. Mahmood SS, Fradley MG, Cohen JV, et al. Myocarditis in patients treated with immune checkpoint inhibitors. J Am Coll Cardiol 2018;71(16): 1755–64.

The Value of T1 Mapping Techniques in the Assessment of Myocardial Interstitial Fibrosis

Hélder Jorge Andrade Gomes, MD[a],
Vinícius de Padua Vieira Alves, MD[b],
Marcelo Souto Nacif, MD, PhD[b,c],*

KEYWORDS

• T1 mapping • Myocardial interstitial fibrosis • Heart failure • Detection

KEY POINTS

• Cardiac fibrosis, characterized by net accumulation of extracellular matrix (ECM) in the myocardium, is a common final pathway of heart failure.
• Tissue characterization is a key capability of CMR imaging that reinforces its role as the best noninvasive tool available, allowing detection of MF.
• The use of CCT for tissue characterization has been validated, with CCT findings showing good correlation with CMR imaging findings.
• T1 mapping should be used to detect incipient changes leading to myocardial damage in several clinical conditions and also in subclinical disease.

INTRODUCTION

Cardiac fibrosis, characterized by net accumulation of extracellular matrix (ECM) in the myocardium, is a common final pathway of heart failure.[1–3] This myocardial fibrosis (MF) is not necessarily the primary cause of dysfunction; it often results from a reparative process activated in response to cardiomyocyte injury. In light of currently available treatments, late-identified MF could be definitive or irreversible, associated with worsening ventricular systolic function, abnormal cardiac remodeling, and increased ventricular stiffness and arrhythmia.[4,5]

Cardiac magnetic resonance (CMR) imaging has evolved significantly in the last decade from a modality restricted to anatomic imaging to one that allows comprehensive assessment of myocardial anatomy and function with unequaled accuracy and reproducibility. Diverse facets of cardiovascular diseases can be assessed in a single examination, which has significant clinical impact.[6,7] Tissue characterization is a key capability of CMR imaging that reinforces its role as the best noninvasive tool available, allowing detection of even small areas of MF by late gadolinium enhancement (LGE).[8–10] In addition, CMR imaging enables differentiation between ischemic and nonischemic patterns according to coherence with the coronary territory and distribution in relation to the subendocardium.[11]

Cardiac computed tomography (CCT) is a significantly faster and more widely available

Conflicts of interest: The authors have nothing to disclose.
[a] Cardiologist and Cardiac Imaging, Hospital Samaritano de São Paulo, São Paulo, Brazil; [b] Radiology Department, Universidade Federal Fluminense, Niterói, Rio de Janeiro, Brazil; [c] Unidade de Radiologia Clínica, Hospital viValle (Rede D'or-São Luiz), São José dos Campos, São Paulo, Brazil.
* Corresponding author. Avenida São João 2400, apto 232 B Belvedere – Jd Colinas, São José dos Campos, São Paulo 12242-000, Brazil.
E-mail address: msnacif@gmail.com

Magn Reson Imaging Clin N Am 27 (2019) 563–574
https://doi.org/10.1016/j.mric.2019.04.007
1064-9689/19/© 2019 Elsevier Inc. All rights reserved.

imaging modality[12] that is tolerated well by patients and has been validated for use in the detection of focal myocardial scarring,[13] calcification, and thrombi.[14] The use of CCT for tissue characterization has been validated recently, with CCT findings showing good correlation with CMR imaging findings.[13]

This article reviews available techniques for MF detection, focusing on noninvasive quantification of diffuse fibrosis and clinical applications.

PATHOGENESIS OF MYOCARDIAL FIBROSIS
Myocardial Interstitial Space Components

Cardiac tissue is made up of highly differentiated cardiomyocytes and stroma (mainly ECM, with tissue fluid and other cells). Cardiac ECM contains fibrillar collagen, especially types I (80%) and III (11%), which provides a structural base for cardiomyocytes and vessels, as well as the consistency required for cardiac tissue resistance to deformation during the cardiac cycle. Collagen fibers also connect adjacent contractile elements and serve as transducers of muscle contraction.[15]

Fibrosis Causes and Subtypes

Microscopically, fibrosis is characterized by an excess of collagen fibers in the ECM caused by the combined increase in collagen synthesis by fibroblasts and myofibroblasts, and decrease or maintenance of collagen degradation by matrix metalloproteinases, leading to the occupation of spaces that should correspond with specialized parenchymal cells.[16] In these coexisting matrices, a constant flux of tissue and collagen turnover is orchestrated by regulatory cytokines, growth factors, enzymes, hormones, and direct cell-to-cell communication induced by mechanical stress, the hormonal environment, and inflammatory responses.[17] Progressive collagen accumulation accounts for a spectrum of ventricular dysfunctional processes that commonly affect diastole first, and subsequently involve systolic performance.

According to the cause of increased interstitial space, fibrosis has 3 subtypes:

1. Reactive interstitial fibrosis (diffuse interstitial or more specifically perivascular distribution). This fibrosis subtype has a progressive onset. It has been described primarily in hypertension, diabetes mellitus, idiopathic dilated cardiomyopathy (DCM), and chronic aortic valve disease, and in remote noninfarcted myocardium after infarction.[18–21] Interstitial fibrosis is an intermediate marker of disease severity that precedes irreversible replacement fibrosis.

2. Infiltrative interstitial fibrosis. This fibrosis subtype is induced by progressive deposition of insoluble proteins (amyloidosis) or glycosphingolipids (Anderson-Fabry disease [AFD]) in the cardiac interstitium.[22,23]

3. Replacement fibrosis: localized (ischemic cardiomyopathy, myocarditis, hypertrophic cardiomyopathy [HCM], sarcoidosis) or diffuse (chronic kidney disease, toxic cardiomyopathies, inflammatory diseases) distribution.[4,24,25] This fibrosis subtype is characterized by the replacement of myocytes after cell damage or necrosis by plexiform fibrosis, composed mainly of type I collagen.

DETECTION BY CARDIAC MAGNETIC RESONANCE IMAGING
Relaxation Times

In CMR imaging, the pixel signal intensity is based on the relaxation of hydrogen nucleus protons in the static magnetic field and on proton density. Such proton relaxation characterizes the longitudinal (spin-lattice; T1) and transverse (spin-spin; T2) relaxation times (in milliseconds). T1 and T2 relaxation times depend on the water molecular environments in tissues and are thus specific to tissue types, varying significantly among tissues but also within the same tissue depending on physiopathologic status (ie, inflammation, edema, or fibrosis).[26]

T1 Terms

T1 values represent the recovery of longitudinal magnetization. Native T1 refers to a value obtained without or greater than or equal to 24 hours after contrast agent application in a patient with normal renal function.[26] A T1 map of the myocardium is a parametrically reconstructed image in which the intensity of each pixel corresponds directly with the T1 value for the corresponding myocardial voxel; a color table is used to facilitate visual assessment.[27]

Gadolinium Enhancement

Gadolinium contrast agents reduce T1 values in adjacent tissue. Thus, local gadolinium tissue concentrations induce differences in signal intensity on T1-weighted images. LGE use for MF visualization is based on the combined increase in contrast agent distribution volume and prolongation of washout related to decreased capillary density in MF tissue.[4]

Extracellular Volume

The myocardial extracellular volume (ECV; percentage) reflects the volume fraction of heart tissue not occupied by cells. The partition coefficient (λ) reflects the relationship between changes in precontrast and postcontrast myocardium and blood T1:

$$\lambda = \Delta R1_{myo} / \Delta R1_{blood}$$

where $R1$ is tissue relaxivity (1/T1) and $\Delta R1$ is $R1_{postcontrast} - R1_{precontrast}$. ECV calculation incorporates correction for the blood plasma volume:

$$ECV = \lambda \, (1 - \text{hematocrit})$$

ECV maps can be generated on a pixel-wise basis when native and postcontrast T1 images are coregistered, quantified, and adjusted for the hematocrit.[26]

T1 Sequences

In a quantitative myocardial T1 sequence, an initial pulse alters the longitudinal magnetization, followed by image acquisition along the relaxation curve and model fitting to derive T1 values.[28] The initial pulse may induce an inversion recovery (IR; modified look-locker inversion recovery [MOLLI],[29–31] shortened MOLLI [ShMOLLI],[32] accelerated and navigator-gated look-locker imaging for cardiac T1 estimation [ANGIE],[33] slice-interleaved T1 [STONE][34]), saturation recovery (SR; saturation recovery single-shot acquisition [SASHA][35]), or combined (saturation pulse–prepared heart rate–independent inversion recovery [SAPHIRE][36]) sequence.

MOLLI[30,31] is the most thoroughly assessed T1 mapping sequence. The original MOLLI sequence used 17 heartbeats with acquisition of 3-3-5 images and 3 heartbeats for recovery between each acquisition [3(3)3(3)5]. Issues with this sequence include its heart rate dependence, long acquisition time, and T1 value underestimation (especially with fast heart rates). To correct for these factors, new combinations of inversion/recovery times and numbers of heartbeats were proposed: native acquisition, 5(3)3 (fewer heartbeats, less heart rate dependence); postcontrast acquisition, 4(1 s)3(1 s)2 (shorter recovery time). These sequences feature rapid acquisition and no heart rate dependence, but the native sequence results in T1 value underestimation because of magnetization transfer effects. Few validation studies for the postcontrast sequence have been conducted. For the blood pool, in which fresh blood enters the image plane, the use of uncorrected T1* images is recommended.

The ShMOLLI sequence[32] requires only 9 heartbeats, using a 5(1)1(1)1 scheme. It has no heart rate dependence and is accurate in precontrast and postcontrast acquisition, but its signal-to-noise ratio is lower than that of MOLLI, it is more artifact prone, and it causes systematic T1 value underestimation at greater than 800 milliseconds (formula corrected).

In the SASHA sequence,[35] 1 image is acquired before saturation, followed by the application of multiple SR pulses with different trigger delay times. This sequence has no T1* effect, heart rate dependence, or T2 sensitivity with a 3-parameter fit, and it is less sensitive to off-resonance effects. However, SR sequences have lower signal-to-noise ratios and less precision when used with a 2-parameter fit compared with IR sequences.

Recently described techniques expand the T1 mapping options. The combined SR/IR SAPHIRE sequence[36] is not sensitive to variations in heart rate but has slightly longer acquisition times. Slavin and colleagues[37] described the SMART1Map SR sequence, in which each R-R interval receives a saturation pulse with the acquisition of longer delay times in the recovery curve, performed across multiple heart beats. This technique obviates T1* correction, as does MOLLI, and is less sensitive to other imaging parameters. Whole-heart T1 mapping with 3D ANGIE[33] and STONE[34] sequences provides full left ventricle (LV) coverage with free-breathing acquisition. In patients with atrial fibrillation, systolic data acquisition using these methods might be more robust than diastolic readout, but it yields lower T1 values.

Specialty societies such as the Society for Cardiovascular Magnetic Resonance/European Association for Cardiovascular Imaging have already made some recommendations that should be followed (**Box 1**).

DETECTION BY CARDIAC COMPUTED TOMOGRAPHY
Delayed Enhancement

Myocardial delayed enhancement (MDE) CMR imaging and MDE computed tomography (CT) have shown good correlation and additional value to its use in clinical practice.[14,38–40] For MF, MDE images are obtained after intravenous administration of iodine contrast using a retrospective electrocardiogram-gating cardiac helical protocol. Senra and colleagues[14] showed that hypoenhancing areas by the presence of calcium on MDE-CMR imaging were better evaluated by multidetector CT using the calcium scoring technique, which shows massive subendocardial calcification, and by MDE-CT, which showed LV apical obliteration with MDE areas associated with calcification. In addition, MDE-CT identified thrombi and calcification matching calcium score images. On MDE-CMR imaging, calcium and thrombi

Box 1
Society for Cardiovascular Magnetic Resonance/European Association for Cardiovascular Imaging recommendations for T1 mapping/extracellular volume calculation

- Native T1 measured in the absence of contrast agent, greater than or equal to 24 hours from last dose in patients with normal renal function.

- Diastolic image acquisition recommended when heart rhythm is regular (specific sequences for tachyarrhythmia are available).

- Review of image quality during acquisition; repeat examination when quality is suboptimal or images are nondiagnostic.

- Hematocrit for ECV calculation obtained immediately or less than or equal to 24 hours before scanning.

- Gadolinium-based contrast doses of 0.1 to 0.2 mmol/kg recommended.

- Postcontrast T1 mapping performed 10 to 30 minutes after contrast administration.

- Native and postcontrast T1 mapping using the same slice prescription.

- For global/diffuse disease, basal and mid short-axis mapping, with optional single long-axis map acquisition. For patchy disease, basal and mid short-axis mapping, with mandatory acquisition of at least 1 long-axis map (4 chamber for amyloid to visualize base-apex gradient, 3 chamber for AFD to assess basal inferolateral scarring).

- For global/diffuse assessment, definition of a single region of interest (ROI) in the septum on midcavity short-axis maps to avoid lung, liver, and vein susceptibility artifacts. Additional ROIs possible for areas of visually abnormal appearance. ROIs can exclude infarcts (ie, include remote myocardium) and include nonischemic LGE.

- Mapping results include absolute numerical values, Z scores (number of SDs by which results differ from local normal mean) when available, and normal reference ranges.

- Interpretations presented as normal or mild, moderate, or severe increase/decrease in ECV.

Data from Messroghli DR, Moon JC, Ferreira VM, et al. Clinical recommendations for cardiovascular magnetic resonance mapping of T1, T2, T2* and extracellular volume: a consensus statement by the Society for Cardiovascular Magnetic Resonance (SCMR) endorsed by the European Association for Cardiovascular Imaging (EACVI). J Cardiovasc Magn Reson 2017;19(1):75.

appear indistinctly as large, dark subendocardial areas. A recent study evaluating the prognostic significance of MF detection by CCT in high-risk patients with HCM with implantable cardioverter-defibrillators (ICDs) showed that patients with more severe MF detected by CCT were more likely to have ventricular fibrillation and tachycardia events that were treated appropriately by ICDs.[39]

Extracellular Volume Measurement

Although ECV imaging by CCT lags behind that by CMR imaging, it is an attractive alternative when CMR imaging is contraindicated.[12,41,42] CCT-based ECV calculation relies on the same principle as CMR imaging-based calculations:

$$ECV \text{ by } CCT = (1 - \text{hematocrit}) \times (\Delta HU_{myo} / \Delta HU_{blood}),$$

where ΔHU is the change in Hounsfield unit attenuation between precontrast and postcontrast. Nacif and colleagues[13] validated CCT-based ECV calculation for humans in 2012; postcontrast images are obtained after a delay of 5 to 10 minutes using the same parameters as for the initial precontrast calcium score scan. ECV measured with CCT shows good reproducibility and correlates well with ECV measured with T1-mapping CMR imaging–determined values ($r = 0.82$; $P<.001$)[13]. In addition, greater ECV values were associated with reduced ejection fractions and increased end-systolic and end-diastolic volumes.[43]

The use of dual-energy CT to quantify myocardial ECV[44,45] might eliminate misregistration errors associated with separate precontrast and post-contrast scans by obviating the need for the precontrast scan.

CT is faster and more widely available, offers greater spatial resolution (particularly in-plane), and permits better isotropic reconstruction than MR imaging. In addition, CCT-based ECV measurement reflects the direct effect of iodine-based contrast agents on the signal (through x-ray absorption), whereas CMR imaging–based assessment relies on measurement of the effect of gadolinium-based contrast agents on protons (assuming the same tissue relaxivity relative to blood, and rapid water exchange between intracellular and extracellular compartments). Furthermore, common contraindications for CMR imaging, such as claustrophobia and some pacemakers, do not apply to CCT.

CLINICAL APPLICATIONS

The ECV may increase with fibrosis, edema, and/or other protein (amyloid) deposition. Increased capillary density and vasodilatation increase the

ECV to a smaller extent. Therefore, ECV changes in isolation require interpretation. Mathematical ECV derivation relies on several assumptions (including the fast-exchange limit), λ measurement, and the patient's hematocrit, representing the cellular fraction of blood.[27]

LGE provides important diagnostic and prognostic information, but T1 mapping and ECV calculation may better quantify the degree of ECM/interstitial expansion.[26] The use of T1 distributions to identify distinct myocardial patterns, such as diffuse MF, specific myopathies, and the periinfarction (gray) zone, should be evaluated in large clinical studies. Applied rigorously,[26] T1 mapping could be ideal for the assessment and quantification of diffuse MF. It could also improve the accuracy of delayed enhancement and MF characterization.

Peculiarities of T1/T1 mapping/ECV calculation in clinical situations of acute (ischemic and inflammatory) and longer-term myocardial damage are briefly described next.

Myocardial Infarction

LGE-CMR imaging has been the gold standard for myocardial infarction (MI) detection and viability assessment,[46] but T1 mapping and ECV assessment provide complementary diagnostic and prognostic information.

In areas of acute ischemia and infarction, native T1 and T2 relaxation times lengthen and the postcontrast T1 time shortens relative to those of remote myocardium.[47] Native T1 may also provide prognostic information through infarct core identification, which is associated inversely with adverse remodeling and all-cause death or first postdischarge hospitalization for heart failure in patients with ST-elevation MI.[48]

Acute and chronic infarcts present distinct T1 changes; precontrast T1 mapping enables acute MI detection, and chronic MIs are associated with adipose tissue deposition, which significantly reduces the T1 relaxation time. The presence of iron after previous bleeding is reflected by a decrease in the T1 value relative to an increase in the surrounding area.[49]

In chronic MI, ECVs reach 60% to 70% without associated microvascular obstruction. T1 mapping with several standard LGEs showed that within 1 week after acute MI the remote region undergoes ECM expansion associated with systolic dysfunction.[28] In patients with chronic total coronary artery occlusion who had undergone revascularization, CMR imaging–based global baseline ECVs less than 30% predicted significant ejection fraction improvement.[50]

Although LGE will remain the mainstay for clinical detection of chronic and acute MIs, T1 mapping and ECV assessment permit further distinct evaluation of remote and periinfarct zones and additional pathophysiologic understanding.

Myocarditis

Clinical and experimental evidence consistently shows the role of T1 mapping in determining the location, extent, and patterns of acute myocarditis, with significantly greater sensitivity than the Lake Louise criteria (85% vs 74%; $P = .025$).[51,52] Native T1 and T2 mapping with LGE significantly improved the diagnostic accuracy of CMR imaging to 96%.[53]

T1 values are significantly increased in patients with acute myocarditis compared with healthy subjects and those with chronic convalescent disease (**Fig. 1**). Hinojar and colleagues[54] proposed T1 relaxation time cutoffs of greater than 5 standard deviations (SDs) to diagnose acute myocarditis and greater than 2 SDs (native T1) for the convalescent phase. Bohnen and colleagues[55] described the use of noncontrast T1/T2 mapping to monitor the course of myocardial inflammation in healing myocarditis.

An important type of myocardial inflammation in South America is Chagas disease. Several

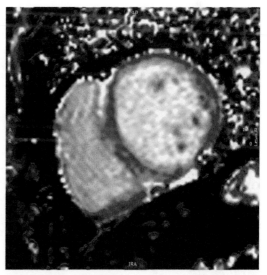

Fig. 1. Acute myocarditis in a 22-year-old man who presented to the emergency room with acute chest pain and positive serum troponin. In this short-axis midventricular slice acquired at 3.0 T, native T1 mapping revealed an increase in T1 values in the midwall portion of the lateral segments, compatible with the diagnosis. An increase in T1 can also be observed in the inferior-septal segments. (*Courtesy of* Juliano de Lara Fernandes, Jose Michel Kalaf Research Insitute, Campinas, Brazil.)

aspects of the pathogenesis are not fully understood, especially in its subclinical phases. On pathology, Chagas heart disease is characterized by chronic myocardial inflammation and extensive MF[56] (**Fig. 2**).

Aortic Stenosis

The LV ejection fraction is not sensitive for the detection of early structural changes in response to pressure overload. LGE-CMR imaging permits the detection of focal replacement fibrosis, and T1 mapping can detect altered ECM possibly reflecting diffuse fibrosis.[57] Increased native T1 time and ECV reflect increased MF in patients with severe aortic stenosis,[58] and a high native T1 value is an independent predictor of adverse outcome in patients with significant aortic stenosis, regardless of the presence of LGE.[59] The T1 map technique may be useful in identifying asymptomatic cases for early intervention.

Arterial Hypertension

Similar to the response to pressure overload in aortic stenosis, T1 mapping has shown slight ECV expansion paralleling LV hypertrophy (LVH) development in patients with arterial hypertension.[60] This expansion is associated with reduced cardiac performance,[61] permitting recognition of

worsening evolution or poor blood pressure control.

Hypertrophic Cardiomyopathy

Myocardial disarray, small vessel disease, and fibrosis are histopathologic hallmarks of familial sarcomeric HCM, and fibrosis detected by CMR imaging or CCT is a risk factor for ventricular fibrillation/tachycardia, heart failure, and sudden cardiac death.[39,62]

Native T1 values are higher in patients with HCM than in controls, even in LV segments without LGE, suggesting that they can be used to detect areas of tissue disorder beyond those detected by LGE.[26] The ECV is increased in patients with typical phenotypes and in asymptomatic positive-phenotype relatives with no clinically relevant finding.[63]

In patients with HCM, the area of ECV exceeding a 30.4% threshold was consistently larger than the area of LGE measured as greater than 2 SDs of remote unenhanced myocardium.[22] In this scenario, T1 mapping and ECV assessment may more accurately characterize disease severity (**Fig. 3**). The clinical and prognostic value of T1 mapping and ECV calculation compared with the standard LGE approach remains to be established.

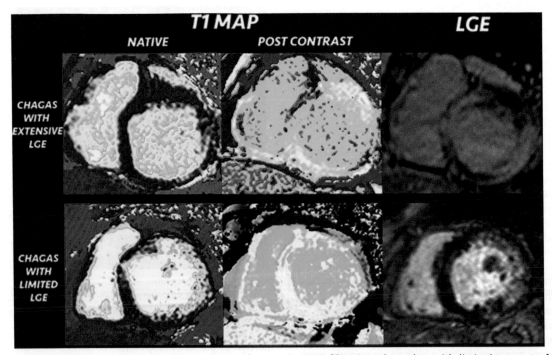

Fig. 2. Two examples of Chagas disease, one with extensive LGE fibrosis and another with limited amount of fibrosis by LGE. T1 maps are able to show the differences between fibrosis tissue and the remote area where some are already affected but are not seen by LGE technique. (*Courtesy of* Carlos E. Rochitte, University of Sao Paulo Medical School, Brazil, São Paulo, São Paulo, Brazil.)

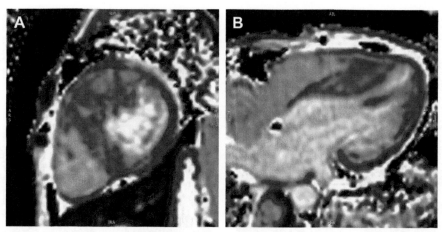

Fig. 3. Short-axis (*A*) and 4-chamber (*B*) views of native T1 images in a patient with HCM, acquired at 3.0 T. The hypertrophic areas in the anteroseptal walls had a high native T1 of 1387 milliseconds, with a diffuse and heterogeneous signal distribution, as can be observed in both images. The native T1 in the apparently normal lateral wall was 1215 milliseconds, within the normal range. (*Courtesy of* Juliano de Lara Fernandes, Jose Michel Kalaf Research Insitute, Campinas, Brazil.)

Amyloidosis

The ventricular myocardium is affected by immunoglobulin light chain (AL) amyloidosis and transthyretin amyloidosis, which has wild-type and mutant subtypes with different natural histories and prognoses. Early recognition and therapy are critical for AL amyloidosis with cardiac involvement (cardiac amyloidosis [CA]), but LGE does not reveal the typical subendocardial tramline pattern or renal impairment.

Native T1 is more sensitive than standard LGE for CA detection (**Fig. 4**). Native T1 mapping permits the differentiation of patients with amyloidosis without cardiac involvement from normal individuals and those with possible and definitive CA.[64,65]

In patients with CA, ECVs are 40% to 50%.[66,67] In those with LVH, amyloidosis generates higher T1 values than do hypertension, HCM, and aortic stenosis. Visual inspection of LGE images obtained with sequential T1 examinations shows the null point of the myocardium before the blood null point in CA, opposite to other LVH causes.[66]

Iron Overload

Iron overload causes severe heart failure and lethal arrhythmia when not diagnosed and effectively treated early. Iron shortens T1, T2, and T2* times, and T2* at 1.5 T (not 3 T) is the gold standard for myocardial iron overload assessment.[26] Native T1 mapping enables differentiation of severe, mild to moderate, and no cardiac iron overload at least as well as T2*.[68] However, in the T2* range of 20 to 30 milliseconds, T1 mapping can detect iron (undetectable by T2*), supporting

suggestions that T1 mapping enables the identification of slight iron accumulation in the heart or in the liver (**Fig. 5**).[69] The clinical significance of low T1 with normal T2* values should be investigated further.

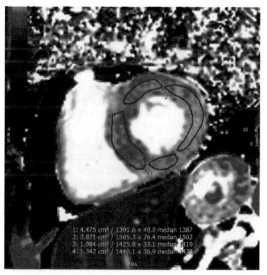

Fig. 4. Native T1 short-axis image from a patient diagnosed with cardiac amyloidosis. The patient had significant chronic renal disease and could not receive gadolinium-based contrast agents because of this constraint. T1 mapping showed a diffuse increase in values throughout the whole myocardium, as noted in the values of the regions of interest measured. The heterogeneous deposition can also be visually appreciated with apparently more intense T1 values in the inferior and lateral walls. (*Courtesy of* Juliano de Lara Fernandes, Jose Michel Kalaf Research Insitute, Campinas, Brazil.)

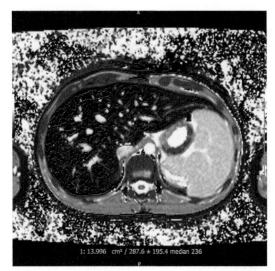

1: 13.996 cm² / 287.6 ± 195.4 median 236

Fig. 5. In this patient with thalassemia major, T1 imaging of the liver was performed in order to assess the liver iron concentration, with a significant reduction in native T1 values as measured in the region of interest shown (T1 = 288 milliseconds). Significant iron concentrations decrease T1 signal, which can be measured using a T1 map like this one, either in the heart or in the liver, as shown in this axial image of the abdomen. Courtesy of Juliano de Lara Fernandes, Jose Michel Kalaf Research Insitute, Campinas, Brazil.

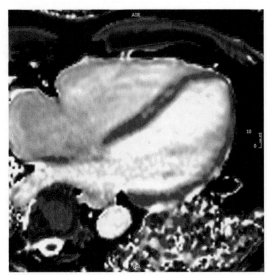

Fig. 6. A patient with heart failure with unknown cause underwent CMR to assess the cause of the disease. Native T1 maps showed high values in the midwall portion of the septal wall, a location typically associated with idiopathic dilated cardiomyopathy. Late gadolinium-enhanced images (not shown) revealed nonischemic scar in this area, further characterizing the hypothesis. (*Courtesy of* Juliano de Lara Fernandes, Jose Michel Kalaf Research Insitute, Campinas, Brazil.)

Anderson-Fabry Disease

AFD is an X-linked lysosomal enzyme disorder associated with intracellular sphingolipid accumulation caused by of α-galactosidase A deficiency. Patients with AFD frequently show characteristic LVH and an LGE pattern in the mid-basal inferolateral wall.[70,71] As in iron overload, native T1 values are low in AFD, in contrast with other LVH causes,[72] because intracellular glycosphingolipid (fat) storage generates a very short (low-value) T1 relaxation time. ECV measurement does not distinguish patients with and without AFD.[73]

Dilated Cardiomyopathy

DCM is associated with diffuse MF development, a prominent feature during disease progression and cardiac remodeling that eludes detection by LGE (**Fig. 6**). Early MF detected by significantly increased native T1 and ECV are potentially useful for differentiating between athletes' heart groups and normal.[74] As in HCM, T1 values and ECVs are high in DCM, even in myocardial segments without LGE,[75] and predict adverse outcomes, allowing for risk stratification and the initiation of timely appropriate management.[76]

Cardiotoxicity

Cardiotoxicity and LV dysfunction are the most common adverse effects of cancer treatment regimens (especially those involving anthracyclines), offsetting the benefits of these lifesaving therapies.[77] Data suggest that anthracycline-induced cardiotoxicity is associated with an early increase in cardiac edema and subsequent increase in MF. The early increase in edema and subacute increase in fibrosis are strongly linked and predictive of late mortality.[78] ECV-based assessment of MF should enable early detection of radiotherapy-induced myocardial damage.[79]

Congenital Heart Disease

Volume and pressure overload are important factors in alterations of myocardial structure and function in congenital heart disease. ECV expansion is associated with a higher incidence of cardiac arrhythmia and greater risk of ventricular dysfunction, even in patients with normal LV ejection fractions and no LGE.[80–82]

Cardiac Allograft Rejection

Acute allograft rejection remains among the most common complications in the first year after transplant. It often results in allograft dysfunction and is a main determinant of mortality and morbidity in the early posttransplant period.[83] Imran and colleagues[84] recently obtained an excellent negative predictive value of 99% using a native T1 value of 1029 milliseconds as a cutoff for the noninvasive diagnosis of clinically significant cardiac allograft rejection.

Masses

Parametric techniques may be used to characterize extracardiac tissues according to fat or water content, with comparison with validated values or remote reference ranges.

LIMITATIONS

Current data confirm the clinical potential of T1 mapping but reveal the lack of T1 value standardization and great variability among T1 acquisition sequences (with significant effects on sensitivity to motion artifacts [arrhythmia], heart rate, and extreme T1 values).[72] Other limitations include the time delay after gadolinium administration, which significantly affects resulting T1 values; the need to account for the presence of LGE areas to determine true T1 values for unaffected myocardium; the need to account for the gadolinium myocardial washout rate, which depends mainly on the patient's glomerular filtration rate; and the need for the hematocrit in calculating λ for the gadolinium contrast agent.

FUTURE PERSPECTIVES

From a technical perspective, next steps will be to shorten the acquisition duration and standardize reference values using multicentric clinical data reflecting healthy and disease states. Sequences enabling possible uniform acquisition despite tachyarrhythmia, with free breathing and no hematocrit (synthetic ECV) requirement, are being developed and refined.[85–87] CCT-based ECV calculation enables assessment of the coronary anatomy and flow, and myocardial tissue characterization using a single modality, with huge implications for imaging workflow, although radiation remains a factor limiting widespread use.

From a clinical perspective, accumulating data indicate the diagnostic and prognostic power of interstitial fibrosis detection by T1 mapping, confirming that it is more sensitive in detecting incipient changes leading to myocardial damage in several clinical conditions; it should thus be useful in daily clinical practice. It also enables the detection of subclinical myocardial changes before the onset of diastolic and systolic dysfunction.

ACKNOWLEDGMENTS

The authors thank Juliano de Lara Fernades and Carlos Eduardo Rochitte for their valuable contributions.

REFERENCES

1. Beltrami CA, Finato N, Rocco M, et al. Structural basis of end-stage failure in ischemic cardiomyopathy in humans. Circulation 1994;89(1):151–63.
2. Beltrami CA, Finato N, Rocco M, et al. The cellular basis of dilated cardiomyopathy in humans. J Mol Cell Cardiol 1995;27(1):291–305.
3. Frangogiannis NG. Cardiac fibrosis: cell biological mechanisms, molecular pathways and therapeutic opportunities. Mol Aspects Med 2019;65:70–99.
4. Mewton N, Liu CY, Croisille P, et al. Assessment of myocardial fibrosis with cardiovascular magnetic resonance. J Am Coll Cardiol 2011;57(8):891–903.
5. Won S, Davies-Venn C, Liu S, et al. Noninvasive imaging of myocardial extracellular matrix for assessment of fibrosis. Curr Opin Cardiol 2013;28(3):282–9.
6. Abbasi SA, Ertel A, Shah RV, et al. Impact of cardiovascular magnetic resonance on management and clinical decision-making in heart failure patients. J Cardiovasc Magn Reson 2013;15:89.
7. Bruder O, Wagner A, Lombardi M, et al. European Cardiovascular Magnetic Resonance (EuroCMR) registry: multi national results from 57 centers in 15 countries. J Cardiovasc Magn Reson 2013;15:9.
8. Ricciardi MJ, Wu E, Davidson CJ, et al. Visualization of discrete microinfarction after percutaneous coronary intervention associated with mild creatine kinase-MB elevation. Circulation 2001;103(23):2780–3.
9. Chibana H, Ikeno F. Usability of cardiac magnetic resonance imaging for procedural myocardial infarction undergoing rotational atherectomy. J Thorac Dis 2018;10(Suppl. 26):S3237–40.
10. Baritussio A, Scatteia A, Bucciarelli-Ducci C. Role of cardiovascular magnetic resonance in acute and chronic ischemic heart disease. Int J Cardiovasc Imaging 2018;34(1):67–80.
11. Mahrholdt H, Wagner A, Judd RM, et al. Delayed enhancement cardiovascular magnetic resonance assessment of non-ischaemic cardiomyopathies. Eur Heart J 2005;26(15):1461–74.
12. Scully PR, Bastarrika G, Moon JC, et al. Myocardial extracellular volume quantification by cardiovascular magnetic resonance and computed tomography. Curr Cardiol Rep 2018;20(3):15.
13. Nacif MS, Kawel N, Lee JJ, et al. Interstitial myocardial fibrosis assessed as extracellular volume fraction with low-radiation-dose cardiac CT. Radiology 2012;264(3):876–83.

14. Senra T, Shiozaki AA, Salemi VM, et al. Delayed enhancement by multidetector computed tomography in endomyocardial fibrosis. Eur Heart J 2008;29(3):347.

15. Lopez Salazar B, Ravassa Albeniz S, Arias Guedon T, et al. Alteraciones del metabolismo del colageno fibrilar en la cardiopatia hipertensiva. Situacion actual y perspectivas (Altered fibrillar collagen metabolism in hypertensive heart failure. Current understanding and future prospects). Rev Esp Cardiol 2006;59(10):1047–57.

16. Zannad F, Rossignol P, Iraqi W. Extracellular matrix fibrotic markers in heart failure. Heart Fail Rev 2010;15(4):319–29.

17. Varo N, Iraburu MJ, Varela M, et al. Chronic AT(1) blockade stimulates extracellular collagen type I degradation and reverses myocardial fibrosis in spontaneously hypertensive rats. Hypertension 2000;35(6):1197–202.

18. Morillas P, Quiles J, de Andrade H, et al. Circulating biomarkers of collagen metabolism in arterial hypertension: relevance of target organ damage. J Hypertens 2013;31(8):1611–7.

19. Markowitz M, Messineo F, Coplan NL. Aldosterone receptor antagonists in cardiovascular disease: a review of the recent literature and insight into potential future indications. Clin Cardiol 2012;35(10):605–9.

20. Zayani Y, El Golli N, Zidi W, et al. Inflammations mediators and circulating levels of matrix metalloproteinases: biomarkers of diabetes in Tunisians metabolic syndrome patients. Cytokine 2016;86: 47–52.

21. Gil-Cayuela C, Rivera M, Ortega A, et al. RNA sequencing analysis identifies new human collagen genes involved in cardiac remodeling. J Am Coll Cardiol 2015;65(12):1265–7.

22. Kellman P, Wilson JR, Xue H, et al. Extracellular volume fraction mapping in the myocardium, part 2: initial clinical experience. J Cardiovasc Magn Reson 2012;14:64.

23. Weidemann F, Niemann M, Breunig F, et al. Long-term effects of enzyme replacement therapy on Fabry cardiomyopathy: evidence for a better outcome with early treatment. Circulation 2009; 119(4):524–9.

24. Maron BJ, Maron MS. Hypertrophic cardiomyopathy. Lancet 2013;381(9862):242–55.

25. Patel MR, Cawley PJ, Heitner JF, et al. Detection of myocardial damage in patients with sarcoidosis. Circulation 2009;120(20):1969–77.

26. Messroghli DR, Moon JC, Ferreira VM, et al. Clinical recommendations for cardiovascular magnetic resonance mapping of T1, T2, T2* and extracellular volume: a consensus statement by the Society for Cardiovascular Magnetic Resonance (SCMR) endorsed by the European Association for Cardiovascular Imaging (EACVI). J Cardiovasc Magn Reson 2017;19(1):75.

27. Radenkovic D, Weingartner S, Ricketts L, et al. T1 mapping in cardiac MRI. Heart Fail Rev 2017; 22(4):415–30.

28. Fernandes JL, Rochitte CE. T1 mapping: technique and applications. Magn Reson Imaging Clin N Am 2015;23(1):25–34.

29. Messroghli DR, Greiser A, Frohlich M, et al. Optimization and validation of a fully-integrated pulse sequence for modified look-locker inversion-recovery (MOLLI) T1 mapping of the heart. J Magn Reson Imaging 2007;26(4):1081–6.

30. Messroghli DR, Radjenovic A, Kozerke S, et al. Modified Look-Locker inversion recovery (MOLLI) for high-resolution T1 mapping of the heart. Magn Reson Med 2004;52(1):141–6.

31. Messroghli DR, Plein S, Higgins DM, et al. Human myocardium: single-breath-hold MR T1 mapping with high spatial resolution: reproducibility study. Radiology 2006;238(3):1004–12.

32. Piechnik SK, Ferreira VM, Dall'Armellina E, et al. Shortened Modified Look-Locker Inversion recovery (ShMOLLI) for clinical myocardial T1-mapping at 1.5 and 3 T within a 9 heartbeat breathhold. J Cardiovasc Magn Reson 2010;12:69.

33. Mehta BB, Chen X, Bilchick KC, et al. Accelerated and navigator-gated look-locker imaging for cardiac T1 estimation (ANGIE): development and application to T1 mapping of the right ventricle. Magn Reson Med 2015;73(1):150–60.

34. Weingartner S, Roujol S, Akcakaya M, et al. Free-breathing multislice native myocardial T1 mapping using the slice-interleaved T1 (STONE) sequence. Magn Reson Med 2015;74(1):115–24.

35. Chow K, Flewitt JA, Green JD, et al. Saturation recovery single-shot acquisition (SASHA) for myocardial T(1) mapping. Magn Reson Med 2014;71(6): 2082–95.

36. Weingartner S, Akcakaya M, Basha T, et al. Combined saturation/inversion recovery sequences for improved evaluation of scar and diffuse fibrosis in patients with arrhythmia or heart rate variability. Magn Reson Med 2014;71(3):1024–34.

37. Slavin GS, Stainsby JA. True T1 mapping with SMART1Map (saturation method using adaptive recovery times for cardiac T1 mapping): a comparison with MOLLI. J Cardiovasc Magn Reson 2013; 15(Suppl 1):P3.

38. Gerber BL, Belge B, Legros GJ, et al. Characterization of acute and chronic myocardial infarcts by multidetector computed tomography: comparison with contrast-enhanced magnetic resonance. Circulation 2006;113(6):823–33.

39. Shiozaki AA, Senra T, Arteaga E, et al. Myocardial fibrosis detected by cardiac CT predicts ventricular fibrillation/ventricular tachycardia events in patients with hypertrophic cardiomyopathy. J Cardiovasc Comput Tomogr 2013;7(3):173–81.

40. Cerny V, Kuchynka P, Marek J, et al. Nutzen der kardialen CT zur Beurteilung verzogerter Kontrastverstarkung bei dilatativer Kardiomyopathie (Utility of cardiac CT for evaluating delayed contrast enhancement in dilated cardiomyopathy). Herz 2017;42(8):776–80.

41. Kurita Y, Kitagawa K, Kurobe Y, et al. Estimation of myocardial extracellular volume fraction with cardiac CT in subjects without clinical coronary artery disease: a feasibility study. J Cardiovasc Comput Tomogr 2016;10(3):237–41.

42. Kurita Y, Kitagawa K, Kurobe Y, et al. Data on correlation between CT-derived and MRI-derived myocardial extracellular volume. Data Brief 2016;7:1045–7.

43. Nacif MS, Liu Y, Yao J, et al. 3D left ventricular extracellular volume fraction by low-radiation dose cardiac CT: assessment of interstitial myocardial fibrosis. J Cardiovasc Comput Tomogr 2013;7(1):51–7.

44. Hong YJ, Kim TK, Hong D, et al. Myocardial characterization using dual-energy CT in doxorubicin-induced DCM: comparison with CMR T1-mapping and histology in a rabbit model. JACC Cardiovasc Imaging 2016;9(7):836–45.

45. Lee HJ, Im DJ, Youn JC, et al. Myocardial extracellular volume fraction with dual-energy equilibrium contrast-enhanced cardiac CT in nonischemic cardiomyopathy: a prospective comparison with cardiac MR imaging. Radiology 2016;280(1):49–57.

46. Kim RJ, Fieno DS, Parrish TB, et al. Relationship of MRI delayed contrast enhancement to irreversible injury, infarct age, and contractile function. Circulation 1999;100(19):1992–2002.

47. Fernandez-Jimenez R, Sanchez-Gonzalez J, Aguero J, et al. Fast T2 gradient-spin-echo (T2-GraSE) mapping for myocardial edema quantification: first in vivo validation in a porcine model of ischemia/reperfusion. J Cardiovasc Magn Reson 2015;17:92.

48. Carrick D, Haig C, Rauhalammi S, et al. Prognostic significance of infarct core pathology revealed by quantitative non-contrast in comparison with contrast cardiac magnetic resonance imaging in reperfused ST-elevation myocardial infarction survivors. Eur Heart J 2016;37(13):1044–59.

49. Baxa J, Ferda J, Hromadka M. T1 mapping of the ischemic myocardium: review of potential clinical use. Eur J Radiol 2016;85(10):1922–8.

50. Chen Y, Zheng X, Jin H, et al. Role of myocardial extracellular volume fraction measured with magnetic resonance imaging in the prediction of left ventricular functional outcome after revascularization of chronic total occlusion of coronary arteries. Korean J Radiol 2019;20(1):83–93.

51. Spartalis M, Tzatzaki E, Doulamis IP, et al. T1-mapping provides superior diagnostic accuracy than late gadolinium enhancement imaging in patients with acute myocarditis. Int J Cardiol 2018;257:341.

52. Pan JA, Lee YJ, Salerno M. Diagnostic performance of extracellular volume, native T1, and T2 mapping versus Lake Louise criteria by cardiac magnetic resonance for detection of acute myocarditis: a meta-analysis. Circ Cardiovasc Imaging 2018;11(7):e007598.

53. Gannon MP, Schaub E, Grines CL, et al. State of the art: evaluation and prognostication of myocarditis using cardiac MRI. J Magn Reson Imaging 2019. [Epub ahead of print].

54. Hinojar R, Nagel E, Puntmann VO. T1 mapping in myocarditis: headway to a new era for cardiovascular magnetic resonance. Expert Rev Cardiovasc Ther 2015;13(8):871–4.

55. Bohnen S, Radunski UK, Lund GK, et al. Tissue characterization by T1 and T2 mapping cardiovascular magnetic resonance imaging to monitor myocardial inflammation in healing myocarditis. Eur Heart J Cardiovasc Imaging 2017;18(7):744–51.

56. Torreão JA, Ianni BM, Mady C, et al. Myocardial tissue characterization in Chagas' heart disease by cardiovascular magnetic resonance. J Cardiovasc Magn Reson 2015;17:97.

57. Delgado V, Bax JJ. Will cardiac magnetic resonance change the management of severe aortic stenosis patients? JACC Cardiovasc Imaging 2018;11(7):984–6.

58. Fehrmann A, Treutlein M, Rudolph T, et al. Myocardial T1 and T2 mapping in severe aortic stenosis: potential novel insights into the pathophysiology of myocardial remodelling. Eur J Radiol 2018;107:76–83.

59. Lee H, Park JB, Yoon YE, et al. Noncontrast myocardial T1 mapping by cardiac magnetic resonance predicts outcome in patients with aortic stenosis. JACC Cardiovasc Imaging 2018;11(7):974–83.

60. Treibel TA, Zemrak F, Sado DM, et al. Extracellular volume quantification in isolated hypertension: changes at the detectable limits? J Cardiovasc Magn Reson 2015;17:74.

61. Rodrigues JC, Amadu AM, Dastidar AG, et al. Comprehensive characterisation of hypertensive heart disease left ventricular phenotypes. Heart 2016;102(20):1671–9.

62. Bruder O, Wagner A, Jensen CJ, et al. Myocardial scar visualized by cardiovascular magnetic resonance imaging predicts major adverse events in patients with hypertrophic cardiomyopathy. J Am Coll Cardiol 2010;56(11):875–87.

63. Ho CY, Abbasi SA, Neilan TG, et al. T1 measurements identify extracellular volume expansion in hypertrophic cardiomyopathy sarcomere mutation carriers with and without left ventricular hypertrophy. Circ Cardiovasc Imaging 2013;6(3):415–22.

64. Karamitsos TD, Piechnik SK, Banypersad SM, et al. Noncontrast T1 mapping for the diagnosis of cardiac amyloidosis. JACC Cardiovasc Imaging 2013; 6(4):488–97.

65. Fontana M, Banypersad SM, Treibel TA, et al. Native T1 mapping in transthyretin amyloidosis. JACC Cardiovasc Imaging 2014;7(2):157–65.

66. White JA, Kim HW, Shah D, et al. CMR imaging with rapid visual T1 assessment predicts mortality in patients suspected of cardiac amyloidosis. JACC Cardiovasc Imaging 2014;7(2):143–56.

67. Mongeon FP, Jerosch-Herold M, Coelho-Filho OR, et al. Quantification of extracellular matrix expansion by CMR in infiltrative heart disease. JACC Cardiovasc Imaging 2012;5(9):897–907.

68. Krittayaphong R, Zhang S, Saiviroonporn P, et al. Detection of cardiac iron overload with native magnetic resonance T1 and T2 mapping in patients with thalassemia. Int J Cardiol 2017;248:421–6.

69. Torlasco C, Cassinerio E, Roghi A, et al. Role of T1 mapping as a complementary tool to T2* for non-invasive cardiac iron overload assessment. PLoS One 2018;13(2):e0192890.

70. Putko BN, Wen K, Thompson RB, et al. Anderson-Fabry cardiomyopathy: prevalence, pathophysiology, diagnosis and treatment. Heart Fail Rev 2015;20(2):179–91.

71. Edwards NC, Teoh JK, Steeds RP. Hypertrophic cardiomyopathy and Anderson-Fabry disease: unravelling septal hypertrophy with T1-mapping CMR. Eur Heart J 2014;35(28):1896.

72. van den Boomen M, Slart R, Hulleman EV, et al. Native T1 reference values for nonischemic cardiomyopathies and populations with increased cardiovascular risk: a systematic review and meta-analysis. J Magn Reson Imaging 2018;47(4): 891–912.

73. Reiter U, Reiter C, Krauter C, et al. Cardiac magnetic resonance T1 mapping. Part 2: diagnostic potential and applications. Eur J Radiol 2018;109:235–47.

74. Mordi I, Carrick D, Bezerra H, et al. T1 and T2 mapping for early diagnosis of dilated non-ischaemic cardiomyopathy in middle-aged patients and differentiation from normal physiological adaptation. Eur Heart J Cardiovasc Imaging 2016;17(7):797–803.

75. Dass S, Suttie JJ, Piechnik SK, et al. Myocardial tissue characterization using magnetic resonance non-contrast T1 mapping in hypertrophic and dilated cardiomyopathy. Circ Cardiovasc Imaging 2012; 5(6):726–33.

76. Puntmann VO, Carr-White G, Jabbour A, et al. T1-mapping and outcome in nonischemic cardiomyopathy: all-cause mortality and heart failure. JACC Cardiovasc Imaging 2016;9(1):40–50.

77. Melendez GC, Hundley WG. Is myocardial fibrosis a new frontier for discovery in cardiotoxicity related to the administration of anthracyclines? Circ Cardiovasc Imaging 2016;9(12) [pii:e005797].

78. Farhad H, Staziaki PV, Addison D, et al. Characterization of the changes in cardiac structure and function in mice treated with anthracyclines using serial cardiac magnetic resonance imaging. Circ Cardiovasc Imaging 2016;9(12) [pii:e003584].

79. Mukai-Yatagai N, Haruki N, Kinugasa Y, et al. Assessment of myocardial fibrosis using T1-mapping and extracellular volume measurement on cardiac magnetic resonance imaging for the diagnosis of radiation-induced cardiomyopathy. J Cardiol Cases 2018;18(4):132–5.

80. Chen CA, Dusenbery SM, Valente AM, et al. Myocardial ECV fraction assessed by CMR is associated with type of hemodynamic load and arrhythmia in repaired tetralogy of Fallot. JACC Cardiovasc Imaging 2016;9(1):1–10.

81. Anderson PA, Sleeper LA, Mahony L, et al. Contemporary outcomes after the Fontan procedure: a Pediatric Heart Network multicenter study. J Am Coll Cardiol 2008;52(2):85–98.

82. Soslow JH, Damon SM, Crum K, et al. Increased myocardial native T1 and extracellular volume in patients with Duchenne muscular dystrophy. J Cardiovasc Magn Reson 2016;18:5.

83. Stehlik J, Edwards LB, Kucheryavaya AY, et al. The Registry of the International Society for Heart and Lung Transplantation: 29th official adult heart transplant report: 2012. J Heart Lung Transplant 2012; 31(10):1052–64.

84. Imran M, Wang L, McCrohon J, et al. Native T1 mapping in the diagnosis of cardiac allograft rejection: a prospective histologically validated study. JACC Cardiovasc Imaging 2019. [Epub ahead of print].

85. Kammerlander AA, Duca F, Binder C, et al. Extracellular volume quantification by cardiac magnetic resonance imaging without hematocrit sampling: ready for prime time? Wien Klin Wochenschr 2018; 130(5–6):190–6.

86. Fent GJ, Garg P, Foley JRJ, et al. Synthetic myocardial extracellular volume fraction. JACC Cardiovasc Imaging 2017;10(11):1402–4.

87. Treibel TA, Fontana M, Maestrini V, et al. Automatic measurement of the myocardial interstitium: synthetic extracellular volume quantification without hematocrit sampling. JACC Cardiovasc Imaging 2016; 9(1):54–63.

Moving?

Make sure your subscription moves with you!

To notify us of your new address, find your **Clinics Account Number** (located on your mailing label above your name), and contact customer service at:

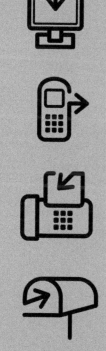

Email: journalscustomerservice-usa@elsevier.com

800-654-2452 (subscribers in the U.S. & Canada)
314-447-8871 (subscribers outside of the U.S. & Canada)

Fax number: 314-447-8029

Elsevier Health Sciences Division
Subscription Customer Service
3251 Riverport Lane
Maryland Heights, MO 63043

*To ensure uninterrupted delivery of your subscription, please notify us at least 4 weeks in advance of move.

Printed and bound by CPI Group (UK) Ltd, Croydon, CR0 4YY

08/05/2025

01864746-0019